Unstable Angina
Recognition and Management

Edited by Allan G. Adelman, MD
and
Bernard S. Goldman, MD

PSG Publishing Company, Inc.
Littleton, Massachusetts

Main entry under title:

Unstable angina.

    Bibliography: p.
    1. Angina pectoris--Congresses. 2. Heart--Surgery--
Congresses. I. Adelman, Allan G., 1936-   II. Gold-
man, Bernard S., 1936-   [DNLM: 1. Angina pectoris--
Diagnosis--Congresses. 2. Angina pectoris--Therapy--
Congresses. WG298 161u 1979]
RC685.A6U57   616.1'22   80-13211
ISBN 0-88416-271-0

This book is dedicated to a truly great Canadian surgeon, Wilfred G. Bigelow, who, as Head of the Division of Cardiovascular Surgery at the Toronto General Hospital, (1952–1977), combined wisdom and foresight with humility and created an environment where new ideas could grow.

CONTRIBUTORS

Allan G. Adelman, MD
Associate Professor
 of Medicine
Division of Cardiology
University of Toronto
Toronto, Ontario
Staff Physician
Division of Cardiology
Toronto General and Mount
 Sinai Hospitals
Canada

Ronald S. Baigrie, MD
Assistant Professor of Medicine
Division of Cardiology
University of Toronto
Director, Coronary Care Unit
Toronto General Hospital
Toronto, Ontario
Canada

Ronald J. Baird, MD
Professor of Cardiovascular
 Surgery
University of Toronto
Head, Division of Cardiovascular
 Surgery
Toronto General Hospital
Toronto, Ontario
Canada

Kulasekaram Balakumaran, MD
Cardiologist
Thoraxcenter, Erasmus University
Academisch Ziekenhuis
Rotterdam
The Netherlands

Jean Bardet, MD
Professeur Agrégé (Cardiologie)
Hôpital Ambroise Paré
Boulogne
France

Jean Pierre Bourdarias, MD
Hôpital Ambroise Paré
Boulogne
France

James W. Butany, MD
Resident in Pathology
University of Toronto
Toronto General Hospital
Toronto, Ontario
Canada

John A. Cairns, MD
Assistant Professor of Medicine
Division of Cardiology
McMaster University
Director, Intensive Care Unit
McMaster University Medical Centre
Hamilton, Ontario
Canada

Brian M. Chesnie, MD
Resident in Cardiology
Toronto General Hospital
Toronto, Ontario
Canada

Sergio Chierchia, MD
Clinical Physiology Laboratory
National Research Council of Italy
Department of Medicine
University of Pisa
Pisa
Italy

George Christakis
Medical Student, University of
 Toronto
Division of Cardiovascular Surgery
Toronto General Hospital
Toronto, Ontario
Canada

Lawrence H. Cohn, MD
Associate Professor of Surgery
Harvard Medical School
Surgeon
Peter Bent Brigham Hospital
Boston, Massachusetts

John J. Collins, Jr., MD
Professor of Surgery
Harvard Medical School
Chief, Division of Cardiothoracic
  Surgery
Peter Bent Brigham Hospital
Boston, Massachusetts

C. Richard Conti, MD
Chief, Division of Cardiology
University of Florida
Chief, Division of Cardiology
JHM Hospital
Gainesville, Florida

R. Charles Curry, MD
Practicing Physician
JHM Hospital
Gainesville, Florida

Robert J. Cusimano
Medical Student
University of Toronto
Division of Cardiovascular Surgery
Toronto General Hospital
Toronto, Ontario
Canada

Jean Christian Farcot, MD
Hôpital Ambroise Paré
Boulogne
France

Bernard S. Goldman, MD
Associate Professor, Department of
  Surgery
University of Toronto
Staff Surgeon
Division of Cardiovascular Surgery
Toronto General Hospital
Head, Division of Cardiovascular
  Surgery
Sunnybrook Hospital
Consultant, Mount Sinai Hospital
Toronto, Ontario
Canada

Max Haalebos, MD
Coronary Care Unit
Thoraxcenter, Erasmus University
Academisch Ziekenhuis
Rotterdam
The Netherlands

Paul G. Hugenholtz, MD
Professor and Head, Department of
  Cardiology
Thoraxcenter, Erasmus University
Head, Division of Cardiology
Academisch Ziekenhuis
Rotterdam
The Netherlands

Wilbert J. Keon, MD
Professor and Chairman, Depart-
  ment of Surgery
University of Ottawa
Chief, Cardiac Unit and Division of
  Cardiothoracic Surgery
Ottawa Civic Hospital
Ottawa, Ontario
Canada

J. Kenneth Koster, Jr., MD
Professor of Surgery
Harvard Medical School
Surgeon
Peter Bent Brigham Hospital
Boston, Massachusetts

Antonio L'Abbate, MD
Associate Professor of Medicine
Institute of Medical Pathology
University of Pisa
Italy

Alan J. Leach, MD
Resident, Department of Medicine
Queen's University
Kingston, Ontario
Canada

Stanley Lee-Son, MD
Department of Anesthesia
Peter Bent Brigham Hospital
Boston, Massachusetts

Jacob Lubsen, MD
Epidemiologist
Research Fellow in Cardiology
Thoraxcenter, Erasmus University
Academisch Ziekenhuis
Rotterdam
The Netherlands

Attilio Maseri, MD
Professor of Cardiovascular
  Medicine
Royal Postgraduate Medical School
University of London
London
England

Peter R. McLaughlin, MD
Assistant Professor of Medicine
University of Toronto
Staff Physician, Division of
  Cardiology
Toronto General Hospital
Toronto, Ontario
Canada

Rolf Michels, MD
Cardiologist, Thoraxcenter,
  Erasmus University
Head, Coronary Care Unit
Academisch Ziekenhuis
Rotterdam
The Netherlands

Henry F. Mizgala, MD
Associate Professor, Department of
  Medicine
University of Montreal
Staff Cardiologist
Montreal Heart Institute
Montreal, Quebec
Canada

John E. Morch, MD
Associate Professor of Medicine
University of Toronto
Associate Director, Cardiovascular
  Unit
Toronto General Hospital
Toronto, Ontario
Canada

Gilbert H. Mudge, MD
Assistant Professor, Cardiovascular
  Division
Peter Bent Brigham Hospital
Boston, Massachusetts

John O. Parker, MD
Professor of Medicine
Queen's University
Chief of Cardiology
Kingston General Hospital
Kingston, Ontario
Canada

Jan Pool, MD
Professor of Cardiology
Thoraxcenter, Erasmus University
Academisch Ziekenhuis
Rotterdam
The Netherlands

Michel Rigaud, MD
Hôpital Ambroise Paré
Boulogne
France

William C. Roberts, MD
Chief, Pathology Branch
Department of Health, Education and
  Welfare
National Institutes of Health
Bethesda, Maryland

Patrick W. Serruys, MD
Coronary Care Unit
Thoraxcenter, Erasmus University
Academisch Ziekenhuis
Rotterdam
The Netherlands

Malcolm D. Silver, MD
Professor and Chairman
Department of Pathology
University of Western Ontario
London, Ontario
Canada

Sallie J. Teasdale, MD
Associate Professor of Anesthesia
University of Toronto
Deputy Anesthetist-in-Chief
Toronto General Hospital
Toronto, Ontario
Canada

Marcel van den Brand, MD
Coronary Care Unit
Thoraxcenter, Erasmus University
Academisch Ziekenhuis
Rotterdam
The Netherlands

Emiel van der Does, MD
Professor of Family Medicine
Erasmus University
Rotterdam
The Netherlands

Stephen Van Devanter, MD
Resident, Thoracic Surgery
Peter Bent Brigham Hospital
Boston, Massachusetts

Renu Virmani, MD
Pathology Branch
National Heart, Lung, and Blood
  Institute
National Institutes of Health
Bethesda, Maryland

Richard D. Weisel, MD
Demonstrator in Surgery
University of Toronto
Staff Surgeon, Division of Cardio-
  vascular Surgery
Toronto General Hospital
Toronto, Ontario
Canada

E. Douglas Wigle, MD
Professor of Medicine
University of Toronto
Head, Division of Cardiology
Toronto General Hospital
Toronto, Ontario
Canada

Robert Zeldin, MD
Resident in Surgery
Division of Cardiovascular Surgery
Toronto General Hospital
Toronto, Ontario
Canada

CONTENTS

INTRODUCTION

Unstable angina has been a focus of attention for internist, cardiologist and cardiac surgeons over the past decade, although the severe anginal pain syndromes — preinfarction angina, impending infarction, intermediate syndrome, angina decubitus, and acute coronary insufficiency — have been recognized as distinct clinical entities for almost half a century. The increased interest in and awareness of these disorders is primarily related to the marked advances in treatment rather than to any major changes in our understanding of the pathophysiology. The introduction of aortocoronary bypass graft surgery in the late 1960s, the beta-blocking agents in the early 1970s, and the use of intensive nitrate therapy in the late 1970s have allowed physicians to treat these severe anginal syndromes more effectively. Prior to this era, the only therapy available for most patients with these conditions was bedrest, analgesics, and sublingual nitroglycerin.

In order to assess the clinical results of these new forms of therapy, it became necessary to classify the severe anginal pain syndromes more accurately. The term "unstable angina" was introduced by Conti to encompass all the previous disorders. Two major subgroups were defined: crescendo angina — angina that is increasing in frequency and severity, usually coming on at rest and relieved in less than 20 minutes by nitroglycerin; and acute coronary insufficiency — severe and usually unprovoked angina that is unrelieved within 20 minutes despite rest and nitrates.

It was essential to exclude definite acute myocardial infarction from these definitions. However, it has only recently been recognized, by radioisotope scintigraphy and CK-MB analysis, that subclinical forms of myocardial damage may coexist with a severe anginal pain syndrome. In fact, there is a spectrum of patients with coronary artery disease and chest pain that ranges from acute myocardial infarction, to angina pectoris with varying degrees of myocardial necrosis, and angina with no myocardial damage at all (Figure I-1). In addition, three patient populations with unstable angina have been identified in a temporal sense. These include previously asymptomatic patients (new onset angina), patients with stable angina who experience a worsening of their symptoms (intensification group), and patients who have a recurrence or onset of severe anginal pain following an acute myocardial infarction (postmyocardial infarction angina).

The pathophysiology of unstable angina is not completely understood. Most studies have shown that the distribution and severity of coronary atherosclerosis in patients with unstable angina is similar to that in patients with stable angina. However, it is possible that the lesions in unstable angina are somewhat more proximal and more severe than those of stable angina (Figure I-2). These differences may not be appreciated by present methods of analyzing coronary angiograms. Furthermore, there may be a paucity of collaterals, or so-called jeopardized collaterals, in these patients (Figure I-3). Again, these may not be fully appreciated at angiography. These subtle differences may explain the severity of symptoms in patients with unstable angina. Another possibility is that these patients have coronary arterial spasm in addition to coronary atherosclerosis. Maseri and colleagues documented by electrocardiographic and hemodynamic monitoring, and by angiography and radioisotope studies, that the majority of patients experience decreased myocardial oxygen supply, rather than increased demand, during ischemic episodes. Although the frequency with which spasm occurs remains to be confirmed, this is perhaps the most exciting inroad to the pathophysiologic mechanisms underlying the severe anginal pain syndromes.

While investigators have debated the functional (vasospastic) or mechanical (occlusive) etiologies in the development or progression of unstable angina occurring in the previously asymptomatic patient, relatively little attention has been paid to altered psychology. Angina pectoris is a subjective symptom and the diagnosis depends wholly on the patient's perception of pain. In our own experience, emotional stress, anxiety, and

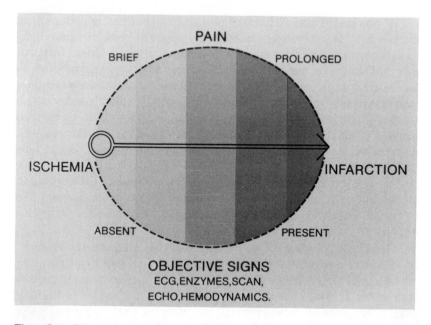

Figure I-1 Schematic representation of the spectrum of myocardial ischemia, from brief angina without objective signs of damage to frank myocardial infarction with definite clinical markers of necrosis.

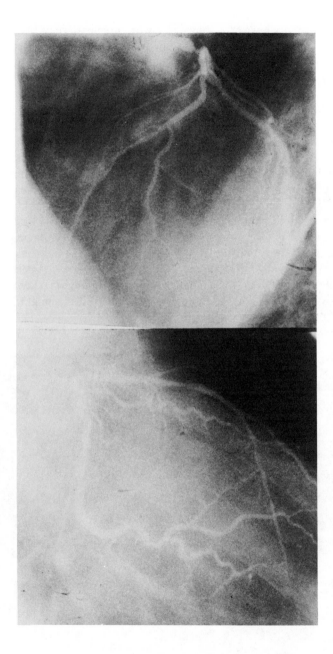

Figure I-2A Coronary angiograms demonstrating severe proximal stenosis in two patients with unstable angina. Left coronary artery in the left anterior oblique (LAO) (top) and right anterior oblique (RAO) (bottom) showing a very tight (95%) stenosis of the main left coronary artery. There is also diffuse disease of the left anterior descending (LAD) coronary artery after the first diagonal branch and significant proximal disease in the circumflex.

patient reactivity have contributed to a worsening pattern of ischemic pain. These factors are implied in the admission to hospital, administration of sedatives, and removal of the patient from a stimulating environment. Anxiety and reactivity are not confined only to patients; cardiologists and angiographers may well heighten the patient's fears by overreaction to either the ECG manifestations of ischemia, or the anatomy delineated at angiography. It is not all that long ago that emergency revascularization surgery was performed upon discovery of significant left main coronary artery stenosis at angiography. In this regard, the enthusiasm and availability of a cardiac surgeon play a role in the aggressive management of unstable angina syndromes. Surgeons have been only too eager in the past to operate immediately on patients with apparently unstable angina, or with severe anatomic lesions. This had two implications: first, patients booked urgently for revascularization are often labelled as having unstable angina, which only confounds and confuses reported results; and second, many patients with early acute myocardial infarction were operated upon urgently for apparent reversible ischemia, resulting in excessive peri-operative infarction rates and mortality. These problems might have been

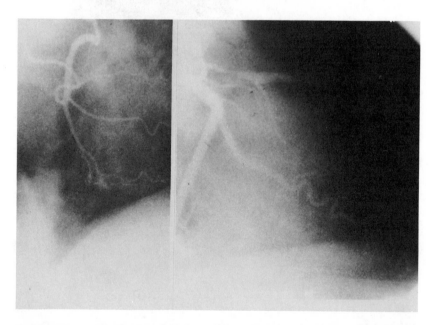

Figure I-2B Left (left) and right (right) coronary arteries in the RAO projection showing a long very tight (95%) stenosis of the LAD proximal to the first septal perforator with a very poor distal filling of the vessel. This is the so-called "widowmaker" lesion. The dominant circumflex and small right are normal. There is no collateral circulation to the LAD from either the circumflex or right coronary arteries.

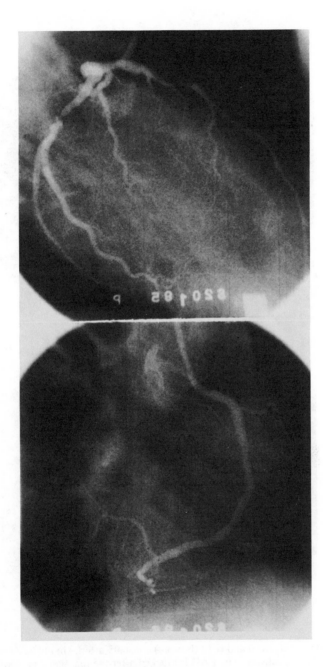

Figure I-3A Coronary angiograms demonstrating lack of collaterals and jeopardized collaterals in two patients with unstable angina. Left (top) and right (bottom) coronary arteries in the RAO projection show a severe (95%) proximal stenosis of the LAD and circumflex coronary arteries. The right coronary artery only shows minor irregularities. There are no collaterals to the affected vessels.

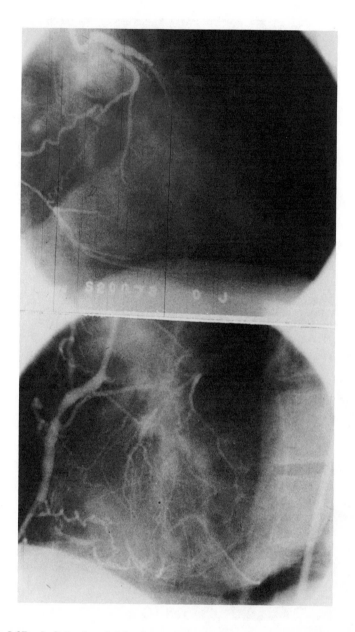

Figure I-3B   Left (top) and right (bottom) coronary arteries in the RAO and LAO projections, respectively. The LAD is blocked after the first septal perforator. The circumflex is a small, nondominant vessel. The right coronary artery has a 90% stenosis proximal to the first acute marginal and is completely blocked distal to the second acute marginal. An extensive collateral circulation has developed from the right to the left anterior descending coronary artery, but this collateral network is jeopardized by the severe proximal stenosis in the proximal right coronary artery.

avoided had a few hours or even days been taken to observe the evolution of the clinical syndrome, the electrocardiographic and laboratory changes, and the response to intensive pharmacologic therapy.

The type of treatment instituted for unstable angina frequently depends on the availability of a bed in an intensive care unit, and if surgery is contemplated, the availability of a cardiovascular surgical team. Thus, local referral patterns, and resources for angiography and cardiac surgery influence therapy and results. A major purpose of this monograph is to present both medical and surgical results of therapy for unstable angina in the light of lessons learned over the past decade. As a result of changes in both classification and management, early infarction and mortality have decreased.

The significant events that altered recognition and management of unstable angina through the 1970s are:

1. Definition and classification
2. Use of beta-blockers
3. Intraaortic balloon pump assist
4. Urgent and emergent aortocoronary bypass grafting
5. National Institutes of Health randomized medical vs surgical trial
6. Improved anesthetic and perioperative management
7. Intraoperative myocardial protection
8. Intensive medical therapy, high-dose nitrates
9. Separation of medical responders from nonresponders
10. Recognition of coronary spasm
11. Recognition of cellular injury within unstable angina
12. Search for redefinition and extended classification

These events resulted in a combined medical and surgical approach to patients. The goal of current therapy is to obtain intensive initial pharmacologic control of the ischemic syndrome, to permit "cooling off," and elective aortocoronary bypass, if indicated or required, reserving both intraaortic balloon pump assist and urgent surgery for nonresponders with resistant pain. The role of spasm and microcellular damage, demonstrable by sophisticated monitoring, nuclear scans, or CK-MB analysis, prompts a fresh look at definitions and subgroups within unstable angina.

In the early 1970s, we considered patients with unstable angina as surgical emergencies and employed the intraaortic balloon pump frequently. We also disrupted elective catheter and surgical schedules considerably. We now tend to institute intensive medical therapy, which in most instances is effective in controlling the anginal pain. We are therefore able to proceed to catheterization and surgery, if indicated, on an elective or semielective basis. This not only reduces the wear and tear of a cardiac surgical service, but protects long elective waiting periods and decreases the risks of emergency surgery in the acutely ischemic patient.

It is really the therapeutic approach to patients with unstable angina that has changed dramatically over the past decade. Much of this monograph deals with the experience of large referral centers in Canada, the United States, and Europe, and with the various forms of medical and surgical treatment currently available to patients with this syndrome. A combined medical and surgical approach to the patient with unstable angina has been effective in the relief of pain, the reduction of infarcts, an increase in physical capacity and, in all likelihood, a prolongation of life. The use of beta-blocking agents in high doses and intensive therapy with oral, sublingual, topical, and, more recently, intravenous nitrates, have become standard coronary-care therapy. The intraaortic balloon pump is available and effective in aborting resistant ischemic pain in patients unresponsive to intensive pharmacologic therapy, or those with morbid anatomy. However, use of this modality has decreased dramatically over the past five years. The 1970s have also witnessed major improvements in the techniques of anesthetic management (particularly during induction), perioperative hemodynamic monitoring, intraoperative myocardial preservation, and increased technical skill in the performance of complete revascularization by multiple coronary bypass grafts with satisfactory patency. With increasing understanding of the role of coronary artery spasm, the availability of nuclear scanning and serial CK-MB sampling in both preoperative and postoperative patients, it is likely that new definitions and subgroups of unstable angina will be defined. The current approach to patients with unstable angina is in keeping with Ashby's Law of Requisite Variety, which, when interpreted in biologic rather than cybernetic terms, states that "a system or organism must exhibit a response repertoire that is equal to the range of the demands of its environment in order to survive." Cardiologists and cardiac surgeons currently have available a therapeutic armamentarium that ensures far greater success in the treatment of patients with unstable angina than in the past.

This monograph is the Proceedings of an International Symposium on Unstable Angina held in Toronto, Ontario, Canada, November 9 and 10, 1979. The contributors presented their works to a large and receptive audience. Both the symposium and this monograph are supported by the Ontario Heart Foundation and the Toronto General Hospital Foundation. The editors wish to express deep appreciation to their numerous medical and surgical colleagues who have been so supportive of this work over the past ten years. We are indebted as well to the countless residents, fellows, and devoted nurses who have assisted in the management and study of these acutely ischemic patients. It is our hope that this monograph will provide them with not only a sense of satisfaction in their own work, but a comparative and meaningful view of similar large series in other parts of Canada, Western Europe, and the United States.

Allan G. Adelman, MD
Bernard S. Goldman, MD

SECTION I

Unstable Angina — An Overview of the Problem: Definition, Prodromata, and Natural History

1 Unstable Angina — An Overview

John A. Cairns, MD

A spectrum of acute symptomatic manifestations of ischemic heart disease lies between the well-defined diagnosis of stable angina pectoris on the one hand and acute myocardial infarction on the other. The term "unstable angina" is the most simple, inclusive, and descriptive that may be applied to this spectrum and is currently in wide use. A variety of terms has been employed, including impending acute coronary artery occlusion,[1] coronary failure,[2] acute coronary insufficiency,[3] slight coronary attacks,[4] intermediate coronary syndrome,[5] crescendo angina,[6] impending myocardial infarction,[7] status anginosus,[8] preinfarction syndrome,[9] preinfarction angina,[10] and unstable angina.[11]

Although the predominant manifestation of all syndromes falling within this spectrum is that of ischemic cardiac pain, each term has tended to focus on different aspects of the symptomatology. The reports concerning these clinical states are difficult to evaluate and compare because of the inconsistent nomenclature and patient selection. Although in the current literature there is consistent use of the term unstable angina, there is significant disagreement as to what syndromes should be included. Accordingly, evaluation and comparison of studies remains difficult. This chapter will discuss the origins of the concept of unstable angina and the delineation of its clinical significance. The evolution of therapy and the changing prognosis will be discussed. The evidence for high-risk subgroups will be reviewed. Problems of definition will be considered, and data from a variety of sources will be discussed in the light of varying definitions. Finally, current working definitions of unstable angina will be reviewed.

Conti et al[12] attempted to describe the spectrum of acute symptomatic manifestations of ischemic heart disease interposed between stable angina pectoris and acute myocardial infarction. They proposed that the term unstable angina encompass the following groups: 1) angina on effort of recent onset, 2) angina on effort with a changing (crescendo) pattern, and 3) angina at rest. The descriptions of these authors and others may be used to define these groups further. Group 1 patients have previously been pain-free and now have a syndrome of typical angina associated with clear precipitating causes (exertion or emotion). Such angina of recent onset is considered to be unstable during the first few weeks it is observed. An arbitrary limit of four weeks is applied in most studies. Group 2 patients have had stable angina for a varying length of time, but within the preceding four weeks there has been abrupt worsening of the pain syndrome. This is generally with a progressive pattern manifested by increased frequency, intensity, duration, or ease of onset, new presence of associated symptoms (sweating, nausea, weakness), or decreased responsiveness to nitroglycerin or cessation of activity. The terms "accelerated" or "crescendo" angina are useful descriptions that have been applied to this pattern of unstable angina. Specifically excluded is a simple, gradual increase in severity of angina over a period of time. Group 3 patients require no stress to provoke episodes of ischemic cardiac pain. Generally the pain is prolonged, arbitrarily at least 15 minutes in most reports, and may respond poorly to oral nitrate therapy. The term "acute coronary insufficiency" is usually reserved for this group in reports employing this term. Frequently with patients in group 3 there is a problem in deciding whether or not a myocardial infarction has occurred. It is therefore necessary to include in the definition of unstable angina laboratory evidence by which acute myocardial infarction may be excluded. Serum enzymes may rise only minimally (under 50% above normal range), and electrocardiograms may not show new Q waves or manifestations of subendocardial infarction (transient ST- and T-wave changes are frequent and represent ischemia). Frequent blood sampling and determination of cardiospecific enzyme[13] indicate that small amounts of necrosis not detected by conventional enzyme sampling protocols may be present in many patients with group 3 unstable angina. Such a conclusion is also suggested by technetium-99m pyrophosphate imaging.[14]

Some variation in nomenclature among studies arises from specifications as to whether the unstable angina pattern is the first manifestation of myocardial ischemia, or whether there is a previous history of ischemic pain. Studies have demonstrated a worse prognosis in patients with previous ischemic pain (stable angina or myocardial infarction). Therefore, if such a history exists, it should be specified, whichever group of unstable angina is presented.[15-17]

A special group of patients who may be considered to have unstable angina are those experiencing recurrent angina during the first month following acute myocardial infarction.[17-19] These early postinfarction angina patients might be designated as group 4 for completeness, although this group is not included in most studies and therapeutic approaches are not so clearly defined as for groups 1, 2, and 3.

Premonitory chest pain, as a sign of impending myocardial infarction, may have been recognized as early as 1799 by Parry,[20] and subsequent references to premonitory pain syndromes were made by Obrastzow and Straschesko,[21] Herrick,[22] Parkinson and Bedford,[23] Levine and Brown,[24] Conner and Holt,[25] and Willius.[26] However, clear recognition of these syndromes and delineation of their clinical importance did not come until 1937 with the publications of Sampson and Eliaser,[1] and Feil.[27]

Sampson and Eliaser reported 29 cases of acute myocardial infarction collected over 2½ years with premonitory signs of "impending acute coronary artery occlusion," consisting of prolonged anginal pain in the majority, and progressively severe exertional pain in the remainder (Table 1-1). They clearly differentiated premonitory symptoms from those of simple angina pectoris and acute myocardial infarction. They referred to an additional study of 27 consecutive cases of acute myocardial infarction in which there was a 48% incidence of premonitory attacks of pain. On this basis, they advocated bedrest for patients with premonitory chest pain syndromes, and referred in this report to six patients treated with complete bedrest whose symptoms resolved within 1 to 3 weeks. They speculated that the development of collateral arterial supply might have forestalled "impending (coronary) occlusion."

Feil noted in 1937 that in approximately 50% of his patients with "coronary thrombosis" the acute attack was "preceded by angina, unrelated to effort or emotion." He reported 15 such patients, all of whom would now be regarded as having group 3 unstable angina (see Table 1-1). He noted that "the pain is more or less constant, of a burning and oppressive character, and is not relieved by rest or nitrates. The pain lasts from a few hours to four weeks." He postulated that a gradually forming thrombus in a stenosed coronary artery was the most probable explanation for the premonitory pain syndrome and advocated efforts to improve coronary flow and reduce cardiac work.

Table 1-1
Retrospective Record Review Studies of Unstable Angina

Author	Year of Publication	Name of Syndrome	Study Population	No. of Patients	Incidence of Prodrome Unstable Angina	Unstable Angina Group*		
						1	2	3
Sampson and Elias[1]	1937	Impending acute coronary artery occlusion	Patients with proven acute myocardial infarction (AMI) who had prodromes	29			29	29
			Patients with proven AMI	27	13/27 (48.1%)			
Feil[27]	1937	Preliminary pain in coronary thrombosis	Patients with proven AMI who had prodromes	15				15
Yater et al[32]	1948	Premonitory, preliminary or prodromal symptoms	Patients with proven AMI	642	60/642 (9.3%)	60	60	60
Mounsey[33]	1951	Prodromal symptoms in myocardial infarction	Patients with proven AMI	139	40/139 (28.8%)		18	22
Smith et al[34]	1951	Pilot attacks of angina	Patients with proven AMI	920	139/920 (15.1%)	139		

*The numbers of patients are repeated when there is an overlap between subgroups.

Master et al[28] published the first large study of premonitory symptoms, based upon the administration of a structured questionnaire to patients with acute myocardial infarction, rather than upon retrospective record reviews (Table 1-2). They found 44% (115/260) of patients had a variety of "premonitory symptoms of acute coronary occlusion" during the four weeks preceding the attack. Angina as a premonitory symptom occurred in 27% (70/260). It is difficult to determine from the report whether or not all the patients with angina had unstable angina by current criteria, but that diagnosis is likely in most since the premonitory symptom was rest pain in 28.5% of patients and 68.5% had pain on mild or moderate activity. There were patients who fit the current criteria for groups 1, 2, and 3 of unstable angina. Master stated that "the anatomic basis for the premonitory symptoms is assumed to be a gradual occlusion of the lumen of the coronary artery by progressive or recurrent intramural hemorrhage or by primary thrombosis on a plaque, which may take hours or days for completion." Although he was pessimistic about the possibility of preventing coronary occlusion by bedrest, he believed that the severity of symptoms and of heart failure following occlusion might be lessened thereby, and mortality reduced.

Master coined the term "acute coronary insufficiency,"[3,29] which he defined as "a deficiency of the coronary circulation due to discrepancy in the demands of the myocardium and its available oxygen and blood supply." Angina pectoris was considered to indicate "a very transient episode of acute coronary insufficiency." Master stressed such precipitating factors as sudden increase in cardiac work (increased blood pressure, heart rate, or cardiac output), decreased coronary blood flow (from decreased blood pressure and decreased cardiac output, as in acute hemorrhage or shock), and interference with oxygenation of the blood (asphyxia, general anesthesia, and pulmonary embolism). In a number of autopsy cases he was able to demonstrate myocardial necrosis in the absence of coronary occlusion, a finding which is now well-recognized in patients with nontransmural myocardial infarction.[30] He believed that small amounts of myocardial necrosis were a common outcome of acute coronary insufficiency. The emphasis in his use of this term was upon readily understood precipitating factors of profound myocardial infarction and coronary occlusion. In later writings he employed the term "impending infarction"[31] for the syndromes now designated as unstable angina, restricting this term to "the syndrome in which anginal pain previously relatively mild and intermittent, abruptly becomes aggravated and acquires new qualities." He specifically excluded patients with acute coronary insufficiency, which he came to regard as virtually synonymous with subendocardial infarction. However, the term "acute coronary insufficiency" became widely used as many subsequent studies employed the term to describe spontaneous unstable angina of the rest-pain type, even though Master's initial descriptions were not of spontaneous reversible pain syndromes.

Table 1-2
Prospective Patient Questionnaire Studies of Prodromes of Acute Myocardial Infarction (AMI)

Author	Year of Publication	Population	No. of Patients	Total Incidence of Prodromes	Incidence of Prodromes Unstable angina	Unstable Angina Group†		
						1	2	3
Master et al[28]	1941	Patients hospitalized with AMI	260	115/260 (44.2%)	70/260 (26.9%)*	50	50	20
Solomon et al[50]	1969	Patients hospitalized with AMI	100	65/100 (65.0%)	59/100 (59.0%)		39	20
Stowers and Short[51]	1970	Patients hospitalized with AMI	180	122/180 (67.8%)	99/180 (55.0%)	43	43	56
Hochberg[52]	1971	Patients hospitalized with AMI	74	62/ 74 (83.8%)	34/ 74 (45.9%)	34	34	34
Freeman and Loughhead[53]	1972	Patients hospitalized with AMI	100		72/100 (72.0%)	40	32	32
Romo[56]	1972	Patients hospitalized with AMI	976	616/976 (63.1%)	309/976 (31.7%)	309	309	309
Alonzo et al[55]	1975	Patients hospitalized with AMI	160	112/160 (70.0%)	75/160 (46.9%)	75	75	75

*Some may not have been unstable.
†The numbers of patients are repeated when there is an overlap between subgroups.

In 1948, Yater et al[32] reported their studies of 866 cases of acute myocardial infarction occurring in army service men under age 40 (see Table 1-1). Among the 642 patients for whom reliable histories were available, the incidence of premonitory symptoms (defined as new symptoms of possible cardiac origin with onset in the three weeks prior to acute myocardial infarction) was 9.3%. In many instances, the symptoms were not those of chest pain, however.

In 1951, Mounsey[33] reported on 139 cases of acute myocardial infarction observed over a 14-year period (Table 1-1). Twenty-nine percent of these patients had prodromal symptoms defined as "history of anginal pain usually with atypical features or intensification or change in the character of previous angina, preceding myocardial infarction by not more than three months." Of these patients, 18 of 40 had pain of crescendo pattern (group 2) and 22 of 40 had rest pain (group 3). The authors stressed the features of crescendo quality, prolonged duration, and the inconstant relation to exertion in delineating the prodromal symptoms. They concluded, "The importance of the clinical diagnosis of this syndrome lies in the prophylactic therapy of myocardial infarction with rest and, possibly, anticoagulant therapy."

Smith et al[34] reported 920 cases of acute myocardial infarction, gathered from the records of the Henry Ford Hospital from 1925 to 1949 (see Table 1-1). Of these patients, 15.1% had developed "pilot attacks of angina," defined as the onset of angina during the month prior to acute myocardial infarction (group 1). It is likely that factors of frequency and severity of ischemic pain were considered, although this is not specified in the paper. The authors advocated hospitalization of patients with the new onset of angina for two weeks with administration of anticoagulants. They formed the impression that this approach had been "beneficial in both the relief of the frequent angina and in the prevention of imminent myocardial infarction," although no data were provided to permit such a conclusion.

In 1956, Levy[6] published the first prospective study of the natural history of patients with unstable angina (Table 1-3). Previous studies had focussed on acute myocardial infarction and had retrospectively examined the incidence of unstable angina. Levy documented 158 patients with a previous history of stable angina and/or myocardial infarction observed in his clinical cardiology practice from 1948 to 1953. Each patient developed either "a sudden alteration of the pattern of angina pectoris after a period of stability of anginal pain" (106/158), or "a sudden recurrence of anginal pain in those with previous angina pectoris and/or coronary thrombosis and in whom a period of relative freedom from pain was present immediately prior to recurrent symptoms" (52/158). Thus, Levy's patients were mainly group 2 unstable angina, although there were likely many who fell into group 3 and some of those with "sudden recurrence of anginal pain" likely remained in group 1. Levy stressed the departure from a well-established pattern of angina. He noted that angina might be more rapidly provoked, occur with greater frequency and severity, or last longer in response to a given stress. He observed broader radiation of the pain, associated signs of nausea, sweating, and vomiting, and less responsiveness to nitroglycerin. In many instances (128/158) the pain occurred at rest.

In general, patients were placed on bedrest at home. A satisfactory follow-up was achieved in approximately 90% of these patients. By three months 58% had developed a stabilization or remission of anginal pain. However, some of these patients experienced minor degrees of myocardial necrosis as evidenced by electrocardiographic (ECG) or erythrocyte sedimentation rate (ESR) changes. A small number (3.2%) had no reduction of their anginal symptoms even after many months. Thirty-nine percent of patients had experienced a myocardial infarction within 12 weeks (if all episodes of sudden death are arbitrarily classed as myocardial infarction), and a total of 32% of patients had died.

In 1961, Vakil[9] reported his follow-up of 251 patients with "intermediate coronary syndrome" selected from his consultant cardiology practice in Bombay, India over a ten-year period (see Table 1-3). The patients all had prolonged and characteristic ischemic pain of greater than 15 minutes duration, transient ECG abnormalities, and absence of clinical, laboratory, or ECG evidence of acute myocardial infarction at entry. Although each case was "subjected to clinical, laboratory, and ECG investigation," treatment was not discussed. After three months, acute myocardial infarction had occurred in 93 of 251 (37%), but death in only 2 of 251 (0.8%).

The increasing recognition of syndromes of ischemia intermediate between stable angina and myocardial infarction led to attempts to improve the prognosis by the use of anticoagulants. Nichol began to treat such patients with anticoagulants in 1947, reporting his initial results in 41 patients in 1950.[35] This work was followed by many other reports of such therapy.[36-40] The conclusion in most of these communications was that anticoagulation reduced the incidence of acute myocardial infarction and sudden death, although by current epidemiologic standards the data are not adequate for meaningful analysis.

Four major trials of anticoagulation therapy in unstable angina, the most recent reported in 1964, unanimously concluded that anticoagulation was efficacious. But not one of them meets the criteria that are essential for such studies,[41] and the conclusions reached must therefore be questioned. Although similar deficiencies have weakened the conclusions of studies of the use of anticoagulants in established myocardial infarction,[41] more recent studies of adequate design indicate benefit in acute myocardial infarction.[42-44]

Table 1-3
Prospective "Natural History" Studies of Unstable Angina – Pre-1970

Author	Year of Publication	Name of Syndrome	Study Population	No. of Patients	Unstable Angina Group†			Acute			Follow-up		
					1	2	3	Time (mo)	AMI*	Death	Time (mo)	AMI	Death
Levy[6]	1956	Changing patterns of angina pectoris	Patients with unstable angina	158		158	158	2	62/158 (39.2%)	51/158 (32.3%)			
Vakil[9]	1961	Intermediate coronary syndrome	Patients with unstable angina	251			251	3	93/251 (37.1%)	2/251 (0.8%)			
Beamish and Storrie[7]	1960	Impending myocardial infarction	Patients with unstable angina, anticoagulant "control"	15		8	7	1.5	12/15 (80.0%)	9/15 (60.0%)	6	14/15 (93.3%)	11/15 (73.3%)
Wood[46]	1961	Acute and subacute coronary insufficiency	Patients with unstable angina, anticoagulant "control"	50			50	2	11/50 (22.0%)	8/50 (16.0%)	6		15/50 (30.0%)
Vakil[47]	1964	Preinfarction syndrome	Patients with unstable angina, anticoagulant "control"	156			156	3	77/156 (49.4%)	37/156 (23.7%)			

*Acute myocardial infarction
†The numbers of patients are repeated when there is an overlap between subgroups.

Nichol and associates[45] used anticoagulant therapy on 318 patients with a diagnosis of impending myocardial infarction on the basis of crescendo and rest-pain features (group 2 and 3) during the period 1947 to 1957. They observed a 30-day infarction rate of 6.6%, with a 1.6% mortality rate. Benefit of therapy was judged by comparison to previous data from untreated patients as there was no control group, and the criteria of infarction were inadequate by present standards.

Beamish and Storrie[7] reported the outcome of 100 patients with unstable angina (group 2 or 3) between 1949 and 1957. Eighty-five patients were hospitalized, put at bedrest, and given anticoagulants. The 15 patients who were not hospitalized because of noncompliance or lack of beds were not given anticoagulants and were considered to be control subjects (see Table 1-3). During the six weeks after diagnosis of acute coronary insufficiency 2 of 85 treated patients suffered acute myocardial infarction, and none died. Of the 15 untreated patients, 12 had infarction (all of them outside of hospital), and nine died. Krauss and associates[15] have observed that bedrest alone may play an important role in the prevention of myocardial infarction in unstable angina. The denial of bedrest and hospital nursing care would be expected to have had an adverse effect on the controls in the study of Beamish and Storrie. Their conclusion that "prompt administration of anticoagulants appears to influence the outcome favorably" is not justified, in view of the inadequacies of the study.

Wood[46] studied 150 patients with unstable angina (group 3) between 1947 and 1957. All were put at bedrest, 100 received anticoagulants and 50 did not (see Table 1-3). During the two months after diagnosis, myocardial infarction occurred in 3% and death in 2% of the treated patients, and in 22% and 16%, respectively, of the control patients. The controlled phase of the study included only the first 40 patients, though even here the treatment regimen was not randomly assigned or double-blind. When there appeared to be an advantage to the first 20 patients who received anticoagulants, there was no further attempt to alternate treated and control patients. The last 30 patients to enter the control group did so because anticoagulants were deemed undesirable for a variety of reasons. The therapeutic regimens appeared to differ only with regard to treatment with anticoagulants, suggesting that anticoagulant therapy was justified in unstable angina. However, the faults with the sampling procedure may have introduced a bias that would invalidate this conclusion.

Vakil[47] reported an anticoagulant trial of 360 patients with "preinfarction syndrome" (group 3) treated between 1949 and 1963. All patients were put at bedrest and sedated. The treated group (190 patients) and the control group (156 patients) were said to be well-matched, but the treatment allocation procedure was not specified (see Table 1-3). Within three months of diagnosis, acute myocardial infarction had occurred in 36.3% of the treated patients (mortality rate 9.5%) and in 49.4% of the control patients (mortality rate 23.7%). Vakil concluded that a statistically significant reduction in acute myocardial infarction and particularly in mortality rate was evident in the treated group. This conclusion may not be justified when one considers the deficiencies in study design, particularly in relation to treatment allocation. A markedly reduced incidence of acute myocardial infarction and death in both control and treated groups in comparison to Vakil's earlier study was not explained in this paper.

The belief, now questioned,[30,48] that coronary artery thrombosis precedes myocardial infarction encouraged the enthusiastic investigation of anticoagulant therapy of the preinfarction syndrome. The impression emerged that anticoagulant therapy is beneficial for patients with unstable angina. However, there is no well-designed and properly controlled study available from which a judgment can be made.

By 1970, patients with unstable angina were regarded as having 1- to 3-month risk of acute myocardial infarction of 21% to 80% and of death of 1% to 60%. These data had emerged from preanticoagulation studies[6,9] and from the control groups in the anticoagulant trials.[7,46,47] Patients had received no long-acting nitrates, no anticoagulants, no beta-blocking agents, and often were not hospitalized. Reduction in activities and nitroglycerin were employed generally. Anticoagulant therapy was regarded as being highly efficacious. Since 1970, a number of series have appeared[15,16,49] describing outcomes in patients treated with varying regimens utilizing long-acting nitrates, anticoagulants, and beta-blocking agents, and thus are not truly natural history studies, but reflect, rather, the outcome of currently popular therapy. The high rates of early acute infarction and death have fallen sharply in these studies, and range from 7% to 15% and 1% to 2%, respectively. The reduction of infarction rate may be in part a result of the changing definition of unstable angina, which now includes patients who are early in their ischemic history. Thus, Fulton and associates[49] included in their study a large number of patients whose only symptom was the onset of angina during the preceding four weeks (group 1), a group not included in many of the earlier studies. On the other hand, Krauss and associates[15] looked only at group 3 patients, yet the incidence of acute myocardial infarction was only 7% in one month. This was a study of patients who arrived in the hospital; therefore patients whose unstable angina progressed to myocardial infarction or death prior to hospitalization were excluded, improving the overall outcome. The reduction in infarction rate in recent studies is likely the result of greater awareness of the significance of the syndrome and an increased tendency to put the patients in the hospital or at bedrest at home. Utilization of anticoagulants and beta-blocking agents may also be a factor. The reduction of mortality rate may reflect the trend to admit these patients to hospital and to monitor them if a myocardial infarction occurs, thereby reducing primary arrhythmic deaths.

The study of Fulton and associates[49] is the most representative of a community experience (Table 1-4). The male patients of a large group of general practitioners in Edinburgh were studied. Patients entered the study if they developed unstable angina typical of groups 1, 2, or 3. They were hospitalized only if they fell into group 2 or group 3, or if myocardial infarction was suspected. No anticoagulants were used. Of 167 patients, 15.5% developed documented or presumed acute myocardial infarction, and 1.8% died within three months, the majority of events occurring within four weeks. Of the 167 patients, 45 were hospitalized, and the acute myocardial infarction rate (20%) and mortality rate (2.2%) in this group were only slightly higher than in the entire group.

The study of Krauss and associates[15] best represents hospital management of unstable angina (see Table 1-4). The study was a retrospective review of 100 patients who had group 3 unstable angina and showed no evidence of myocardial infarction over the first 48 hours in the coronary care unit. The medical management was not standardized. About half the patients received an anticoagulant, one-third a long-acting nitrate, and one-sixth propranolol. The incidence of myocardial infarction in the hospital was low, only 7%. All but one of these myocardial infarctions occurred in the group of 36 patients who continued to experience prolonged ischemic pain after 12 hours of bedrest. The hospital mortality rate was only 1%, the single death occurring suddenly in an elderly man with a presumed infarct late in his hospital course. The patients were followed after hospital discharge, and during the first year; a significant incidence of myocardial infarction and death ensued. There were six further documented myocardial infarctions (two of whom died), seven sudden deaths presumed secondary to myocardial infarction, and three noncardiac deaths. Thus, the myocardial infarction rate after one year was 20%, and the mortality rate 15% of the 88 patients available for follow-up.

The study of Gazes and associates[16] is of interest because it is the first reported long-term follow-up study of unstable angina (see Table 1-4). They prospectively followed for ten years 140 patients in whom they diagnosed preinfarction angina group 2 or 3 prior to 1961. Patients were treated with bedrest, nitrates, sedatives, analgesia, low-calorie and low-fat diets, and 91 of 140 were treated with anticoagulants. Beta-blocking drugs were used only late in the follow-up study. At three months, acute myocardial infarction had developed in 20.7%, and death in 10%. The authors identified a subgroup of 54 patients whose pain persisted after 48 hours of bedrest, among whom the three-month myocardial infarction rate was 35%, and the mortality rate 26%. Of the total group, 18% were dead at the end of one year, whereas in the subgroup, 43% were dead. The mortality rates for the total group and subgroup were, respectively, at five years 39% and 73%, and at ten years 52% and 81%. Fifty-one of the 54 patients with persisting pain had had stable angina prior to the diagnosis of preinfarction angina.

Table 1-4
Prospective "Natural History" Studies of Unstable Angina — Post-1970

Author	Year of Publication	Name of Syndrome	Study Population	No. of Patients	Unstable Angina Group			Acute			Follow-up		
					1	2	3	Time (mo)	AMI*	Death	Time (mo)	AMI	Death
Krauss et al[15]	1971	Acute coronary insufficiency	Patients hospitalized with unstable angina, no acute myocardial infarction or death in 48 hr	100			100	1	7/100 (7.0%)	1/100 (1.0%)		20/100 (20.0%)	13/88 (14.8%)
			Subgroup with pain after 12 hr	36				1 (16.7%)	6/36	0			
Gazes et al[16]	1973	Preinfarction (unstable) angina	Patients hospitalized with unstable angina, no acute myocardial infarction or death in 48 hr	140		140	140	3	29/140 (20.7%)	14/140 (10.0%)	12	25/140 (17.9%)	
			Subgroup with pain after 48 hr	54		54	54	3	19/54 (35.2%)	14/54 (25.9%)			23/54 (42.6%)
Fulton et al[49]	1972	Unstable angina	Patients developing unstable angina in community	167	88	79	79	3	26/167 (15.6%)	3/167 (1.8%)			
			Subgroup requiring hospitalization	45		45	45	3	9/45 (20.0%)	1/45 (2.2%)			

*Acute myocardial infarction

Important high-risk groups of unstable angina were identified by these recent studies. It had been previously stated in several reports that patients whose unstable angina was superimposed on stable angina or previous myocardial infarction had a worse prognosis. Krauss[15] noted excess mortality rates during the 20 months' follow-up in such patients. Gazes[16] found that persisting pain in the hospital most frequently occurred in these patients, and there were excess rates of acute myocardial infarction and death in the early (three months') and late (ten years') follow-up. Gazes also found that those patients who demonstrated transient ECG abnormalities in association with pain had a worse prognosis. The highest risk group in each study included those patients whose pain persisted in the hospital on medical therapy. Acute infarction and death were much more frequent in this group of patients. In the Gazes study the excess infarction and mortality rates persisted through the ten-year follow-up.

Much of the clinical significance of unstable angina arises from the resultant risk of myocardial infarction. Unstable angina has therefore been recognized as a prodrome of acute myocardial infarction. The initial reports of prodromata in acute myocardial infarction were retrospective. Sampson and Eliaser[1] and Feil[27] examined patients with acute myocardial infarction who had experienced prodromes, attempting to delineate the features of prodromal symptoms. Yater,[32] Mounsey,[33] and Smith et al[34] attempted to determine the incidence of prodromes from retrospective reviews of the records of patients who had experienced acute myocardial infarction. The hazards of retrospective reviews are now well-recognized and prompted a series of prospective studies directed at better delineation of the prodromes of acute myocardial infarction.

Solomon et al[50] administered a structured questionnaire to 100 consecutive patients with subsequently proven acute myocardial infarction admitted to the coronary care unit of the New York Hospital from 1967 to 1968 (see Table 1-2). "Prodromata" were defined as "a constellation of new symptoms of presumed cardiac origin, or worsening of existing cardiac symptoms, which precede acute myocardial infarction by a period not exceeding two months." Sixty-five percent of patients had such prodromata, and 59 of 65 (91% of those with prodromata) consisted of chest pain with or without symptoms. Those patients with non–chest-pain prodromes experienced burning of the chest, dyspnea, vertigo, weakness, or fatigue. Prodromes were recurrent in 56 of 65 patients, and 43 of 65 had a progressive or crescendo syndrome of increasing frequency, severity, or duration before culminating in acute myocardial infarction. The episodes occurred mainly with exertion or emotion, although 19 of 65 patients had their symptoms only at rest, and 8 of 65 had both rest and exertional symptoms. It is apparent that 59 of 100 patients with chest-pain prodromes had what we would now call unstable angina. This prospective study pointed out the high incidence of unstable angina preceding acute myocardial infarction.

A further group of studies confirmed Solomon's observations. Stowers and Short[51] interviewed 180 patients with proven acute myocardial infarction while they were in the hospital (see Table 1-2). Of 180 patients, 122 (68%) had a history of "unusual symptoms beginning during the two months before admission" for acute myocardial infarction. In 99 of 180 (55%) the outstanding symptom was the onset or intensification of attacks of pain or discomfort at the site of origin, or greatest intensity of the pain that subsequently led to their admission. In 43 of 99 patients the pain occurred only on effort and was relieved by rest, in 37 of 99 the pain occurred mainly on effort, though sometimes at rest, and in 19 of 99 the pain occurred mainly at rest. The authors advised that patients with exertional prodromata should rest at home and those with rest pain should receive anticoagulants. They stressed the need for physicians to recognize prodromal symptoms and considered the desirability of educating the public in this field.

Hochberg[52] reported a study of 74 consecutive coronary care patients with acute myocardial infarction who were interviewed with respect to prodromes. They occurred in 62 of 74 (84%) patients but consisted of chest pain in only 34 of 62. Comparison with other studies is difficult because prodromes were defined simply as "one or more of a set of symptoms which were present at least 24 hours before admission and were not the immediate reason for seeking medical attention." The onset was "within the last few weeks or months," and in 32% the duration was greater than one month.

Freeman and Loughhead[53] administered a standardized questionnaire to 100 consecutive coronary care patients with proven acute myocardial infarction who survived at least 24 hours. Seventy-two percent of these patients had a recognizable prodrome, 90% of these having the prodromal symptoms for less than four weeks. The prodrome consisted of the onset of angina in 40 of 56 patients who had experienced no previous angina, and a change in anginal pattern with increased severity of attacks in 32 of 44 patients with a past history of angina. The authors pointed out the potential advantages of hospitalizing patients with prodromal symptoms, possibly reducing the incidence of infarction and sudden death.

Studies of the incidence of prodromal symptoms preceding sudden death (presumed coronary death) have been more difficult to conduct. Recent investigators have attempted to delineate the incidence of prodromes of sudden death by conducting structured interviews with the relatives and close associates of victims. The victim may not have expressed his symptoms, the person interviewed may have forgotten reported symptoms in the emotional trauma of the death, or he may have falsely reported symptoms as a result of suggestions arising from the interview. It is therefore not surprising that greater variation and ambiguity is present in the studies of sudden death prodromes than in those of acute myocardial infarction.[54]

Alonzo et al,[55] reported a series of 160 patients hospitalized for acute myocardial infarction and 138 patients who died suddenly (within 24 hours of onset of symptoms of the terminal event) of acute coronary heart disease outside of the hospital. Seventy percent (112/160) of acute myocardial infarction patients experienced prodromal symptoms (median duration, 10.5 days) (see Table 1-2). Sixty-four percent (88/138) of the sudden death victims had such symptoms (median duration, 30 days) (Table 1-5). Of those, acute anginal symptoms were the most frequent, occurring in 67%. Chest pain was much less frequently reported (35%) in the sudden death victims. Fatigue, weakness, and dyspnea were common prodromal symptoms in both groups.

Romo[56] in Finland, carried out a large study of patients experiencing sudden death or acute myocardial infarction. He found that 63% of patients (616/976) with acute myocardial infarction experienced new (prodromal) symptoms during the four weeks preceding the attack (see Table 1-2), whereas 53% (127/239) experiencing sudden death had such symptoms (see Table 1-5). An anginal prodrome, defined as "angina pectoris of recent onset, or a change in pattern of previous angina pectoris" occurred in 32% of patients (309/976) with acute myocardial infarction and in 16% of victims (38/239) of sudden death.

The study of Kuller et al[57] from Baltimore reported 240 patients experiencing sudden death with atherosclerotic heart disease (see Table 1-5). In the two weeks preceding death 37% (77/240) had chest pain but many patients had a history of atherosclerotic heart disease and only 13% (28/240) had an increase in frequency of their pain during the preceding two weeks. A variety of other symptoms were reported.

The problem is to define prodromes of myocardial infarction and sudden death with sufficient clarity that public and professional education programs might be undertaken in the attempt to reduce mortality.[54] Prodromal symptoms of myocardial infarction are most frequently those of unstable angina,[50-53] and the educational endeavors indicated are clear. The reduced incidence of acute myocardial infarction and sudden death observed in recent prospective studies of unstable angina[15,16,49] supports the value of recognizing these prodromes. However, although sudden death is preceded by prodromal symptoms about as frequently as is acute myocardial infarction, symptoms are less specific. Unstable angina precedes sudden death with less than half the frequency that it precedes acute myocardial infarction. The predominant symptoms are usually fatigue, weakness, and dyspnea. An effective approach to the perception of prodromes of sudden death and to management awaits development.

As the syndromes of unstable angina have been recognized and defined, potential outcomes have been delineated. Therapeutic regimens have been tested and standardized approaches to management have evolved.[58,59] Effort-induced angina of recent onset (group 1) is assessed for precipitating

Table 1-5
Prospective Patient Questionnaire of Associated Studies of Prodromes of Sudden (Coronary) Death

Author	Year of Publication	Population	No. of Patients	Total Incidence of Prodromes	Incidence of Prodromes Unstable angina	Unstable Angina Group*		
						1	2	3
Kuller et al[57]	1972	Death within 24 hr of symptoms	240		28/240 (11.7%)		28	
Romo[56]	1972	Death within 1 hr of symptoms	239	127/239 (53.1%)	38/239 (15.9%)	38	38	38
Alonzo et al[55]	1975	Death within 24 hr	138	88/138 (63.8%)	31/138 (22.5%)	31	31	31

*The numbers of patients are repeated when there is an overlap between subgroups.

and aggravating factors and is generally treated by modification of the patient's activities and with nitroglycerin therapy. Angina that occurs rarely and only in association with heavy exertion or severe emotional upset may require no other drug therapy. If angina is more readily precipitated, therapy with propranolol, perhaps supplemented by long-acting nitrates, is usually instituted with appropriate consideration of side effects and contraindications. As long as the angina remains predictable, stable, and minimally limiting to the patient, further therapeutic interventions are not usually undertaken, although the intensity of investigation varies somewhat among cardiologists.

If there is a progressive character to angina of recent onset, the patient is considered to fall into group 2. If this is the case, or if a patient shows crescendo angina (group 2) or prolonged rest angina (group 3), management is more vigorous and aimed at preventing acute myocardial infarction and sudden death. Accordingly, the patient is admitted to a coronary care unit for electrocardiographic monitoring. Serial enzymes are determined, and ECGs are obtained to detect any myocardial infarction that may have already occurred. An attempt is made to reduce the oxygen demands of the myocardium as much as possible by instituting bedrest and adequate sedative and analgesic therapy. If there are no contraindications, propranolol or another beta blocker is usually given orally, particularly if ischemic pain is recurrent in the hospital. There has been no controlled study of the use of propranolol in unstable angina, but a number of reports have appeared[12,60-64] and beta blockade has become standard therapy for unstable angina in most centers. A progressively increased dose is employed until appropriate beta blockade is achieved.[62] Long-acting nitrates are also given, although reports of their efficacy are scarce.[64,65] With the recognition that coronary artery spasm may be causative in some patients, long-acting nitrates may be heavily relied upon and beta blockade may even be considered deleterious. Calcium antagonists such as verapamil, nifedipine, and perhexaline have been utilized and may be particularly effective in patients suspected of having coronary artery spasm.[66] The role of anticoagulants remains ill-defined.

Studies have demonstrated that the risk of acute myocardial infarction and death is increased in patients with ECG abnormalities accompanying their pain and with recurrent episodes of rest pain in the hospital on optimal medical therapy.[15,16] Such patients are managed with the most vigorous medical therapy, but the small group who continue to have pain while receiving full medical therapy in the hospital generally undergo coronary angiography and aortocoronary bypass surgery, although no clear proof of efficacy is available.

Current medical therapy results in control of symptoms in the majority of patients hospitalized with unstable angina. The National Institutes of Health (NIH) study[67] has shown that urgent surgical treatment is not necessary and is probably not desirable for these patients. However, the role of surgery in ongoing management remains controversial. Major medical centers generally employ one of the following approaches. In the first approach, the majority of patients undergo catheterization relatively soon after the episode of unstable angina and aortocoronary bypass surgery is performed on every possible patient, whether or not angina recurs. A second approach is to carry out coronary angiography on the majority of patients, but in the absence of pain recurrence, to operate only on those patients with certain distributions of coronary artery lesions (particularly left main coronary artery stenosis or proximal three-vessel disease) known to carry a high risk of death in patients with stable angina.[68,69] A third, more conservative approach is to maintain vigorous medical therapy, reserving coronary angiography and surgical therapy for patients whose symptoms recur.[70] These approaches await systematic evaluation.

Although current medical therapy offers a good prognosis in the first one to three months after the onset of unstable angina, and the NIH study indicates that urgent surgery does not further improve prognosis, the incidence of death during the first year after diagnosis (mean 17% from several studies),[15,16,17] is a persisting source of concern. In comparison, among patients who survive for at least one month after an acute myocardial infarction, the mortality for the remainder of the year is about 9.5%.[72] The annual mortality in stable angina is about 4%,[73] and for men aged 35 to 65 years it is 1%.[74] Attempts to reduce the disproportionate mortality in unstable angina persist.

Unstable angina may be defined as a spectrum of acute myocardial ischemic pain syndromes lying between the well-defined diagnosis of stable angina pectoris on the one hand and acute myocardial infarction on the other. Review of the numerous studies employing a variety of terms to describe the syndromes and to emphasize certain features indicates that the term unstable angina should encompass the following presentations:

Angina of recent onset (previous four weeks)

Angina with a progressively severe (crescendo) pattern (previous four weeks)

Angina of prolonged duration (> 15 min) at rest

Angina occurring in the early period (four weeks) after myocardial infarction.

Whichever group the patient falls into, it should be specified whether the pain syndrome is the first presentation of myocardial ischemia or whether there was previous stable angina or myocardial infarction. It should also be specified whether the pain originates at rest or on exertion (including emotion, arrhythmia, and other precipitants of increased myocardial oxygen consumption). Myocardial necrosis must be ruled out, particularly in group 3 patients, by serial determination of myocardial enzymes and recording of ECGs. Generally the patient may be classified in only one group. If features characteristic of more than one group are present, generally, group 2 will predominate over group 1, and group 3 over either group 1 or 2. The time frame for designation of a given syndrome as unstable angina is generally four weeks. Prolonged rest angina is generally considered to be unstable without regard to date of onset. Patients with brief rest angina (< 15 min) are being recognized and may have transient coronary artery spasm. In the present system they would be included in group 2 if the onset had been within the past four weeks. The value of considering prolonged rest angina separately (group 3) is that the prognosis is worse, and in a significant number of these patients the presenting pain is the manifestation of an acute myocardial infarction.

Analysis of the literature indicates that all four groups listed above may be legitimately included within the definition of unstable angina. However, it is essential in evaluating the literature to discern which groups have been included in a given study. The tables in this chapter list the groups included in each study. It is also important that investigators designing new studies clearly define which groups are to be included. The prognosis is different among the four groups. Group 1 includes every patient who develops angina, yet the majority will be found, after a period of observation, to have a stable pattern and a relatively good prognosis. Group 3 includes patients with recurrent episodes of rest pain in hospital, the group most likely to have ECG abnormalities, and with the highest risk of infarction and death.[15,16] It may be concluded that group 2 patients have a somewhat better prognosis, although studies have not been specifically designed to reveal such a difference.[58] Group 4 patients have not been well studied but are generally regarded as having a rather poor prognosis.

There has been a tendency in recent studies of surgical therapy of unstable angina to focus on patients with a worse prognosis. Thus the recent NIH study[67] entered patients whose chest pain was "sufficiently severe to warrant admission to a coronary care unit within seven days of the last episode of pain, when the physician suspects impending infarction." Transient ECG changes associated with the pain were required for inclusion in the study. This requirement decreases the likelihood of a false diagnosis of ischemic pain, but it also selects a group of patients at relatively high risk of acute myocardial infarction and sudden death.[16] Eighty-four percent of the patients entering the NIH study had recurrences of pain in the CCU on full medical therapy, a further indication of the high-risk group under consideration.[15,16] Seldon et al[75] conducted a randomized trial of medical vs surgical therapy in 40 patients with group 3 unstable angina. Entry required recurrences of angina after 24 hours of hospital bedrest and the observation of reversible ST- and/or T-wave changes on the ECG. Recent epidemiologic investigations have indicated that some high-risk patients may not necessarily show a high level of response to therapies being investigated[76]; therefore these high-risk patients may not necessarily be the only ones that should be assessed in such studies.

It is essential that investigators continue to specify which groups of unstable angina patients from the target population of a given study and what entry requirements will be applied. Interpretation of the study results and their application to subsequent clinical problems demands clear knowledge of the entry criteria, since the term unstable angina includes a variety of ischemic syndromes with different prognoses.

There are several purposes in defining unstable angina with its various groups. Interpretation of the literature requires clear definition of the term and particularly of the four groups, if the development of therapeutic approaches and assessment of outcomes are to be evaluated. Clinically, the diagnosis of unstable angina is an operative definition that prompts immediate therapy for a condition that may presage acute myocardial infarction or sudden death or may itself be a manifestation of an acute (usually small) myocardial infarction. Delineation of the various groups within the definition is a powerful prognostic tool. The design of any new study of unstable angina demands clear definitions that are consistent with those now available in the literature.

This chapter has reviewed the development of the concept that a group of myocardial ischemic pain syndromes (eventually designated as unstable angina) lies intermediate between stable angina and acute myocardial infarction. A broad definition of unstable angina has been presented. Stress has been laid upon the responsibility of the investigator to define which groups of unstable angina patients constitute a study population. Interpretation and application of the results depends upon such definitions.

REFERENCES

1. Sampson, J.J., and Eliaser, M. The diagnosis of impending acute coronary artery occlusion. *Am Heart J.* 13:676, 1937.

2. Blumgart, H.L., Schlesinger, M.J., and Zoll, P.M. Angina pectoris, coronary failure, and acute myocardial infarction: the role of coronary occlusion and collateral circulation. *JAMA.* 116:91, 1941.

3. Master, A.M., Gubner, R., Dack, S. et al. Differentiation of acute coronary insufficiency with myocardial infarction from coronary occlusion. *Arch Intern Med.* 67:647, 1941.

4. Papp, C., and Smith, K.S. Electrocardiographic patterns in slight coronary attacks. *Br Heart J.* 13:17, 1951.

5. Graybiel, A. The intermediate coronary syndrome. *US Armed Forces Med J.* 6:1, 1955.

6. Levy, H. The natural history of changing patterns of angina pectoris. *Ann Intern Med.* 44:1123, 1956.

7. Beamish, R.E., and Storrie, V.M. Impending myocardial infarction. Recognition and management. *Circulation* 21:1107, 1960.

8. Papp, C., and Smith, K.S. Status anginosus. *Br Heart J.* 22:259, 1960.

9. Vakil, R.J. Intermediate coronary syndrome. *Circulation* 24:557, 1961.

10. Resnick, W.H. Preinfarction angina. I. The transaminase test—a diagnostic aid. *Mod Concepts Cardiovasc Dis.* 31:751, 1962.

11. Fowler, N.O. Preinfarction angina. *Circulation* 44:755, 1971.

12. Conti, C.R., Brawley, R.K., Griffith, L.S.C. et al. Unstable angina pectoris: morbidity and mortality in 57 consecutive patients evaluated angiographically. *Am J Cardiol.* 32:745, 1973.

13. Klein, M.S., Ludbrook, P.A., Mimbs, J.W. et al. Perioperative mortality rate in patients with unstable angina selected by exclusion of myocardial infarction. *J Thorac Cardiovasc Surg.* 73:253, 1977.

14. Willerson, J.R., Parkey, R.W., Boute, F.J. et al. Technetium stannous pyrophosphate myocardial scintigrams in patients with chest pain of varying etiology. *Circulation* 51:1046, 1975.

15. Krauss, K.R., Hutter, A.M., Jr., and DeSancitis, R.W. Acute coronary insufficiency. Course and follow-up. *Circulation* 45(suppl 1):I-66, 1972.

16. Gazes, P.C., Mobley, E.M., Jr., Faris, H.M., Jr. et al. Preinfarctional (unstable) angina—a prospective study—ten year followup. Prognostic significance of electrocardiographic changes. *Circulation* 48:331, 1973.

17. Bertolasi, C.A. Tronge, J.E., Carreno, C.A. et al. Unstable angina—prospective and randomized study of its evolution with and without surgery. Preliminary report. *Am J Cardiol.* 33:201, 1974.

18. Levine, F.H., Gold, H.K., Leinbach, R.C. et al. Management of acute myocardial ischemia with intraaortic balloon pumping and coronary bypass surgery. *Circulation* 58 (suppl I):1-69, 1978.

19. Levine, F.H., Gold, H.K., Leinbach, R.C. et al. Safe early revascularization for continuing ischemia after acute myocardial infarction. *Circulation* 60 (suppl I):I-5, 1979.

20. Parry, C.H. *An Inquiry into the Symptoms and Causes of Syncope Anginosa, Commonly Called Angina Pectoris.* London: Cadell and Davies, 1799, p. 28.

21. Obrastzow, W.P., and Straschesko, N.D. Zur Kenntnis der thrombosie der Koronararterien des herzens. *Ztschr Klin Med.* 71:116, 1910.

22. Herrick, J.B. Clinical features of sudden obstruction of the coronary arteries. *JAMA.* 59:2015, 1912.

23. Parkinson, J., and Bedford, D.E. Cardiac infarction and coronary thrombosis. *Lancet* 1:4, 1928.

24. Levine, S.A., and Brown, C.L. Coronary thrombosis: its various clinical features. *Medicine* 8:245, 1929.

25. Conner, L.A., and Holt, E. The subsequent course and prognosis in coronary thrombosis. *Am Heart J.* 5:705, 1930.

26. Willius, F.A. Certain factors influencing survival and death in coronary artery disease. *Proceedings of the Staff Meetings, Mayo Clinic* 11:414, 1936.

27. Feil, H. Preliminary pain in coronary thrombosis. *Am J Med Sci.* 193:42, 1937.

28. Master, A.M., Dack, S., and Jaffe, H.L. Premonitory symptoms of acute coronary occlusion; a study of 260 cases. *Ann Intern Med.* 14:115, 1941.

29. Master, A.M., Dack, S., Grishman, A. et al. Acute coronary insufficiency: an entity. Shock, hemorrhage and pulmonary embolism as factors in its production. *Mt Sinai J Med NY.* 14:8, 1947.

30. Roberts, W.C., and Buja, L.M. The frequency and significance of coronary arterial thrombi and other observations in fatal acute myocardial infarction. *Am J Med.* 52:425, 1972.

31. Master, A.M. The treatment of "impending infarction" (premonitory phase of coronary occlusion). *Chest* 43:302, 1963.

32. Yater, W.M., Traum, A.H., Brown, W.G., et al. Coronary artery disease in men eighteen to thirty-nine years of age. Report of eight hundred sixty-six cases, four hundred fifty with necropsy examinations. *Am Heart J.* 36:334, 1948.

33. Mounsey, P. Prodromal symptoms in myocardial infarction. *Br Heart J.* 13:215, 1951.

34. Smith, F.J., Keyes, J.W., and Denham, R.M. Myocardial infarction: a study of the acute phase in 920 patients. *Am J Med Sci.* 221:508, 1951.

35. Nichol, E.S. The use of anticoagulants in acute coronary insufficiency or impending myocardial infarction. *South Med J.* 43:565, 1950.

36. Jaffe, H.L., Halperin, H., and Nelson, L.M. Evaluation of anginal pain in the various stages of coronary artery disease. *NY State J Med.* 47:1382, 1947.

37. Smith, K.S., and Papp, C. The prevention of impending cardiac infarction by anticoagulant treatment. *Br Heart J.* 14:467, 1951.

38. Engelberg, H. Heparin therapy of severe coronary atherosclerosis with observation of its effect on angina pectoris, 2-step electrocardiogram and ballistogram. *Am J Med Sci.* 224:487, 1952.

39. Maurice, P., Beaumont, J.L., Leupin, A. et al. Premonitory period of myocardial infarction. *Arch Mal Coeur.* 48:551, 1955.

40. Anderson, G.M. Anticoagulant therapy in coronary artery insufficiency. *J Louisiana Med Soc.* 108:59, 1957.

41. Gifford, R.H., and Feinstein, A.R. A critique of methodology in studies of anticoagulant therapy for acute myocardial infarction. *N Engl J Med.* 280:351, 1969.

42. Holzman, D., Paraskos, J.A., and Lyon, A.F. Committee Report: Veterans Administration Hospital Investigators. Anticoagulants in acute myocardial infarction: results of a cooperative clinical trial. *JAMA.* 225:724, 1973.

43. Arnott, W.M., Biggs, R., and Gilchrist, A.R. Assessment of short-term anticoagulant administration after cardiac infarction: Report of the Working Party on Anticoagulant Therapy in Coronary Thrombosis to the Medical Research Council. *Br Med J.* 1:335, 1969.

44. Chalmers, T.C., Matta, R.J., Smith, H. Jr. et al. Evidence favoring the use of anticoagulants in the hospital phase of acute myocardial infarction. *N Engl J Med.* 297:1091, 1977.

45. Nichol, E.S., Phillips, W.C., and Casten, G.C. Virtue of prompt anticoagulant therapy in impending myocardial infarction: experiences with 318 patients during a 10-year period. *Ann Intern Med.* 50:1158, 1959.

46. Wood, P. Acute and subacute coronary insufficiency. *Br Med J.* 1:1779, 1961.

47. Vakil, R.J. Preinfarction syndrome – management and follow-up. *Am J Cardiol.* 14:55, 1964.

48. Chandler, A.B., Chapman, I., Erhardt, L.R. et al. Coronary thrombosis in myocardial infarction. Report of a workshop on the role of coronary thrombosis in the pathogenesis of acute myocardial infarction. *Am J Cardiol.* 34:823, 1974.

49. Fulton, M., Lutz, W., Donald, K.W. et al. Natural history of unstable angina. *Lancet* 1:860, 1972.

50. Solomon, H.A., Edwards, A.L., and Killip, T. Prodromata in acute myocardial infarction. *Circulation* 40:463, 1969.

26

51. Stowers, M., and Short, D. Warning symptoms before major myocardial infarction. *Br Heart J.* 32:833, 1970.

52. Hochberg, H.M. Characteristics and significance of prodromes of coronary care unit patients. *Chest* 59:10, 1971.

53. Freeman, J.W., and Loughhead, M.G. Prodromal angina preceding acute myocardial infarction. *Med J Aust.* 1:325, 1972.

54. Feinleib, M., Simon, A.B., Gillum, R.F. et al. Prodromal symptoms and signs of sudden death. *Circulation* 52 (suppl III):III-155, 1975.

55. Alonzo, A.A., Simon, A.B., and Feinleib, M. Prodromata of myocardial infarction and sudden death. *Circulation* 52:1056, 1975.

56. Romo, M. Factors related to sudden death in acute ischemic heart disease. A community study in Helsinki. *Acta Med Scand.* (suppl 547), 1972.

57. Kuller, L., Cooper, M., and Perper, J. Epidemiology of sudden death. *Arch Intern Med.* 129:714, 1972.

58. Cairns, J.A., Fantus, I.G., and Klassen, G.A. Unstable angina pectoris. *Am Heart J.* 92:373, 1976.

59. Cairns, J.A. Current management of unstable angina. *Can Med Assoc J.* 119:477, 1978.

60. Papazoglov, N.M. Use of propranolol in preinfarction angina. *Circulation* 44:303, 1971.

61. Mizgala, H.F., Khan, A.S., and Davies, R.O. The effect of propranolol in acute coronary insufficiency: a preliminary report (abstr). *Clin Res.* 17:637, 1969.

62. Fischl, S.J., Herman, M.V., and Gorlin, R. The intermediate coronary syndrome: clinical angiographic and therapeutic aspects. *N Engl J Med.* 288:1193, 1973.

63. Master, A.M., and Jaffe, H.L. Propranolol vs saphenous vein graft bypass for impending infarction (preinfarction syndrome). *Am Heart J.* 87:321, 1974.

64. Mizgala, H.F., Theroux, P., Convert, G. et al. Prospective randomized trial of perhexiline maleate, isosorbide dinitrate and propranolol in unstable angina (abstr). *Circulation* 56 (suppl III):III-225, 1977.

65. Willis, W.H., Russell, R.O., Jr., Mantle, J.A. et al. Hemodynamic effects of isosorbide dinitrate vs nitroglycerine in patients with unstable angina. *Chest* 69:15, 1976.

66. Maseri, A., Mimmo, R., Chierchia, S. et al. Coronary artery spasm as a cause of acute myocardial ischemia in man. *Chest* 68:625, 1975.

67. Unstable Angina Pectoris Study Group. Unstable angina pectoris national cooperative study group to compare surgical and medical therapy. II. In-hospital experience and initial follow-up results in patients with one, two and three-vessel disease. *Am J Cardiol.* 42:839, 1978.

68. Takaro, T., Hultgren, H.N., Lipton, M.J. et al. VA cooperative randomized study of surgery for coronary arterial occlusive disease. 2. Subgroup with significant left main lesion. *Circulation* 54 (suppl III):3-107, 1976.

69. Task Force on Coronary Artery Surgery. Coronary artery surgery. 1. Manifestations and natural history of coronary artery disease: development and evaluation of aortocoronary bypass surgery. *Can Med Assoc J.* 117:451, 1977.

70. Plotnick, G.D., and Conti, C.R. Unstable angina: angiography, short- and long-term morbidity, mortality and symptomatic status of medically treated patients. *Am J Med.* 63:870, 1977.

71. Schroeder, J.S., Lamb, I.H., and Harrison, D.C. Patients admitted to the coronary care unit for chest pain: high risk subgroup for subsequent cardiovascular death. *Am J Cardiol.* 39:829, 1977.

72. Pell, S., and D'Alonzo, C.A. Immediate mortality and five-year survival of employed men with a first myocardial infarction. *N Engl J Med.* 270:915, 1964.

73. Kannel, W.B., Feinleib, M. Natural history of angina pectoris in the Framingham study. Prognosis and survival. *Am J Cardiol.* 29:154, 1972.

74. Weinblatt, A.B., Frank, C.W., Shapiro, S. et al. Prognostic factors in angina pectoris—a prospective study. *J Chronic Dis.* 21:231, 1968.

75. Seldon, R., Neill, W.A., Ritzman, L.W. et al. Medical versus surgical therapy for acute coronary insufficiency: a randomized study. *N Engl J Med.* 293:1329, 1975.

76. Gent, M., and Sackett, D.L. The qualification and disqualification of patients and events in long-term cardiovascular clinical trials. Edited by M. Verstraete, J. Vermylen, and H. Roberts. In *The Challenge of Clinical Trials in Thrombosis.* Stuttgart: Schattauer Verlag, 1979.

2 Acute Coronary Events in the Community: Significance of Unstable Angina as a Prodromal Symptom

Jacob Lubsen, MD, Jan Pool, MD,
Emiel van der Does, MD, and
Paul G. Hugenholtz, MD

Instances of an acute coronary event (ie, acute myocardial infarction [AMI] or sudden cardiac death) are a major cause of disability and death in most industrialized countries.[1] The fatality rate is high, especially in the first few hours after the attack, and attempts to decrease the early mortality have not been successful. The question of whether or not the occurrence of an acute coronary event can be predicted on the basis of prodromal symptoms or other phenomena that precede the event is, therefore, of great interest. If such a prediction is possible with an acceptable degree of certainty, a more timely institution of treatment could in principle be envisioned.

The notion that prodromal symptoms frequently precede an acute coronary event is primarily based on case-history studies.[2] Such studies have suggested the presence of a wide variety of symptoms ranging from unusual fatigue to "classical" unstable angina in a large proportion of patients before an acute coronary event occurs. Case-history studies are limited by the possibility that the information in the cases is distorted because of the disease event itself. This is a particularly difficult problem in the context of the relationship between prodromal symptoms and acute coronary events. Case-history studies, therefore, have not given much insight into questions of the predictability of such events, and a working group of the World Health Organization (WHO)[3] concluded in 1971 that follow-up studies were needed.

A number of follow-up studies have been reported. Many of them are reviewed in Chapter 1, which also discusses the problem of definition and its consequences in the interpretation of the results. Most of the studies, such as those of Vakil[4] and of Lie et al,[5] were limited to hospitalized patients. Although the WHO[3] has advocated more comprehensive studies, these have rarely been carried out, and only the study by a group of investigators working in Edinburgh, Scotland[6] involved patients irrespective of hospitalization. This study was concerned with the prognosis of patients with unstable angina referred to a special clinic by general practitioners. It has yielded valuable information on the prognosis of unstable angina in the community but failed to answer several important questions. For instance, the Edinburgh study[6] did not attempt to show how often an acute coronary event is preceded by recognized unstable angina or to what extent unstable angina is a better predictor of a future acute coronary event than less "typical" symptoms.

The Imminent Myocardial Infarction Rotterdam (IMIR) study[7] was similar in objective and design to the Edinburgh study, but its scope was more comprehensive in that it included not only patients consulting their physician for unstable angina but also patients with other unstable (ie, recent or recently worsened) symptoms without apparent extracardiac cause. Based on data from this study, which gave a comprehensive picture of the occurrence of acute coronary events in an industrialized community in The Netherlands, this chapter will attempt to answer some of the questions left open by earlier studies.

THE IMIR STUDY

Methods

In 14 general practices situated in and around the city of Rotterdam, instances of patient-physician contact were registered from October, 1972 through May, 1974 whenever the patient complained of recent or recently increased chest pain and/or recent and unexplained dyspnea, palpitations, upper abdominal pains, dizziness, syncope, mood changes; "recent" referred to the last four weeks and "unexplained" to "without apparent extracardiac cause." Also, all instances of sudden cardiac death, defined as death within 24 hours after the onset of the attack and without apparent extracardiac cause, were registered upon notification by the physician. Inclusion was restricted to men aged 20 years and older and women aged 25 and older. Management of patients was left to the physician's discretion, although common opinion led to the adoption of some general policies.

After verifying that the inclusion criteria were met, the physician took a detailed history and performed a simple physical examination, using a standardized questionnaire for recording data. Then, a provisional inclusion diagnosis was recorded. Finally, the physician decided whether or not immediate hospitalization was necessary and gave, if applicable, the indications for it.

If no immediate hospitalization followed the initial contact, the patient was seen directly either at home or at a special clinic by a technician. The technician completed an additional questionnaire, recorded a standard 12-lead electrocardiogram, and took a blood sample to assess serum levels of the enzymes alpha-hydroxybutyric dehydrogenase (a-HBDH), glutamic oxaloacetic transaminase (GOT), and creatinine phosphokinase (CPK). For these investigations, technicians were kept available on a 24-hour basis. When the patient was hospitalized, test results and other clinical information were obtained from the hospital.

After inclusion, there was a ten-month follow-up period for the collection of further data on the clinical course of the patient. ECG and enzyme studies were repeated after three days and after one week; another ECG was recorded one month after inclusion. At all these occasions, a short questionnaire on the current status of the patient was also completed.

At the conclusion of follow-up, ie, ten months after entry into the study, an ECG was recorded, and a detailed questionnaire was completed on current symptoms and medical events during follow-up. In addition, information was obtained from the patient's physician and, if applicable, from consulting specialists or from hospitals. Acute coronary events at inclusion or during follow-up were classified as either "definite" or "possible" AMI or as "sudden cardiac death." A modified version of the World Health Organization criteria for AMI[8] was used, details of which are available from the authors upon request.

Results

Of the 1387 patients included, 43 were registered as "sudden cardiac death." Of the remaining 1344, 130 (10%) patients had either "definite" or "possible" acute myocardial infarction at inclusion (Table 2-1).

Of the 1214 patients free of AMI at inclusion, 82 (7%) sustained an acute coronary event during follow-up. Of these events, 19 (23%) were classified as "sudden cardiac death." Of the remaining 64 instances of "definite" or "possible" AMI, four were fatal (see Table 2-1). Four patients were excluded from further analysis because of incomplete data. One of these sustained an acute coronary event during the first month of follow-up. Age and sex data for the remaining 1210 patients are given in Table 2-2. A total of 252 (21%) patients had unstable exertional angina at inclusion, which was "worsening" in 134 patients and "new" in the remaining 118. In another 841 patients (69%), other (nonanginal) chest pain was among the symptoms recorded at inclusion while in the remaining 117 (10%) patients, unstable symptoms other than chest pain were present (Table 2-3).

Worsening angina was associated with the highest rate—9% (12/134)—of acute coronary event within one month after inclusion. This rate was lowest, fewer than 1% (1/117), in patients without symptoms of chest pain. Unstable angina and other chest pain were associated with one-month acute coronary event rates of 8% (20/252) and 3% (22/841), respectively. Of the 43 patients who sustained an acute coronary event within a

Table 2-1
Acute Coronary Events at Inclusion and During Follow-up

	Total No. of Patients	Sudden Cardiac Death	Definite AMI*	Possible AMI	No AMI
Inclusion	1387	43	93	37	1214
Follow-up	83	19	34†	30‡	—

*Acute myocardial infarction.
†Three fatal.
‡One fatal.

Table 2-2
Age and Sex Distribution of Patients Free of Acute Myocardial Infarction (AMI) at Inclusion by Event During Follow-up

	Events During Follow-up	
Variable	*Acute Coronary Event**	*No Acute Coronary Event*
Total number of patients	82 (100%)	1128 (100%)
Men	56 (68%)	609 (54%)
Age (yr)		
median, men	62	51
range, men	22–88	21–88
median, women	71	56
range, women	39–84	25–92

*"Definite" AMI, "possible" AMI, or sudden cardiac death.

month after inclusion, fewer than half, 20, had unstable angina at entry into the study, and only one patient had symptoms other than chest pain at that time (see Table 2-3).

Patients with unstable angina had a ten-month rate of acute coronary event of 13% (33/252). Within this group, a higher rate, 16% (22/134), was associated with "worsening" than with "new" angina, which had a ten-month rate of 9% (11/118). However, the difference was not statistically significant ($p < 0.1$, see Table 2-3). In patients who did not have angina, a ten-month rate of 5% (49/958) was observed. Their prognosis did not depend on the presence of chest pain at inclusion (see Table 2-3).

DISCUSSION

In the IMIR study, a patient was included if he consulted the physician for symptoms recognized as fulfilling the inclusion criteria. Among the patients included by this mechanism, a number of cases of "definite" or "possible" acute myocardial infarction were found to be present on the basis of electrocardiograms and enzyme studies. But after exclusion of such cases, a group of symptomatic patients without AMI remained who had a ten-month acute coronary event rate of 7% (83/1214, see Table 2-1). Such a rate is considerably higher than the rate that would obtain among the general population.

Table 2-3
Symptoms at Inclusion and Acute Coronary Events During Follow-up in Patients Free of Acute Myocardial Infarction (AMI) at Inclusion

Symptoms at Inclusion	No. of Patients at Risk	Acute Coronary Events* Within 1 Month	1–10 Months	Total Acute Coronary Events	
Worsening† angina	134	12	10	22	$p < 0.1$
New angina‡	118	8	3	11	
Other chest pain	841	33	20	42	$p < 0.6$
Other than chest pain	117	1	6	7	
Total	1210	43	39	82	

$p < 0.0003$§ (bracketing the two grouped pairs)

*"Definite" AMI, "possible" AMI, or sudden cardiac death.
†Exercise-induced chest pain, relieved within 10 min by stopping exercise, present longer than four weeks, and increasing in severity during the four weeks prior to inclusion.
‡As "worsening angina" but present less than four weeks.
§p values are based on a two-sided modified Fisher-exact test.[10]

Unstable angina has received much attention as a prodromal symptom of an acute coronary event.[9] In the present study, patients free of AMI who had unstable angina according to our criteria, had an 8% (20/252) at one-month and a 13% (33/252) at ten months acute coronary event risk. For all other patients taken together, the ten-month acute coronary event risk was 5% (49/958) or only about one third of the risk associated with the presence of unstable angina (see Table 2-3). Consequently, the presence of unstable angina identified a subgroup that was indeed at elevated risk. In this context, one finding seems of particular practical interest. Of 43 patients free of acute myocardial infarction who sustained an acute coronary event during one month of follow-up, fewer than half (20) had unstable angina at inclusion (see Table 2-3).

This finding, together with the fact that a number of acute coronary events were already present at inclusion, indicates that patients who eventually sustain an acute coronary event are infrequently seen for unstable angina shortly before the event takes place. Therefore, the absence of unstable angina cannot be taken by the physician as necessarily meaning that no short-term risk of an acute coronary event exists. In dealing with the problem of impending coronary events, the physician cannot confine his attention to patients with unstable angina.

The only other community study that seems to have been done apart from this one was carried out in Edinburgh, Scotland.[6] Men under 70 years of age, suffering from unstable angina, were followed for six months; a 16% (39/251) acute coronary event rate was reported for that period.[6] This study was concerned with both "new" and "worsening" angina. The diagnosis was made by a cardiologist; 171 of the 251 patients had ST-depression or T-wave changes on the ECG, and only 28 patients had a completely normal ECG. Eighty-seven patients were admitted to the hospital, but their prognosis did not differ significantly from the nonhospitalized patients; nor did the prognosis depend significantly on whether the angina was "new" or "worsening." In the IMIR study, an even lower acute coronary event rate was observed for patients with either "new" or "worsening" angina; these patients had a 13% (33/252, see Table 2-3) ten month rate. In comparing these two studies, it must, however, be remembered that the IMIR also studied women, who have a lower acute coronary event risk. In the IMIR the diagnosis of "unstable angina" was based on a questionnaire rather than on the physician's impression, as was the case in the Edinburgh study.[6]

Apart from information on the prognosis of unstable angina, the IMIR also supplied information on other aspects of the prodromata of acute coronary events. Patients who were sustaining an acute coronary event at the time of inclusion did not have prodromal symptoms of such a nature or severity that they consulted a physician and were consequently included into the study before the event occurred. Since 77% of these patients did not have a history of a previous myocardial infarction, it is evident that many patients who sustain an acute coronary event do not have prodromal symptoms for which a physician is consulted or even a history of a previous event.

REFERENCES

1. Vedin, J.A., Wilhelsson, C., Elmfeldt, D. et al. Sudden death: identification of high risk groups. *Am Heart J.* 86:124–132, 1973.

2. Gillum, R.F., Feinleib, M., Margolis, J.R. et al. The pre-hospital phase of acute myocardial infarction and sudden death. 1. Prodromata of acute coronary events. *Prev Med.* 5:408–413, 1976.

3. World Health Organization, Regional Office for Europe. *The Prodromal Symptoms of Myocardial Infarction and Sudden Death*. Report of a working group. Copenhagen, 1971.

4. Vakil, R.J. Preinfarction syndrome – management and follow-up. *Am J Cardiol.* 14:55–63, 1964.

5. Lie, L.I., Wellens, H.J.J., and Durrer, D. Een prospectieve studie van het dreigende hartinfarct. *Ned Tijdschr Geneeskd.* 118:1218–1220, 1974.

6. Duncan, B., Fulton, M., Morrison, S.L. et al. Prognosis of new and worsening angina pectoris. *Br Med J.* 1:981–985, 1976.

7. Van der Does, E., Lubsen, J., Pool, J. et al. Acute coronary events in general practice: objectives and design of the I.M.I.R. study. *Hart Bull.* 7:91–98, 1976.

8. World Health Organization, Regional Office for Europe. *Ischaemic Heart Disease Registers*. Report of the 5th working group. Copenhagen, 1971.

9. Cairns, J.A., Fantus, I.G., and Klassen, G.A. Review: unstable angina pectoris. *Am Heart J.* 92:373–386, 1976.

3 The Natural History of Unstable Angina Pectoris

John O. Parker, MD, and
Alan J. Leach, MD

The introduction of new medical and surgical methods for treating symptomatic coronary artery disease has made knowledge of the natural history of stable and unstable angina important. Interest in angina arose in large part from studies of patients with myocardial infarction or sudden death. These studies revealed that many such patients have prodromal symptoms over a period of a few hours to several weeks before the occurrence of such cardiac events.[1-7] Alonzo and co-workers,[6] in their retrospective study of patients hospitalized with myocardial infarction or with sudden cardiac death, found that prodromal symptoms had been present in 70% of the infarction group and 64% of those dying suddenly. New or accelerated angina was the most frequently reported symptom in the infarction group, while nonspecific complaints such as fatigue, weakness, and dyspnea were more common in those with sudden death. In the series of Harper and co-workers[7] 577 consecutive patients with acute myocardial infarction were studied. Fifty-eight percent of the patients with a history of chronic angina noticed worsening of their symptoms in the month prior to infarction, and 21% of all patients had new onset angina in the month before infarction. Of the 577 patients, 39% had unstable angina prior to infarction. Both Solomon and co-workers[4] and Harper and associates[7] found that patients with a history of chronic angina were more likely to have a period of unstable angina prior to infarction than patients without previous symptoms.

The term unstable angina covers a clinical spectrum situated between chronic stable angina and myocardial infarction. Four subgroups of unstable angina are recognized: 1) New onset angina, 2) Crescendo angina—increasingly frequent and prolonged exertional pain or onset of rest pain lasting less than fifteen minutes, 3) Acute coronary insufficiency—prolonged pain at rest associated with transient electrocardiographic changes, and 4) Postinfarction angina. Additional subgroups may also be considered that would include patients with variant angina and patients who fail to improve following institution of medical therapy while in the hospital. Patients with unstable angina may evolve from one subgroup to another.

This chapter will review the literature regarding the natural history of unstable angina, recognizing that this is not the true natural history, as the majority of patients will have received medical therapy. The best that we may accomplish is an outline of the clinical course of patients treated nonsurgically with forms of medical therapy that have varied depending on when the patients were studied. It is probable that the prognosis differs among the various subgroups of patients,[8] and thus we have reviewed the natural history of the major subgroups of unstable angina. Unfortunately, many studies do not permit such an analysis, as data for the subgroups are not provided. The subgroups of postinfarction angina and variant angina have either been excluded from or not analyzed in the reported natural history studies and will not be included in this review. Those subgroups are discussed in other chapters.

ANGINA OF RECENT ONSET

All patients with angina have had a first episode. Thereafter, angina may disappear, may continue as stable exertional angina, may become increasingly frequent or severe, may occur at rest, or may progress to myocardial infarction. Most studies of unstable angina include recent onset angina in their admission criteria. One study[9] required only the recent onset of angina, while others have required that the angina must not only be of recent onset but must demonstrate either a progressive pattern or become severe enough to require hospital admission to rule out myocardial infarction.[10-14]

The study of Fulton and co-workers[9] included a large number (87 of 167) with angina occurring for the first time within the previous four weeks. Unfortunately, this large group of patients was not described further, and the events in this particular subgroup were not analyzed separately. Kraus and associates[10] followed 100 patients with acute coronary insufficiency. In that group 33 patients had no previous symptoms suggestive of angina. Over the mean follow-up period of 20 months there were fewer cardiac deaths among these patients than in the patients with a history of previous angina. Ten of the 13 patients who died suddenly, and all nine who died with myocardial infarction, were in the group with previous angina. Gazes and associates[11] subdivided the patients with unstable angina into three types: type 1, patients with recent onset angina that was progressive and who had pain at rest lasting less than 15 mintues; type 2, patients who were similar to those of type 1 but had a history of chronic angina; type 3, patients with rest pain greater than 15 minutes in duration. They also recognized a separate "high-risk" group of patients who had persisting symptoms following hospitalization. Fifty-one of the 54 patients in the high-risk subgroup had prior stable angina. Only 1 of 27 patients with recent onset angina developed a myocardial infarction in the three-month follow-up, compared with 22 of the 109 patients with previous angina. Over the same period there were no deaths in patients with recent onset angina, compared with nine (8%) in the group with previous angina.

Alison and associates[12] included patients with recent onset effort-induced angina in the unstable group only if they had progression in the pattern of effort-induced angina or developed pain at rest. Of the 188 patients with unstable angina, 47 had angina of recent onset meeting these criteria. These patients had a good short-term prognosis as all of the in-hospital complications occurred in the group with previous angina. Others[13,14] suggest that the prognosis may not be as favorable for such patients with recent onset angina. For instance, 25% of Skjaeggestad's patients[13] with recent onset angina developed myocardial infarction or death within two months compared with 12% of those with previous angina or infarction. From the available data we cannot resolve whether patients with recent onset crescendo angina or recent onset coronary insufficiency fare better or worse than those with similar symptoms developing on a background of chronic stable angina.

Chahine[8] feels that patients with recent onset, mild to moderate exertional angina should not be considered as having unstable angina unless the angina is progressive or occurs at rest. Should the group of patients with recent onset angina be stratified further into those patients with recent onset but stable or improving angina, recent onset and crescendo angina, and recent onset angina with acute coronary insufficiency? Statistics pertaining to the early course of patients with recent onset, mild to moderate exertional angina are not available. The Framingham study[14] does, however, indicate that over a long term, patients with de novo angina have an annual mortality rate of 4%. Inclusion of such patients in the study by Fulton and associates[9] may have influenced morbidity and mortality for the overall group of patients with unstable angina.

CRESCENDO ANGINA

There are few data concerning the natural history of this subgroup of patients as most studies do not subdivide the clinical presentations of unstable angina adequately. In reviewing the literature there are only two studies in which the prognosis for crescendo exertional angina and acute coronary insufficiency are analyzed. Bertolasi and co-workers in 1974[16] and 1976[17] pointed out that there was a significant difference in the prognosis of patients with crescendo angina and those with acute coronary insufficiency. This prospective study compared the evolution of such patients treated medically or surgically. The study contained few medically treated patients, only 27 with crescendo angina and 24 with acute coronary insufficiency. Followed for an average of 32 months, the patients with crescendo angina had a 7% infarction rate compared with 38% in the patients with acute coronary insufficiency. The mortality rates for the two groups were 7% and 46%, respectively. The criteria for acute coronary insufficiency allowed minor enzyme elevation, which may have led to the inclusion of some patients with myocardial infarction. This study points out that patients with crescendo angina are a low-risk group in terms of morbidity and mortality relative to those with acute coronary insufficiency. All patients had coronary angiography, and the group with crescendo angina tended to have a better developed collateral circulation than the group with acute coronary insufficiency. The presence of collaterals could conceivably play a role in determining whether a patient presented with crescendo exertional angina or acute coronary insufficiency, and could be responsible for the more benign clinical course of patients with crescendo angina.

Gazes and co-workers[11] studied 140 patients with unstable angina, 113 of whom were followed to time of death or 120 months. We will consider them in this subgroup, as, by our criteria, only four had coronary insufficiency, the remainder crescendo angina. The mortality rate for the entire group was 10% at three months, 18% at one year, 25% at two years, 39% at five years, and 52% at ten years. Myocardial infarction occurred in 17% during the acute phase and in 21% by three months.

ACUTE CORONARY INSUFFICIENCY

Many of the studies of unstable angina concern the group of patients we would classify as having acute coronary insufficiency. In this subgroup of patients the reported infarction rates range from 1%[18] to 19%[19] in the acute stage, with mortality of up to 35%[16] at 8.3 months. Early infarction rates vary from 3%[20] to 62%.[19] The wide range in the reported complications is probably due in part to the variability of admission criteria for the studies and to differences in the medical management. Vakil[18] reported 360 patients who had prolonged chest pain lasting longer than 15 minutes. Their treatment included bedrest and sedation, and 190 patients received anticoagulant therapy. There were four early deaths (three days) for an early mortality rate of only 1%, but this rose to 16.4% at three months and at that time the infarction rate was 40.6%. Berk and co-workers,[19] on the other hand, studied 21 patients with severe chest pain at rest associated with either ST-segment elevation (ten patients) or ST-segment depression ≥ 2 mm (ten patients) or deep precordial T-wave inversion (one patient). Their treatment included oxygen, bedrest, sublingual nitrates, and propranolol. Of the 21 patients, 13 had myocardial infarction an average of four days after entering the study, and almost one third of these were fatal. Three of the 21 patients died in the hospital, and one shortly following discharge. Kraus and co-workers[10] observed 100 patients who had prolonged chest pain within 24 hours of hospital admission, most associated with new ECG changes. Seven patients developed myocardial infarction in the acute phase, with one death. Over the 20-month average follow-up, 22 of the 100 patients died of cardiac causes, 13 suddenly, and nine with myocardial infarction. In addition there were 14 nonfatal myocardial infarctions. The mortality and infarction rates were both approximately 1% per month in this study. Skjaeggestad[13] followed 132 patients admitted to hospital with acute coronary insufficiency. Over the two-month follow-up period the mortality rate was 2.5% per month and the nonfatal myocardial infarction rate 7.5% per month. The majority of these complications were early, with only three of the 22 events occurring after three weeks. Excluding the first two days the clinical course was comparable to that of 163 patients with uncomplicated myocardial infarction followed for two months. There was a 9.8% incidence of serious complications in the former group compared with a 6.1% incidence in the latter.

The results of the National Cooperative Study Group to compare medical and surgical therapy in unstable angina were recently published.[21] Admission criteria for the study included unstable angina severe enough to warrant hospital admission to rule out myocardial infarction, coronary artery stenosis of greater than 70% in at least one vessel, and suitability for aortocoronary bypass surgery both from the point of coronary anatomy and adequacy of left ventricular function. Patients with greater than 50% stenosis of the left main coronary artery were excluded from the study. It is important to note that 90% of the patients had angina at rest while in the hospital, although rest pain was not one of the admission criteria. The patients were followed for a mean period of 30 months. There were 147 patients treated medically, and their early and late mortality and infarction rates were compared with 141 patients treated surgically. The overall in-hospital mortality rate for the medical group was 3%, and the cumulative late mortality 10%. The in-hospital myocardial infarction rate was 8%, and the cumulative late infarction rate 19%. At one year there was a 7% mortality in the medical group, with the two-year mortality rate estimated at 9%.

PATIENTS WITH PERSISTING ANGINA
FOLLOWING HOSPITALIZATION

Several authors have analyzed the course of patients whose unstable angina did not respond to medical therapy after a period of hospital treatment. Criteria applied for inclusion in this subgroup of patients varied from those with pain recurring after more than 12 hours in the hospital,[10] to pain recurring four or more days after hospital admission.[14]

Gazes and co-workers[11] followed 54 patients with unstable angina who had persisting pain after more than 48 hours in the hospital. During the first three months of follow-up, 19 (35%) developed myocardial infarction, which was fatal in 63%. There were 14 deaths in this group of 54 (26%) during the first three months of follow-up. These figures are in contrast to the infarction rate of 21% and mortality rate of 10% for the entire group of patients with acute coronary insufficiency. Thus, two thirds of the myocardial infarctions and all the fatal myocardial infarctions occurred in the group of patients whose symptoms persisted despite hospital treatment. In this subgroup patients with ischemic ST depression, prior myocardial infarction, or prior stable angina were at greater risk of serious complications in the first three months.

Kraus[10] and co-workers examined patients with pain occurring after 12 hours in the hospital and concluded that such patients had a high incidence of major complications. All early myocardial infarctions and the single early death occurred in the subgroup of patients with persisting symptoms.

In the study by Heng and associates[14] 46 patients had symptoms persisting after hospitalization. Therapy in most cases included the administration of nitroglycerin and beta-blocking drugs. Twelve (26%) of this group died or had a myocardial infarction during their hospitalization, which was in contrast to the 10% incidence of such complications in patients without persisting symptoms.

However, the poor prognosis of patients with persisting symptoms in the hospital has not been regularly demonstrated. Selden and co-workers[22] included only patients who had continued episodes of pain at rest after 24 hours of bedrest, and all such patients had electrocardiographic changes suggestive of ischemia. Of the 19 medical patients, 14 received propranolol. Despite the poor prognosis reported by others[10,11,14] only two of their patients developed myocardial infarction over a four-month follow-up period and there were no deaths. With the exception of this study[22] the literature favors the view that patients with unstable angina whose symptoms persist despite medical therapy in the hospital are at high risk for serious complications.

STUDIES OF UNSTABLE ANGINA
WITHOUT SEPARATION INTO SUBGROUPS

Many studies of unstable angina provide data for the entire spectrum without analyzing each subgroup separately. For example, the study of Fulton and co-workers[9] on the natural history of 167 patients with unstable angina included patients with recent onset angina, crescendo angina, and acute coronary insufficiency. Sixteen percent were followed for less than three months, while 84% were followed from three to six months. In the total follow-up at six months 26 patients (16%) had major complications. Twenty-three patients (14%) had myocardial infarctions, and four (2%) died. Seventeen of the 26 serious complications occurred within four weeks, the latest complication developing at 13 weeks. Only 45 (27%) of the patients were hospitalized in this study. Eight of these patients (18%) had a myocardial infarction in the hospital, and one died shortly after discharge.

Heng and co-workers[14] reported the natural history of 158 patients with crescendo angina or acute coronary insufficiency. Patients with myocardial infarction within four weeks of their presentation with unstable angina were excluded. Within the first three weeks, 20 patients (13%) sustained myocardial infarctions, and there were six deaths (4%). Over the subsequent six-year follow-up the average annual mortality was approximately 5%. Significant risk factors for late mortality included age over 60 years, cardiomegaly, and pulmonary congestion at the time of admission to hospital. Although not statistically significant, previous myocardial infarction, hypertension, and persisting pain in the hospital tended to be associated with increased risk of late mortality.

Hultgren and co-workers[23] included patients with crescendo angina and acute coronary insufficiency in their patient population. Patients with myocardial infarction within the previous three months were not included.

Considering the medical group of 66 patients, nonfatal myocardial infarctions occurred in 17%, and there was a mortality rate of 21% over a mean follow-up period of 18 months. Most major complications occurred more than one month after hospital admission. Two-thirds of the nonfatal infarctions and three-quarters of the deaths occurred during the late follow-up period. No data are provided, but it is stated that there were no significant differences between patients with major complications and the entire medical group in terms of the presence of crescendo angina or acute coronary insufficiency, ECG evidence of previous myocardial infarction, severity of ECG changes with pain, enzyme changes, or persistence of chest pain for more than 48 hours after hospitalization.

In a recent study[24] by Armstrong and associates 199 patients with unstable angina admitted to a coronary care unit were followed for an average of 13.6 months. During their hospitalization the patients had daily electrocardiograms, daily blood sampling for creatine kinase (CK, also, creatine phosphokinase—CPK) analysis in the hospital laboratory, and blood sampling every four hours for 48 hours for CK analysis in a research laboratory. The CK analysis done in the hospital laboratory must have remained within the normal range and must not have shown a greater than 50% increase for patients to be included in the study. Of the entire group 19% were found to have a significant CK rise with serial sampling, which had been missed by daily sampling. Patients without ECG changes or CK elevation by serial sampling were found to have a relatively benign course (2% mortality, no infarctions) while those with ECG changes and CK elevation had the worst prognosis (15% mortality, 10% infarction rate). Those with either ECG changes or CK elevation had an intermediate prognosis. These observations may provide another explanation for the varying prognosis reported in patients with unstable angina. Patients may show similar clinical presentations; yet those who have ECG changes and enzyme changes detected by serial sampling techniques appear at increased risk of major complications.

CORONARY ANATOMY AND UNSTABLE ANGINA

The severity of coronary artery disease as defined by coronary arteriography is known to play a major role in the prognosis of patients with coronary artery disease. Studies in patients with coronary artery disease have shown that the risk of cardiac death increases with the number of vessels involved regardless of the severity of symptoms. Burggraf and Parker[25] found that the annual mortality from coronary artery disease was 5% in a group of patients without angina or a history of previous myocardial infarction. This is compared with a 6% mortality in a group of patients having either of these clinical features. In this study the distribution of single-, double-, and triple-vessel disease was similar in those patients with mild angina (grades 1 and 2) and those with angina occurring at rest (grade 4). The mortality rate for any degree of coronary artery disease was similar in asymptomatic patients and in those with angina at rest. Oberman and associates[26] followed the clinical course of 246 patients with coronary artery disease undergoing coronary angiography and found that angina pectoris, nocturnal angina, and unstable angina did not independently affect the long-term prognosis. The criteria for unstable angina in the latter series included chest pain either occurring at rest, lasting 15 minutes or more during a single episode, or onsetting within three months of admission to hospital. It is not clear from the study how many patients underwent angiography during the acute stages of unstable angina. As this study took place between 1965 and 1970 when angiography was not commonly performed in patients with unstable angina, it is probable that a selected group of patients who survived the acute course of unstable angina was studied.

Alison and associates[12] recently addressed themselves to the correlation between the coronary anatomy as defined by coronary arteriography and the clinical course of patients with unstable angina. Their study population included those with recent onset exertional angina, crescendo angina, and acute coronary insufficiency, all developing within three months of hospitalization. The 188 patients were subdivided into two groups on the basis of the arteriographic findings. Group A (156 patients) had severe coronary artery disease, including 20 patients with 50% or more narrowing of the main left coronary artery. Group B (32 patients) had either normal coronary arteries (20 patients) or mild to moderate disease (12 patients). In the 136 patients of group A who did not have main left coronary artery disease, all but one had pain at rest. The distribution of disease in these patients was single-vessel disease in 36%, double-vessel disease in 38%, and triple-vessel disease in 26%. In the 20 patients with left main coronary artery disease 15% had no other disease, 15% had involvement of one other vessel, 25% two other vessels, and 45% had triple-vessel disease in addition to the main left disease. The in-hospital mortality was 4.5%, and the myocardial infarction rate 7.7%. These complications all occurred in the patients of group A. Eleven of the 12 patients who had myocardial infarctions and/or death had triple-vessel disease, six had left main disease, and one had severe anterior descending disease with minimal right coronary artery narrowing. Six myocardial infarctions (3.2% of patients) and three deaths (1.6% of patients) occurred within 24 hours of the cardiac catheterization. Of note, 10.6% of the patients who met the clinical criteria for unstable angina were found to have normal coronary arteriography and an equal number had severe left main disease.

Plotnick and Conti[20] followed 32 patients with unstable angina and angiographically documented coronary artery disease. Over 48 months, five of the six deaths occurred in patients with triple-vessel disease and four of these patients had poor left ventricular function. The mortality of patients with "operable" disease from the point of view of suitable coronary disease and good ventricular function had a first-year mortality of 9.5% compared to 18% for those with "inoperable" disease. The mortality in patients with poor ventricular function was 29% in the first year.

In the cooperative study on unstable angina[21] 24% of the medical group had single-vessel disease, 37% double-vessel disease, and 39% triple-vessel disease. In patients with single-vessel disease the anterior descending

Table 3-1
Summary of Natural History Studies in Unstable Angina

Authors	Subgroup	No. of Patients	Angiography					Early (Mo)
			S	D	T	LM	N	
Fulton et al[9]	Combined	167			No			2% (3)
Hultgren et al[23]	Combined	66	19%	27%	54%			5% (1)
Alison et al[12]	Combined	188	26%	28%	18% (n = 188)	11%	17%	4% (H)
Gazes et al[11]	C, ACI	140			No			10% (3)
Heng et al[14]	C, ACI	158			No			4% (H)
Vakil[18]	ACI	360			No			1% (H)
Kraus et al[10]	ACI	100			No			1% (H)
Skjaeggestad[13]	ACI	132			No			5% (2)
Selden et al[22]	ACI	19			All*			0% (H)
Bertolasi et al[16]	C	27	11%	48%	41% (n = 27)			4% (H)
Bertolasi et al[17]	ACI	24	25%	37.5%	37.5% (n = 24)			21% (H)
Berk et al[19]	ACI	21			None			19% (3-H, week after discharge)
Plotnic and Conti[20]	ACI	32	28%	22%	50% (n = 32)			9% (H)
Cooperative Study[21]	ACI	147	24%	37%	39% (n = 147)			3% (H)

S = Single. D = Double. T = Triple-vessel disease. LM = Left main disease. N = Normal or moderately diseased coronary arteries. (Mo) = Months of follow-up. CAD = Coronary artery disease. BBB = Bundle branch block. MI = Myocardial infarction. C = Crescendo angina. ACI = Acute coronary insufficiency. H = In hospital (usually ≤ 1 month). LV = Left ventricle.
*Details not stated

coronary artery was the most frequently involved. In patients with double-vessel disease a combination of anterior descending and right coronary disease was as common as anterior descending and circumflex disease, with right coronary artery and circumflex disease the least common combination. While 6% of those with single-vessel disease died in the hospital, only 4% with double-vessel disease, and none with triple-vessel disease died in the hospital. This trend persisted during the late follow-up period with mortality of 11%, 6%, and 5% for single-, double-, and triple-vessel disease,

Table 3-1 *(continued)*

Mortality	Myocardial Infarction		
Late (Mo)	Early (Mo)	Late (Mo)	Risk Factors for Complications
	14% (3)		Increased C:T ratio
21% (18)	6% (1)	17% (18)	
	6% (H)		Severity of CAD Highest catheterization risk in those with left main.
18% (12) 39% (60) 52% (120)	21% (3)		Recurrent symptoms in hospital especially if prior BBB, prior angina, MI, or ischemic T changes.
5% (72) annually	13% (H)		Early — Recurrent symptoms in hospital. No previous ischemic heart disease. Late — Pulmonary congestion, cardiomegaly, age $\geq$ 60 years.
16% (3)		41% (3)	
22% (20)	7% (H)	23% (20)	Previous angina. Recurrent symptoms in hospital.
	13% (2)		
	0% (H)	11% (4)	
7% (32)	4% (H)	7% (32)	Severity of CAD and LV dysfunction.
46% (32)	25% (H)	38% (32)	Severity of CAD and LV dysfunction.
	62% (H)		
19% (48)	3% (H)	19% (48)	Severity of CAD and LV dysfunction.
10% (30)	8% (H)	19% (30)	Severity of CAD.

respectively. The early and late myocardial infarction rate, however, was greater for patients with triple-vessel disease than in patients with single- or double- vessel disease.

Thus, the mortality of patients with unstable angina in most studies[12,20,26] appears related to the extent of coronary artery disease and left ventricular dysfunction. As pointed out by the study of Alison et al,[12] there are patients with normal coronary arteriograms who are clinically inseparable from patients with severe coronary disease. The patients with normal coronary arteriograms are expected to have an excellent prognosis regardless of their symptom presentation[27]; therefore, their inclusion in any series will affect the long-term results. It is essential that studies on the natural history of unstable angina include diagnostic coronary arteriography to exclude such patients.

In summary, the term "unstable angina" represents a spectrum of clinical presentations (Table 3-1). The reported natural history of medically treated patients with unstable angina varies depending upon the definition of the population studied and the treatment received. Of patients presenting with unstable angina, those with acute coronary insufficiency and those with persisting symptoms of unstable angina after hospital treatment appear to be at highest risk of major complications. The electrocardiogram and frequent CK analysis may also provide important prognostic information. The prognosis is most accurately defined, however, by the extent of the underlying coronary artery disease and left ventricular dysfunction found at angiography.

Studies of the natural history of unstable angina should include precise definition of the patient population. Otherwise it is very difficult to evaluate and compare modification of the course of patients with unstable angina by either medical or surgical intervention.

REFERENCES

1. Sampson, J.J., and Eliaser, M. The diagnosis of impending acute coronary occlusion. *Am Heart J.* 13:675–686, 1937.

2. Feil, H. Preliminary pain in coronary thrombosis. *Am J Med Sci.* 193:42–48, 1937.

3. Mounsey, P. Prodromal symptoms in myocardial infarction. *Br Heart J.* 13:215–226, 1951.

4. Solomon, H.A., Edwards, A.L., and Killip, T. Prodromata in acute myocardial infarction. *Circulation* 40:463–471, 1969.

5. Stowers, M., and Short, D. Warning symptoms before major myocardial infarction. *Br Heart J.* 32:833–838, 1970.

6. Alonzo, A.A., Simon, A.B., and Feinbeib, M. Prodromata of myocardial infarction and sudden death. *Circulation* 52:1056–1062, 1975.

7. Harper, R.W., Kennedy, C.K., DeSanctis, R.W. et al. The incidence and pattern of angina prior to acute myocardial infarction: a study of 577 cases. *Am Heart J.* 97:178–183, 1979.

8. Chahine, R.A. Unstable angina. The problem of definition. *Br Heart J.* 37:1246–1249, 1975.

9. Fulton, M., Lutz, W., Donald, K.W. et al. Natural history of unstable angina. *Lancet* 1:800–865, 1972.

10. Kraus, K.R., Hutter, A.M., and DeSanctis, R.W. Acute coronary insufficiency course and follow-up. *Circulation* 45 & 46(suppl):166–171, 1972.

11. Gazes, P.C., Mobly, F.M., Faris, H.M. et al. Pre-infarctional (unstable angina) — a prospective study — 10 year follow-up. Prognostic significance of electrocardiographic changes. *Circulation* 48:331–337, 1973.

12. Alison, H.W., Russel, R.O., Mantle, J.A. et al. Coronary anatomy and arteriography in patients with unstable angina. *Am J Cardiol.* 41:204–209, 1978.

13. Skjaeggestad, Ö. The natural history of intermediate coronary syndrome. *Acta Med Scand.* 193:533–536, 1973.

14. Heng, M.K., Norris, R.M., Singh, B.N. et al. Prognosis in unstable angina. *Br Heart J.* 38:921–925, 1976.

15. Kannel, W.B., and Feinbeib, M. Natural history of angina pectoris in the Framingham study, prognosis and survival. *Am J Cardiol.* 29: 154–163, 1972.

16. Bertolasi, C.A., Tronge, J.E., Carreno, C.A. et al. Unstable angina — prospective and randomized study of its evolution with and without surgery. Preliminary report. *Am J Cardiol.* 33:201–207, 1974.

17. Bertolasi, C.A., Tronge, J.F., Riccitelli, M.A. et al. Natural history of unstable angina with medical or surgical therapy. *Chest* 70:596–605, 1976.

18. Vakil, R.J. Pre-infarction syndrome — management and follow-up. *Am J Cardiol.* 14:55–63, 1964.

19. Berk, G., Kaplitt, M., Padmanabhan, V. et al. Management of pre-infarction angina evaluation and comparison of medical vs. surgical therapy in 43 patients. *J Thorac Cardiovasc Surg.* 71:110–117, 1976.

20. Plotnic, G.D., and Conti, D.R. Unstable angina: angiography, short and long-term morbidity, mortality and symptomatic status of medically treated patients. *Am J Med.* 63:870–873, 1977.

21. Russel, R.O., Moraski, R.E., Kouchoukos, N. et al. Unstable angina pectoris: National Cooperative Study Group to compare surgical and medical therapy. II. In-hospital experience and initial follow-up results in patients with one, two and three vessel disease. *Am J Cardiol.* 42:839–848, 1978.

22. Selden, R., Neill, W.A., Ritzmann, L.W. et al. Medical versus surgical therapy for acute coronary insufficiency — a randomized study. *New Engl J Med.* 293:1329–1333, 1975.

23. Hultgren, H.N., Pfeifer, J.F., Angell, W.W. et al. Unstable angina: comparison of medical and surgical management. *Am J Cardiol.* 39:734–740, 1977.

24. Armstrong, P.W., Chiong, M.A., and Parker, J.O. The spectrum of unstable angina (abstract). *Ann R Coll Phys Surg Can.* 28, 1979.

25. Burggraf, G.W., and Parker, J.O. Prognosis in coronary artery disease. Angiographic hemodynamic and clinical factors. *Circulation* 51:140–156, 1975.

26. Oberman, A., Jones, U.B., Riley, C.P. et al. Natural history of coronary artery disease. *Bull Nat Acad Med.* 48:1109–1125, 1972.

27. Brushke, A.V.G., Proudfit, W.L., and Sones, F.M., Jr. Clinical course of patients with normal and slightly or moderately abnormal coronary arteriograms. A follow-up study on 500 patients. *Circulation* 47:936–945, 1973.

SECTION II

Pathophysiology of Unstable Angina

4 The Amount of Coronary Narrowing in the Four Major Epicardial Coronary Arteries in Unstable Angina Pectoris: The Quantitative Approach

William C. Roberts, MD, and
Renu Virmani, MD

It has been recognized that patients with angina pectoris usually have considerable narrowing of one or more of their major epicardial coronary arteries.[1-4] However, the exact amount of luminal narrowing in any one or in each of the four major epicardial coronary arteries has not been described. Accordingly, the degree of cross-sectional luminal narrowing in each 5-mm segment of each of the four major epicardial coronary arteries was determined in 22 patients who died shortly after aortocoronary bypass operations for relief of clinically isolated unstable angina pectoris and the observations in them were compared to those in 20 control subjects.

PATIENTS AND METHODS

A total of 22 necropsy patients with clinically isolated unstable angina pectoris with death within three days of aortocoronary artery bypass operation were included in this study. Certain clinical and cardiac morphologic observations in them are summarized in Table 4-1.

Table 4-1

QUANTITATION OF CORONARY NARROWING IN UNSTABLE ANGINA PECTORIS:
Clinical Observations and Non-Coronary Cardiac Findings in 22 Patients and in 20 Control Subjects

Group	No. Pts.	Age (Years) Range (Mean)	Sex M	Sex F	DM	SH	Duration (Months) Angina Range (Mean)	c Done	c >200	T Done	T >200	C Values (mg/dl) Range (Mean)	Heart Weight (gm) Range (Mean)	Increased[a] Heart Weight	LV N	LV F
Angina	22	37-59 (48)	13 (59%)	9 (41%)	4 (18%)	10 (45%)	2-120 (18)	19	16* (84%)	8	3	148-420 (266)*	240-520 (384)*	6 (27%)	4[b]	6[b] (27%)
Controls	20	39-65 (51)	11 (55%)	9 (45%)	0	0	0	17	3**	5	2	106-245 (171)**	190-390 (302)**	0	0	0

Abbreviations: c = serum cholesterol (mg/dl); DM = diabetes mellitus; F = fibrosis; LV = left ventricle; N = necrosis; SH = Systemic hypertension (systolic blood pressure >140 and/or diastolic >90 mm Hg); T = serum triglyceride (mg/dl).

* to ** p<.001

[a]Weight >400 Gm in men and >350 Gm in women.

[b]None had clinical evidence of acute myocardial infarction.

Unstable angina was defined as anterior thoracic pain of recent onset (less than one month before clinical evaluation) or a recent change in the pattern of the pain in terms of frequency, severity, intensity, and ease of provocation. Nocturnal or rest angina or prolonged angina within three months of death was considered unstable. There was no electrocardiographic or enzymatic evidence of recent acute myocardial infarction in any of the hospitalized patients with unstable angina.

Clinically isolated was defined as absence of clinical evidence, at any time, of acute myocardial infarction and of congestive cardiac failure. None of the patients had associated valvular, congenital, primary myocardial (hypertrophic cardiomyopathy), or pericardial heart disease.

Controls

Control subjects had the following characteristics:

1. Similar age and sex to that of the study patients
2. Death from a noncardiac condition
3. Absence of symptoms suggesting or indicating myocardial ischemia or cardiac dysfunction during life
4. Absence of systemic hypertension ($>$ 140 mm Hg systolic and/or $>$ 90 mm Hg diastolic
5. Absence of therapeutic mediastinal irradiation
6. Absence of cardiomegaly ($>$ 400 gm for men and $>$ 350 gm for women) at necropsy

Twenty subjects, who fulfilled the above criteria, were selected as controls. Eight died of carcinoma (breast, three; pancreas, two; ovary, 2; tongue, one), four of leukemia, seven of lymphoma, and one from multiple myeloma.

The coronary arteries in all patients and in control subjects were studied in similar fashion. The hearts were fixed for at least one day in formalin. The four major epicardial coronary arteries then were excised intact, x-rayed, and fixed for at least another day. Following decalcification (if necessary), each of the four major coronary arteries was cut transversely to its longitudinal axes into approximately 5-mm long segments and each segment was labeled sequentially from either its aortic ostium or from its origin from the left main. The number of 5-mm segments examined in the study patients and control subjects is summarized in Table 4-2. The 5-mm segments were labeled, dehydrated (alcohol and xylene), embedded in paraffin, and two histologic sections were cut and stained from each paraffin block. The Movat stain was used on one histologic section and all determinations of luminal narrowing were based on examination of the

Movat-stained sections because it clearly outlines the internal elastic membrane of the arteries. The degrees of narrowing were based on histologic examination of each cross-section magnified 25 to 50 times. The judgment regarding the degree of luminal narrowing of each 5-mm segment was based on the degree of luminal obliteration within the luminal circle bordered by the internal elastic membrane. The circle was visually subdivided into four equal-sized quadrants, and the percent of cross-sectional area luminal narrowing in each 5-mm segment was classified as follows: 0% to 25%, 26% to 50%, 51% to 75%, and 76% to 100%.

In addition to sectioning the major epicardial coronary arteries, at least three histologic sections extending from endocardium to epicardium and for at least 2 cm in circumferential dimension were prepared from left ventricular myocardium from each patient and stained by hematoxylin and eosin. Gross myocardial fibrosis (see Table 4-1) was confirmed histologically in six patients (26%) and 4 had transmural left ventricular myocardial coagulation necrosis. No control subjects had either myocardial fibrosis or necrosis by histologic examination.

RESULTS

Among the 22 patients with unstable angina, 85 major coronary arteries were examined. (The left main was not examined in three patients.) Among the 20 control subjects, 77 coronary arteries were examined. (The left main was not examined in three subjects.) All 22 study patients had 76% to 100% cross-sectional area luminal narrowing by atherosclerotic plaque in at least one of their four major coronary arteries, and five (25%) of the 20

Table 4-2

NUMBER OF 5-mm LONG SEGMENTS OF MAJOR EPICARDIAL CORONARY ARTERY
EXAMINED PER PATIENT:

Unstable Angina Pectoris (AP) (22 Patients) versus Controls (C) (20 Subjects)

Coronary Artery	Number (Range [Mean]) of Segments Per Patient	
	AP (22 Patients)	C(20 Subjects)
Left Main	1- 4 (2.1)	1- 3 (1.6)
Left anterior descending	6-34 (16.0)	8-31 (17.2)
Left circumflex	4-33 (12.0)	5-19 (9.7)
Right	9-29 (17.7)	11-37 (19.4)
Total Segments of 4 Coronary Arteries Per Patient	21-75 (47.6)	28-69 (47.7)

control subjects had this degree of narrowing (Table 4-3). Of the 22 study patients, 21 (95%) had two or more of their four major coronary arteries narrowed > 75% in cross-sectional area by atherosclerotic plaque, whereas only two (10%) of the 20 control subjects had two or more arteries narrowed to this degree. Of the 22 study patients, ten (45%) had > 75% narrowing by atherosclerotic plaque of all four major coronary arteries; eight (36%) other patients had three arteries narrowed to this degree; three (14%) had two arteries narrowed to this extent; and only one patient had only one of the four arteries > 75% narrowed. Thus, of the possible 88 major coronary arteries in the 22 study patients (actually only 85 arteries were examined), 71 (81%) were > 75% narrowed in cross-sectional area by atherosclerotic plaque for an average of 3.2 coronary arteries per study patient. If the left main coronary artery was excluded, 61 (93%) of the other 66 major (right, left anterior descending, and left circumflex) coronary arteries were narrowed > 75% in cross-sectional area by atherosclerotic plaque, for an average of 2.8 coronary arteries per study patient. Of the five control subjects with > 75% cross-sectional area narrowing of one or more coronary arteries by atherosclerotic plaque, none had all four major coronary arteries narrowed to this degree, one had three arteries so narrowed, one had two arteries so narrowed, and three had one artery so narrowed.

Table 4-3

NUMBER OF 22 PATIENTS WITH UNSTABLE ANGINA PECTORIS (AP)
AND 20 CONTROL SUBJECTS (C) SHOWING MAXIMUM LUMINAL NARROWING
OF ONE OR MORE MAJOR EPICARDIAL CORONARY ARTERIES BY
ATEROSCLEROTIC PLAQUES

| Coronary Artery | Percent Cross-Sectional Area Luminal Narrowing | | | | | | | | Totals | |
| | 0-25 | | 26-50 | | 51-75 | | 76-100 | | AP | C |
	AP	C	AP	C	AP	C	AP	C		
R	0	0	0	0	0	1	1	1	1	2
LAD	0	0	0	0	0	1	0	2	0	3
R, LAD	0	0	0	0	0	4	2	1	2	5
LAD, LM	0	0	0	0	0	0	1	0	1	0
LAD, LC	0	0	0	0	0	2	0	0	0	2
R, LAD,LC	0	0	0	1	0	5	8	1	8	7
R,LM*,LAD,LC	0	0	0	0	0	1	10	0	10	1
Totals (%)	0	0	0 (0)	1 (5)	0 (0)	14 (70)	22 (100)	5 (25)	22 (100)	20 (100)

*Sections of LM not examined in 3 anginal patients and in 3 control subjects.

Abbreviations: R = Right; LM = Left Main; LAD = Left anterior descending; LC = Left circumflex.

Thus, of the possible 80 major coronary arteries in the 20 control subjects (actually, only 77 arteries were examined), eight (10%) were narrowed > 75% in cross-sectional area by atherosclerotic plaque for an average of 0.4 coronary arteries per control subject. If the left main coronary artery was excluded, eight (13%) of the 60 other major (right, left anterior descending, and left circumflex) coronary arteries were narrowed > 75% in cross-sectional area by atherosclerotic plaque for an average of 0.4 coronary arteries per control subject. Thrombus was absent in the coronary arteries in all 22 patients and in all 20 controls.

The results of the quantitative analysis of the 5-mm long coronary segments in both study patients and control subjects are summarized in Figure 4-1. Of the 1049 5-mm long segments of major coronary arteries examined in the 22 study patients, 497 segments (47%) were 76% to 100% narrowed in cross-sectional area by atherosclerotic plaque (controls = 1%), 304 (29%) were 51% to 75% narrowed (controls = 29%), 129 (12%) were 26% to 50% narrowed (controls = 48%) and 119 (11%) were 0% to 25% narrowed (controls = 22%). The mean percent of 5-mm coronary segments narrowed 0% to 25%, 26% to 50% and 76% to 100% was significantly different (p < 0.05) between study patients and control subjects at each of the four levels of narrowing. The mean percent of 5-mm segments of left main, left anterior descending, left circumflex, and right coronary arteries narrowed 0% to 25%, 26% to 50%, and 76% to 100% was significantly different (p < 0.05) between study patients and control subjects at each of the four levels of narrowing (Figure 4-1). The mean percent of 5-mm segments of the left main, left anterior descending, left circumflex, and right coronary arteries at each of the four levels of narrowing was similar in the study patients (Figure 4-2A). The mean percent of segments of each of the four major coronary arteries narrowed to varying degrees in the control subjects was similar (Figure 4-2B).

The mean percent of 5-mm segments narrowed 76% to 100% in cross-sectional area in the proximal half of the left anterior descending and left circumflex coronary arteries was greater than the mean percent of 5-mm segments similarly narrowed in the distal halves of these arteries (p < 0.01) (Figure 4-3), but the amount of severe narrowing in the proximal and distal halves of the right coronary artery was not significantly different.

The seven patients 45 years of age and younger had a higher percentage of 5-mm segments severely narrowed than did the 15 patients aged 46 to 65 years (63 ± 6 vs 41 ± 6%) (p < 0.05) (Table 4-4). Sex, heart weight and the presence or absence of a healed left ventricular infarct (clinically silent) did not alter the percentage of coronary segments severely (> 75%) narrowed.

DISCUSSION

Many thousands of autopsies during this century have demonstrated severe narrowings in one or more major epicardial coronary arteries of patients with coronary heart disease. However, until recently there has been no attempt to quantitate the degree and extent of coronary luminal narrowing in these patients. The present study provides quantitative information on the degree and extent of luminal narrowing in each of the four major epicardial coronary arteries in patients with clinically isolated unstable angina pectoris. Approximately 24 cm (1049 5-mm segments) of the four major (right, left main, left anterior descending, and left circumflex) epicardial coronary arteries were examined in each of 22 patients or a total of 525 cm of major coronary artery. Each 1-cm segment was divided into equal-sized halves and a histologic section examined from each 5-mm segment. Of the 22 patients studied, in nearly one half (47%) of the entire

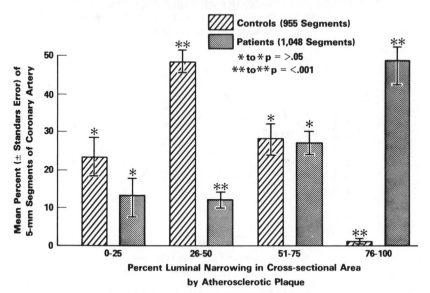

NUMBER OF 5-mm SEGMENTS OF ALL 4 MAJOR CORONARY ARTERIES NARROWED TO VARIOUS DEGREES IN *UNSTABLE ANGINA PECTORIS* (22 PATIENTS AGED 37 - 59 [AVG 48]) AND IN CONTROLS (20 SUBJECTS AGED 39 - 65 [AVG 51])

Figure 4-1   Percent of 5-mm segments of all four major coronary arteries narrowed to various degrees in the 22 study patients and in the 20 control subjects.

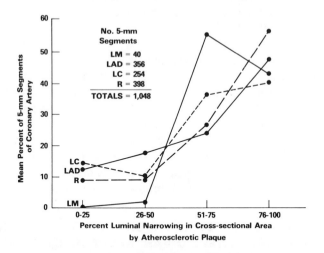

MEAN PERCENT OF 5-mm SEGMENTS OF EACH OF THE
4 MAJOR CORONARY ARTERIES NARROWED TO
VARIOUS DEGREES IN *UNSTABLE ANGINA PECTORIS*
(22 PATIENTS AGED 37 - 59 [AVG 48])

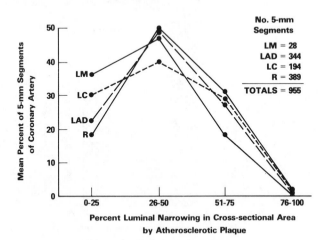

PERCENT OF 5-mm SEGMENTS OF EACH OF THE 4
MAJOR CORONARY ARTERIES NARROWED TO
VARIOUS DEGREES IN 20 *CONTROL SUBJECTS*
(AGED 39 - 65 [AVG 51])

Figure 4-2 Mean percent of 5-mm segments of each of the four major coronary arteries narrowed to various degrees in the 22 study patients (**A**) and in the 20 control subjects (**B**). In the study patients the amount of narrowing at each of the four levels of narrowing is similar in each of the four major coronary arteries. The same is true for the control subjects. LM = left main; LAD = left anterior descending; LC = left circumflex; R = right.

lengths of the four major epicardial coronary arteries studied, the lumens were > 75% narrowed in cross-sectional area by atherosclerotic plaque. In addition, another 29% of the major coronary arteries had luminal narrowing between 51% and 75% in cross-sectional area. Thus 76% of the lengths of the four major epicardial coronary arteries in the 22 study patients were > 50% narrowed in cross-sectional area by atherosclerotic plaque. (A 75% cross-sectional area narrowing is equivalent to a 50% diameter reduction on luminogram.[5]) In contrast, only 30% of the lengths of the four major coronary arteries in the control subjects were narrowed > 50% ($p < 0.001$).

MEAN PERCENT OF 5-mm LONG SEGMENTS OF THE PROXIMAL AND THE DISTAL HALVES OF THE RIGHT, LEFT ANTERIOR DESCENDING AND LEFT CIRCUMFLEX CORONARY ARTERIES NARROWED >75% IN CROSS SECTIONAL AREA BY ATHEROSCLEROTIC PLAQUE IN 22 PATIENTS WITH *UNSTABLE ANGINA PECTORIS*

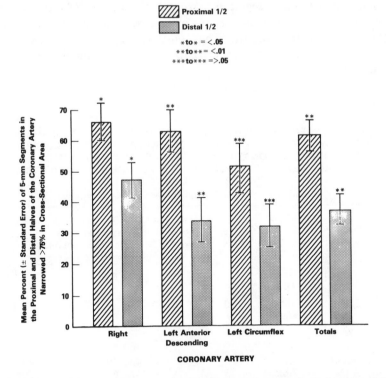

Figure 4-3 Mean percent of 5-mm segments of the proximal and distal halves of the right, left anterior descending, and left circumflex coronary arteries in the 22 study patients. The mean percent of 5-mm segments narrowed greater than 75% in cross-sectional area by atherosclerotic plaque in the proximal halves of these three arteries is greater than that in the distal halves.

Not only was severe narrowing widespread in the study patients, but some degree of narrowing was present in virtually every 5-mm segment of coronary artery. Of the coronary arterial segments studied, 89% were narrowed over 25% in cross-sectional area, and not a single 5-mm segment in a single patient was entirely normal. Thus, coronary atherosclerosis in necropsy patients with clinically isolated unstable angina pectoris is diffuse, involving, for practical purposes, all segments of all four major epicardial coronary arteries.

Fortunately, from an operative standpoint, the degree of severe (> 75%) narrowing in the distal halves of the left anterior descending and left circumflex coronary arteries in the 22 study patients was significantly less than in the proximal halves of these two arteries. The distal half of the right was not significantly less narrowed than was the proximal half.

Surprisingly among the study patients, no significant differences were found in the degree of severe narrowing of the left main, left anterior descending, left circumflex, or right coronary arteries. In addition, the percent of 5-mm coronary segments narrowed 0% to 25%, 26% to 50%, and 76% to 100% in cross-sectional area by atherosclerotic plaque was similar in each of these three arteries. Thus, unstable angina is associated with a high frequency of severe (> 75%) narrowing of the left main as well as the other coronary arteries.

Table 4-4

MEAN PERCENT OF TOTAL 5-mm SEGMENTS IN THE 4 MAJOR (RIGHT, LEFT MAIN, LEFT ANTERIOR DESCENDING, AND LEFT CIRCUMFLEX) EPICARDIAL CORONARY ARTERIES NARROWED > 75% IN CROSS-SECTIONAL AREA BY ATHEROSCLEROTIC PLAQUE IN 22 PATIENTS WITH UNSTABLE ANGINA PECTORIS:
Comparison of Four Clinical or Morphologic Parameters

Parameter Analyzed		No. Pts.	Mean Percent (± Standard Error) of 5-mm Coronary Segments Narrowed > 75% in Cross-Sectional Area by Atherosclerotic Plaque	p Value
Age (Years)	≤ 45	7	63 ± 6	< .05
	46 - 65	15	41 ± 6	
Sex	Men	13	48 ± 6	ns
	Women	9	48 ± 8	
Heart Weight	Increased*	6	52 ± 11	ns
	Normal	16	48 ± 5	
Healed Infarct,** Left Ventricle	Present	6	48 ± 10	ns
	Absent	16	47 ± 6	

* > 400 gms in men: > 350 gm in women.
** Clinically silent.

The amount of severe (> 75%) coronary narrowing present in the study patients was greater in the patients 45 years of age and under than in those over age 45. But the percent of coronary segments > 75% narrowed was similar in men and women, in those with increased compared to those with normal sized hearts, and in those with myocardial scars (healed infarcts) compared to those without.

SUMMARY

A quantitative analysis of the degree and extent of coronary arterial narrowing by atherosclerotic plaques in the entire lengths of each of the four major epicardial coronary arteries in 22 patients with unstable angina pectoris is described at necropsy and the observations are compared to those in 20 control subjects. Of 1049 5-mm long segments of the left main, left anterior descending, left circumflex, and right coronary arteries examined in the 22 patients (average 48 per patient), 497 (47%) were 76% to 100% narrowed in cross-sectional area by atherosclerotic plaques (controls = 1%); 304 (29%) were 51% to 75% narrowed (controls = 29%); 454 (48%) were 26% to 50% narrowed and only 119 (11%) segments were less than 26% narrowed (controls = 22%). The amount of severe (> 75%) narrowing of the right, left main, left anterior descending, and left circumflex coronary arteries by atherosclerotic plaques was similar. The amount of severe (> 75% narrowing in the distal half of the right and left anterior descending coronary arteries was significantly less (p < 0.05) than in the proximal halves of these two arteries.

REFERENCES

1. Zoll, P.M., Wessler, S., and Blumgart, H.L. Angina pectoris. Clinical and pathologic correlations. *Am J Med.* 11:331, 1951.

2. Lenegre, J., and Himbert, J. Critical study of the relationship between angina pectoris and coronary atherosclerosis. *Am Heart J.* 58:539, 1959.

3. Guthrie, R.B., Vlodaver, Z., Nicoloff, D.M. et al. Pathology of stable and unstable angina pectoris. *Circulation* 51:1059, 1975.

4. Roberts, W.C. The coronary arteries and left ventricle in clinically isolated angina pectoris. A necropsy analysis. *Circulation* 54:388, 1976.

5. Arnett, E.N., Isner, J.M., Redwood, D.R. et al. Comparison of degrees of coronary arterial narrowing in coronary heart disease by cineangiography during life to the degree observed histologically at necropsy. *Ann Intern Med.* (In press).

5 The Myocardium in Stable and Unstable Angina

Malcolm D. Silver, MD, and
James W. Butany, MD

This study correlates clinical and pathologic findings in 35 patients who had stable or unstable angina pectoris. The individuals were selected for study because their history immediately before death was known. They had been studied by cardiologists, and their form of angina had been classified clinically before they died. Furthermore, they either died suddenly or their death occurred during or within 48 hours of coronary surgery. The mode of death, we believed, would make it possible to distinguish morphologically between preexisting myocardial lesions and those that might have been caused by surgery or other procedures. Each patient was in the hospital two or more days before death and had no clinical, enzymatic, or electrocardiographic evidence of an acute myocardial infarction in that period. Our particular objective was to determine if any form of myocardial damage might account for the change in pattern of angina known clinically as unstable angina.

MATERIALS AND METHODS

Definitions

Angina pectoris was defined as a syndrome characterized by chest pain that is, most often, a presenting manifestation of ischemic heart disease but which may occur in other conditions characterized by myocardial ischemia, for example, aortic valve stenosis or anemia.[1] Patients with angina pectoris were divided into two groups. They were classed as having stable angina if they had anterior thoracic pain related to effort, the attacks lasted three to ten minutes, the pattern of recurrence did not change, and the pain was promptly relieved by rest and/or nitroglycerin. Patients with unstable or preinfarction angina, on the other hand, had either a rapid progression of their original symptoms or change in the pattern of stable angina. Individuals in this group were further subdivided.[2] In those with crescendo angina, the original attacks came with increasing frequency, with or without provocation, lasted less than 15 minutes, and were relieved promptly by coronary vasodilators. During such attacks transient electrocardiographic changes of ischemia could be recorded, but no patient developed electrocardiographic signs of a myocardial infarct. Acute coronary insufficiency was typified by attacks of angina that lasted more than 20 minutes and were only partially or not relieved by coronary vasodilators. Again, patients with this form of unstable angina could have transient electrocardiographic changes of ischemia during an attack of pain, but they did not develop electrocardiographic signs of myocardial infarction and their serum enzyme levels remained normal.

Patient Data

Of the 35 patients who had angina pectoris, 29 had had aortocoronary bypass surgery and died within 48 hours of the operation, the majority (27) less than 24 hours postoperatively; five others died suddenly in the hospital while awaiting bypass surgery, and one died 24 hours after cardiac catheterization.

None of the patients had a congenital heart lesion or valvular heart disease. The clinical chart of each patient was reviewed to gather information regarding the history of major symptoms and their duration, the family and social history, and the clinical examination. In each case the diagnosis of one of the forms of angina defined above had been made by a cardiologist and was confirmed by our review.

Morphological Studies

The heart of each patient was weighed, opened following the course of blood flow, and gross findings were noted with a photographic record. Coronary artery and vein bypass grafts were sectioned at 3- to 4-mm intervals along their length and the findings recorded. Histologic sections were prepared from each of the vascular segments and stained by hematoxylin and eosin and a combined Verhoeff elastic-Masson trichrome stain. Histologic blocks of myocardium that included all of the surface area of slices made parallel to the atrioventricular groove at the apex, mid-ventricular level, and base were sectioned and stained with hematoxylin and eosin.

The histologic material was reviewed by both pathologists together at a double-headed microscope, with the cases divided in a random fashion and their identification known to a third person. In all cases 12 myocardial sections and up to 80 vascular sections were examined from each heart.

Definition of histologic lesions   The degree of luminal stenosis caused by coronary atherosclerosis was estimated visually on histologic sections and graded on a scale of 1 to 5 with grade 1 representing 0% to 25% stenosis, grade 2, 26% to 49%, grade 3, 50% to 74%, grade 4, 75% to 99% stenosis, and grade 5, complete occlusion. Lesions causing $\geq$ 50% stenosis are referred to as "significant" atherosclerosis in the text. Areas of occlusion were classified as "recent" if composed of thrombus, or "old" if composed of fibrous connective tissue with or without small blood vascular channels.

Myocardial lesions were defined as "scars" if mature, collagenous, connective tissue replaced muscle fibers; as "healed necrosis" if cellular connective tissue replaced myocardial fibers; as "acute" if the muscle fibers showed contraction band change,[3] acidophilia, or marked vacuolation; or as "infarcts" if they showed coagulation necrosis with or without a polymorphonuclear leukocyte infiltrate. Such myocardial lesions might be focal or affect a large area. They could involve the subendocardial half of the left ventricular wall or be transmural. To tabulate lesions the left ventricular wall was divided into anterior, septal and posterior segments.

Statistical Analysis

The tests of significance used to determine differences between groups were the chi square test, Student's t-test, and Fischer's exact procedures for comparing two proportions based on small samples.

RESULTS

Patient Data

Patient data are given in Table 5-1. Twenty-five patients were men (71%) and ten women. There were significantly more men than women in the group as a whole (p < 0.5) and the subgroup that had stable angina (p < 0.1), while approximately equal numbers of men and women had unstable angina and both of its subtypes. No difference in mean age was apparent between patients suffering from stable as compared to unstable angina or between those with either form of unstable angina. Nor was there any difference in the age grouping of the sexes. Thirty-one percent of the patients had a family history of myocardial infarction. Two individuals with stable angina had such a history compared to nine in the unstable group (not statistically significant). No patient with angina had valvular heart disease. More people with unstable angina had had a previous myocardial infarct clinically, with more men than women in both groups having had such an event. However, the difference in numbers between the groups was not statistically significant. Overall, 37% of the patients had had a previous myocardial infarct. In considering risk factors one patient with stable angina and one with unstable angina had diabetes mellitus. The first was a 64-year-old man whose diabetes had been controlled by lente insulin for many years; the second, with acute coronary insufficiency, was a man of 51 years who was obese and had had his diabetes controlled by diet alone. He died after cardiac catheterization and before coronary artery surgery was done. Fourteen patients (40% of the total with angina) had hypertension, four with stable angina and ten unstable angina (differences not statistically significant). Eighty percent of all patients smoked more than ten cigarettes a day. The number of smokers did not differ significantly between the groups. Only one patient, a 32-year-old woman with hypertension and crescendo angina who died suddenly while awaiting operation, had a hyperlipoproteinemia (type IV).

On the average, patients with unstable angina had their symptoms approximately six months longer than those with stable angina while a change in pattern of angina had been apparent for six and a half weeks in those with acute coronary insufficiency and for nine weeks in those with crescendo angina. In neither instance was this difference statistically significant.

Mode of Death

The mode of death is shown in Table 5-2. No patient with stable angina died while awaiting coronary artery surgery whereas five with unstable angina did. Of these, one developed electrocardiographic evidence

Table 5-1
Patient Data

Category of Angina	No. of Patients	Mean Age (yr)	Sex		Patients with Family History of Myocardial Infarction		Patients with Evidence of Previous Myocardial Infarction		Patients with Hypertension (diastolic) >90 mm Hg		Patients who Smoked >10 Cigarettes per Day		Average Duration of Symptoms (mo)
			M	F	M	F	M	F	M	F	M	F	
Stable	12	52 ± 11	11	1	1	1	3	0	4	0	9	1	46
Unstable	23	56 ± 13	14	9	6	3	7	3	5	5	11	7	53
Acute coronary insufficiency	11	55 ± 14	9	2	4	1	5	2	3	2	7	2	52
Crescendo	12	54 ± 13	5	7	2	2	2	1	2	3	4	5	55

of an acute myocardial infarction immediately before death and the other four died suddenly. Approximately equal numbers of the groups with stable and unstable angina died during surgery or postoperatively. All dying during an operation "could not be weaned off bypass." Of patients with stable angina dying postoperatively, nine had persistent arrhythmias and one a "low output syndrome." Among those with unstable angina two had operative complications, five a "low output syndrome," three persistent arrhythmias, two metabolic problems and one a cardiac arrest 48 hours after surgery.

Table 5-2
Mode of Death

Catetory of angina	Preoperative death	Intraoperative death	Postoperative death	Total
Stable	0	2	10	12
Unstable	5	5	13	23
Acute coronary insufficiency	4	1	6	11
Crescendo	1	4	7	12

Morphological Findings

Heart weight   The average heart weight among patients with the different categories of angina is shown in Table 5-3. The differences are not statistically significant. Left ventricular hypertrophy, judged as a heart weight greater than 350 gm in women and 450 gm in men, was present in 77% of patients with angina pectoris; in 67% of those with stable angina; in 83% of those with unstable angina; in 83% of those with acute coronary insufficiency; and in 83% of those with crescendo angina.

Table 5-3
Heart Weight

Category of Angina	Average Heart Weight (gm)
Stable	509 ± 96
Unstable	528 ± 148
Acute coronary insufficiency	563 ± 174
Crescendo	496 ± 118

Coronary atherosclerosis   The numbers of patients in each group that had significant atherosclerosis (defined as $\geqslant$ 50% stenosis) in their coronary arteries is shown in Table 5-4. The majority in all groups had significant triple-vessel disease, usually with many foci of atherosclerosis causing $\geqslant$ 50% stenosis along the course of the vessels. The severity of atherosclerosis ($\geqslant$ 50% stenosis) found in a single coronary artery did not differ between the groups, but more patients with stable angina had severe atherosclerosis in the left anterior descending coronary artery and circumflex coronary artery systems, while the left anterior descending and the right coronary arteries seemed particularly affected in patients with unstable angina.

Table 5-4
Coronary Atherosclerosis

Category of Angina	No. of Patients with Significant ($>$ 50%) Atherosclerosis in Coronary Arteries vs No. of Patients without Severe Atherosclerosis		
	Right	*Left anterior descending*	*Circumflex*
Stable	9/3	11/1	11/1
Unstable	20/3	23/0	17/6
Acute coronary insufficiency	10/1	11/0	8/3
Crescendo angina	10/2	12/0	9/3

Coronary artery occlusions   Data about coronary occlusions are provided in Table 5-5. Twenty of the 35 patients with angina (57%) had occlusions in their coronary arteries. There was no statistical difference between the groups in the likelihood of finding an occlusion versus no occlusion. In each group any occlusion found seemed more likely to be present in the left anterior descending and right coronary arteries than in the circumflex vessel. In the angina group as a whole this finding was significant with a $p < 0.01$. In the group with unstable angina only, the finding was significant at the 5% level. In all other groups there was no significant difference.

Twelve recent and 16 old occlusions were found in the vessels. The likelihood of an old versus a recent coronary occlusion being present in the coronary artery did not differ significantly between the groups. Patients with angina often had more than one occlusion in their coronary arteries, a total of 28 being found; but when the groups were compared, no statistical difference could be demonstrated in the likelihood of this occurring.

Table 5-5
Coronary Occlusions

Category of Angina	Patients With/Without Occlusion in Coronary Artery System	Total Occlusions	Type of Occlusion					
			Right Coronary Artery Recent/Old		Left Anterior Descending Coronary Artery Recent/Old		Circumflex Coronary Artery Recent/Old	
Stable	7/5	9/7	2	1	3	3	0	0
Unstable	13/10	19/13	3	5	2	6	2	1
Acute coronary insufficiency	8/3	12/8	2	3	1	3	2	1
Crescendo angina	5/7	7/5	1	2	1	3	0	0

Myocardial lesions   All but three hearts showed some form of myocardial lesion as defined above.

Old scars   Data concerning old scars are shown in Table 5-6. Twenty-two hearts showed old scars (63%). Statistically, no group of patients was more or less likely to show old scars. Such old scars could be focal in nature or involve large areas of myocardium. In the latter instance they were regarded as previously healed myocardial infarcts. Patients with unstable angina seemed more likely to exhibit focal scars, healed infarcts, or both types of lesions than those with a stable angina, but no difference was obvious statistically between the groups of patients. Old scars, both focal and healed infarcts, were subendocardial more often than transmural, but the frequency at these sites was not statistically different when the groups were compared. Again, both types of scars were found in the anterior, septal, or posterior walls of the left ventricle with equal frequency in all groups.

Healing scars   Data about healing scars are presented in Table 5-7. Fourteen patients with angina had healing lesions (40%) interpreted as indicating myocardial necrosis in the days or weeks preceding surgery or death. The lesions were found with equal frequency in the hearts of patients with stable or unstable angina.

Healing scars could be focal or extensive. In the latter instance we regarded them as healing infarcts. Focal healing scars were found more frequently than healing infarcts in the hearts of patients with stable and unstable angina, but we could demonstrate no statistical difference in the frequency of the lesions between the groups of patients. Again, both types of healing scars seemed more likely to be subendocardial than transmural, but no statistical difference in their location was demonstrable between the groups. Both types of lesions seemed to affect individual walls of the left ventricle equally.

Acute lesions   These lesions were found in 22 hearts (63%) (see Table 5-8). No statistical difference was obvious between the groups of patients with regard to the presence or absence of the lesion and, when present, they occurred with equal frequency in all groups. Three of the five patients who died suddenly showed these lesions, but only one had developed ECG signs of an infarct immediately before death (no coagulation necrosis was evident histologically). The other 19 patients who had them all died postoperatively and the lesions were judged an operative complication.

Acute lesions were predominantly subendocardial in location, being transmural in only one patient. They likely represent areas of myocardium that had been subject to ischemic insult and then reperfused, and were as likely to be present in all walls of the left ventricle as confined to only one (12 diffuse/10 single wall affected). In the latter instance one wall of the left ventricle was affected as often as another.

Table 5-6
Myocardial Damage: Old Scars

Category of Angina	No. of Patients with Old Scars/No Scars	Type and Location of Old Scars in 22 Patients		
		Hearts with Healing/ Focal Scarring	Hearts with Both Lesions	Hearts with Subendocardial/ Transmural Lesions
Stable	6/6	2/4	0	6/0
Unstable	16/7	14/2	7	10/6
Acute coronary insufficiency	9/2	8/1	6	5/4
Crescendo angina	7/5	6/1	1	5/2

Table 5-7
Myocardial Lesions: Healing Scars

Category of Angina	No. of Patients with Healing Scar/No Healing Scar	Type and Location of Healing Scar in 14 Patients		
		Healing Infarct/ Focal Healing Scar	Both Lesions	Subendocardial/ Transmural Lesions
Stable	5/7	1/4	0	4/1
Unstable	9/14	2/7	1	8/1
Acute coronary insufficiency	6/5	1/5	1	5/1
Crescendo angina	3/9	1/2	0	3/0

Table 5-8
Myocardial Lesions: Acute Lesions and Infarcts

Category of Angina	Acute Lesions No. of Patients Where Present/Absent	Myocardial Infarcts No. of Patients Where Present/Absent
Stable	9/3	4/8
Unstable	13/10	4/19
Acute coronary insufficiency	7/4	3/8
Crescendo angina	6/6	1/11

Myocardial infarcts   Eight patients had acute myocardial infarcts (23%) (see Table 5-8). All infarcts were subendocardial with approximately equal numbers occurring in each wall of the ventricle. There was no statistical difference between groups with regard to the likelihood of finding or not finding an infarct, and the lesions occurred with approximately equal frequency in each group of patients.

Each of the infarcts showed coagulation necrosis associated with a slight to moderate polymorphonuclear leukocyte infiltrate and were judged to be between 12 and 24 hours old. All occurred in patients who died in the postoperative period and four were associated with occlusive thrombi in the supplying coronary artery. Two occurred in patients with stable angina and two among those with unstable angina. All infarcts were judged to have occurred during or immediately after operation and to have caused the patient's death.

DISCUSSION

The patients studied were predominantly men in their mid-50s; cigarette smokers; and had significant coronary atherosclerosis, as is usual in patients with clinically evident coronary artery disease or angina pectoris.[4,5] The percentage of our patients affected by systemic hypertension (40%) falls between those of the groups studied by Zoll et al (60%)[6] and Guthrie et al (31%)[7]; but none of our patients had valvular heart disease. Nevertheless, as in previous studies, severe coronary atherosclerosis alone or severe coronary atherosclerosis combined with systemic hypertension were the findings most often associated with angina pectoris. Smoking more than ten cigarettes per day was also common in these patients.

The main morphologic findings in our group of patients were: 77% of their hearts were hypertrophied; the majority had significant triple-vessel coronary artery disease; 57% had old or recent occlusions in their coronary arteries, mainly in the left anterior descending and right vessels; 63% had old scars in the myocardium; and 40% had healing scars. All of these forms of myocardial damage seemed more likely to be found in the subendocardial zone than to be transmural. It might be thought that the healing scars, found in 40% of our patients and indicating myocardial necrosis occurring in the days or weeks preceding surgery or death, could be a trigger to change the clinical pattern of angina pectoris; but no statistical differences in these findings could be demonstrated among the groups of patients with different clinical forms of angina pectoris. Thus, we could neither distinguish morphologically between hearts of patients with the different forms of angina pectoris nor delineate myocardial changes that could account for the change in the clinical behavior of angina, experienced by individuals with unstable angina.

Roberts and Spray[8] have described the morphologic features in 27 patients with "pure" angina pectoris (the clinical condition was not further defined as stable or unstable angina) who died during or shortly after cardiac catheterization or cardiac operations to increase myocardial oxygenation. In their group 78% were men. The anginal symptoms had existed on the average of 25 months; 41% had intermittent, systemic hypertension; 77% smoked cigarettes; the majority had severe ($\geq$ 75% stenosis) triple-vessel coronary artery disease with diffuse involvement; and 52% showed scarring in the left ventricular wall with the scars being mainly subendocardial and small. The findings in the coronary arteries in our series are comparable, but more of our patients (63%) had myocardial scarring, again mainly subendocardial. The latter difference probably reflects the different selection of the patients in each of the investigations. Neither the patients in the series of Roberts and Spray[8] nor any of those in our series had valvular heart disease.

The study of Guthrie and colleagues[7] is the one most closely comparable to this. However, more of their patients had diabetes mellitus and/or abnormalities of their serum lipids; more had a history of previous myocardial infarction; several had valvular lesions; and a greater number survived for a longer period following bypass surgery. Those authors found that "the pathological profile including distribution and severity of coronary disease, left ventricular hypertrophy and antecedent myocardial infarction did not differ appreciably" among patients with stable or unstable angina. Our study confirms that opinion. Differences were noted by Guthrie et al[7] with regard to the frequency of a coronary thrombus and/or an acute myocardial infarction that made the authors suggest that many cases "classified as having unstable angina pectoris may actually be suffering an acute myocardial infarction that is undetected by the usual clinical tests." We cannot support that point of view. Twelve of our patients had recent thrombotic occlusions (compared to 17 in their series), five in the stable group (four infarcts), and seven in the unstable angina group (four infarcts); but histologically we estimated that the infarcts had developed at or immediately after surgery. Again, if we related recent coronary occlusions and healing scars, no matter whether they were focal or represented healed infarcts, to explain the changes in patients' symptoms, no significant difference between groups was demonstrable.

The clinical profile of the patients resembles that of the clinical population with angina pectoris, but the group we studied was a select one. Therefore, we cannot be certain that our patients truly represent the population with angina pectoris. Nevertheless, we conclude, from the group studied, that changes in the clinical pattern of angina pectoris producing the clinical syndromes known as acute coronary insufficiency or crescendo angina are not mirrored by recognizable, distinct morphologic changes in the myocardium. In other words, a recognizable change in myocardial morphology does not precede the change in the clinical picture of angina pectoris. Rather, the cause must lie elsewhere: for example, progression of coronary atherosclerosis; partial or complete obstruction of a coronary artery,[9] although this concept is not supported by our evidence; a change in collateral supply[10]; spasm of coronary arteries[11]; or these or other factors alone or in combination. Nevertheless, our findings do not exclude the possibility that a change in the pattern of angina pectoris may eventually lead to a patient developing a myocardial infarction, as is recognized clinically.[12-14]

We thank Professors A. Csima and M. Halliday, Department of Preventive Medicine and Biostatistics, University of Toronto, for the statistical analyses. This study was supported by a grant from the Ontario Heart Foundation.

REFERENCES

1. Ross, R.S. Ischemic heart disease. Edited by M.W. Wintrobe, G.W. Thorn, R.D. Adams et al. In *Harrison's Principles of Internal Medicine* 6th ed. New York: McGraw-Hill Book Co., 1970.

2. Williams, W.G., Aldridge, H., Silver, M.D. et al. Preinfarction angina what is it? Edited by J.C. Norman. In *Coronary Artery Medicine and Surgery: Concepts and Controversies.* New York: Appleton-Century-Crofts, 1975.

3. Reichenbach, D.D. and Benditt, E.P. Catecholamines and cardiomyopathy: the pathogenesis and potential importance of myofibrillar degeneration. *Hum Pathol.* 1:125, 1970.

4. Fowler, N.O. Clinical diagnosis. *Circulation* 47:1079, 1972.

5. Fulton, M. and Julian, D.G. Unstable angina. Edited by D.G. Julian. In *Angina Pectoris.* New York: Churchill-Livingstone, 1977.

6. Zoll, P.M., Wessler, S., and Blumgart, H.L. Angina pectoris: clinical and pathologic correlations. *Am J Med.* 11:331, 1951.

7. Guthrie, R.B., Vlodaver, Z., Nicoloff, D.M. et al. Pathology of stable and unstable angina pectoris. *Circulation* 51:1059, 1975.

8. Roberts, W.C., and Spray, T.L. Pure angina pectoris: morphological features. Edited by D.G. Julian. In *Angina Pectoris.* New York: Churchill-Livingstone, 1977.

9. Neill, W.A., Ritzman, L.W., and Selden, R. The pathophysiologic basis of acute coronary insufficiency: observations favoring the hypothesis of intermittent reversible coronary obstruction. *Am Heart J.* 94:439, 1977.

10. Fischl, S.J., Herman, M.V., and Gorlin, R. The intermediate coronary syndrome. *N Engl J Med.* 288:1193, 1973.

11. Maseri, A., Severi, S., De Nes, M. et al. "Variant" angina: one aspect of a continuous spectrum of vasospastic myocardial ischemia. *Am J Cardiol.* 42:1019, 1978.

12. Levy, H. The natural history of changing patterns of angina pectoris. *Ann Intern Med.* 44:1123, 1956.

13. Fulton, M., Lutz, W., Donald, K.W. et al. Natural history of unstable angina. *Lancet* 1:860, 1972.

14. Gazes, P.C., Mobley, E.M., Duncan, R.C. et al. Preinfarctional (unstable) angina: a prospective study; ten year follow up. *Circulation* 48:331, 1973.

6 Vasospastic Myocardial Ischemia

Attilio Maseri, MD,
Antonio L'Abbate, MD, and
Sergio Chierchia, MD

Our understanding of the pathogenic mechanisms of ischemic heart disease is rapidly expanding as a result of the growing interest in this field. A series of observations demonstrates that myocardial ischemia may be caused by different pathogenic mechanisms and may manifest itself with variable pictures. Independent of its cause, transient ischemia may result in signs of left ventricular failure and/or arrhythmias, and it may or may not be associated with chest pain.

For many years progress in our understanding of the pathogenic mechanisms of angina pectoris has been hampered by descriptive classifications that were based on clinical features. The terms exertional, emotional, and decubitus angina could only be taken to indicate the occasion of the onset of symptoms. More recently the terms "stable" and "unstable" angina gained wide acceptance because they appeared to carry a prognostic implication. Implicitly, our thinking was heavily conditioned by the classic definition of angina pectoris as given by C.K. Friedberg[1] (and also recorded in the Glossary of the National Heart, Lung and Blood Institute's Task Force Report on Arteriosclerosis[2,3]). This definition led to the extrapolated notion that the only important variable in the development of acute transient myocardial ischemia is coronary atherosclerotic stenosis resulting in a limited blood supply, which is unable to meet excessive increases in myocardial demand. In his textbook of cardiology, Friedberg[1] states that "the occurrence of the pain or pressure with effort is an essential element of the syndrome although it does not occur invariably with the same exertion. The pain of angina pectoris may occur at rest, but if it does not also occur with effort or cannot be reproduced by bodily exertion the diagnosis of angina pectoris may be questioned." Thus, although recognizing that angina may occur with variable levels of exertion and even at rest, implicitly he 1) attributed the variable threshold of angina only to different levels of myocardial demand for the same heart work, and 2) practically denied the very existence of angina at rest with unimpaired exercise tolerance and the possible role of a functional variability of myocardial blood supply.

A large body of evidence now indicates that angina may be caused by reduced coronary blood flow rather than by an increase in myocardial metabolic demand beyond the possibility of supply. Therefore it appears totally arbitrary to assume, without objective demonstration, that a variable threshold of angina is related to a variable level of myocardial demand for similar levels of heart work.

The stimulus to challenge the traditional concept that increased demand in the presence of limited supply was the only respectable cause of angina has come from studies of "variant" angina,[4] which have now expanded to other forms of angina at rest. Variant angina has been shown not to be caused by increased myocardial demand, but by coronary vasospasm.[5,6] This is now considered a proved hypothesis.[7] On the basis of observations performed on a large number of patients, we have come to the conclusion that variant angina is frequent when appropriately looked for and adequately investigated.[8] Variant angina is not a discrete syndrome, but rather represents one extreme of a continuous spectrum of acute myocardial ischemia caused by coronary vasospasm. Indeed, our observations suggest that coronary vasospasm may result in different degrees of ischemia with variable electrocardiographic changes with or without typical chest pain.[8,9] Coronary vasospasm may also cause sudden coronary death[9] and may evolve into myocardial infarction.[10] These views seem to be gaining acceptance.[11]

STUDIES ON THE MECHANISMS OF ANGINA AT REST

The availability of new technologies and especially new interest and unbiased approaches applied to the study of anginal patients, are making it increasingly clear that the relationship between atherosclerosis and symptoms of ischemic disease is not a linear one. A list of a few nonlinearities will illustrate the point.

- Only one in ten persons with coronary atherosclerosis is symptomatic.[12,13]
- Severity of symptoms correlates poorly with the severity of coronary atherosclerosis. Some patients have severe atherosclerosis with mild symptoms; others have minimum atherosclerotic lesions with severe clinical symptoms.[14]
- Approximately 10% of patients with angina pectoris or myocardial infarction have normal or nearly normal coronary arteries.[15]
- The severity of coronary atherosclerosis is often similar in patients with either stable or unstable angina, despite the generally recognized fact that unstable angina carries a much greater risk of complications, infarction, and sudden death.[15-17]
- About 10% of patients with electrocardiographically proved "unstable" angina had to be excluded from randomized surgical trials because their coronary lesions were not severe enough (Conti, R. Personal communication).[18,19]

On the basis of these incongruities, and starting in 1973, we approached the problem by studying patients with angina at rest — "unstable" angina — because they usually have frequent anginal attacks and therefore can be observed more readily.

Hemodynamic Studies (Figure 6-1)

A first series of studies with hemodynamic monitoring was undertaken at our laboratory.[5,20] These studies showed that there was no increase in myocardial oxygen consumption preceding (and thus causing) the ischemic attacks in patients with variant angina in agreement with previous findings.[21] Angiographically we could demonstrate that the ischemia was due to coronary artery spasm. At that time, however, our findings were questioned on the basis that angiographically demonstrated coronary artery spasm could be catheter-induced.

We had also observed that patients with variant angina sometimes showed ischemic episodes with S-T segment depression rather than elevation, and others who usually showed episodes with S-T segment depression sometimes showed S-T segment elevation. The hemodynamic pattern was similar in these episodes. They were never preceded by an increase in the determinants of myocardial oxygen consumption; the degree of left ventricular function impairment was greater in the episodes with S-T segment elevation, suggesting a greater severity of ischemia.[20,22] Accordingly, in none of the patients exhibiting only S-T segment depression that we have studied so far, did we detect an increase in heart rate, systolic blood pressure, or left ventricular dp/dt prior to the onset of the S-T segment changes. Similar findings were reported by others.[23] The occurrence of pain followed by minutes the onset of ischemia; thus anginal pain is only a late marker of ischemia and obviously an increase in blood pressure and heart rate detected at the moment of pain cannot be considered the cause of the ischemia as usually thought[24,25] because ischemia had already begun minutes earlier.

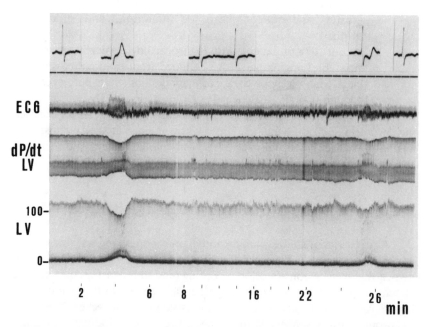

Figure 6-1 Playback of hemodynamic recording performed in a patient who had myocardial ischemic episodes with both S-T segment elevation and depression. Two successive episodes are reported here, the first characterized by S-T segment elevation and positivization of the T wave, the second by S-T segment depression. Both the episodes were asymptomatic and they are not preceded by any increase in heart rate, systolic blood pressure, or dp/dt. The electrocardiographic changes are associated with increase in diastolic and reduction in systolic left ventricular pressure and impairment of dp/dt. The hemodynamic changes during the S-T segment depression are relatively less pronounced. (Maseri et al. *Am J Cardiol.* 1979 [in press]. Reproduced with permission.)

Regional Myocardial Perfusion Studies (Figure 6-2)

In the attempt to establish whether or not the transient ischemic attacks at rest were indeed caused by a reduction of coronary blood supply we performed a second series of studies in the same type of patients with variant angina.[6,25] Using myocardial thallium-201 scintigraphy, we were able to demonstrate, following the injection of the tracer during the ischemic attack, massive transmural deficits in myocardial perfusion. These deficits correlated well with the regions from which S-T segment elevations had been recorded during episodes of pain. In addition, they corresponded to the vascular territory shown to have undergone vasospasm at angiography during those same attacks. These observations have recently been confirmed by studies using other methods.[26,27]

Similar massive transmural deficits in tracer uptake were also seen in patients with only transient normalization of previously inverted T waves, or with only peaking of T waves with or without anginal pain. In episodes characterized by ST-segment depression, the deficits in thallium-201 uptake were more diffuse but not transmural, a pattern compatible with diffuse subendocardial ischemia.[28] Patients who had attacks of angina with ST-segment depression both spontaneously at rest and during an effort test showed much more evident regional deficits in thallium uptake during spontaneous attacks than during exercise-induced attacks. We believe that these differences may be related to a reduction in regional myocardial perfusion during spontaneous angina and to an inadequate increase in perfusion during exertional angina occurring at a higher level of double product, ie, approximately twice that recorded at the beginning of spontaneous attacks.[29]

A sudden severe drop in oxygen saturation in the great cardiac vein was consistently observed in episodes of spontaneous angina before the onset of left ventricular dp/dt and ST-segment changes in the anterior leads. Conversely, when ST-segment changes occurred in inferior leads (indicating ischemia of the inferior wall drained by the posterior cardiac vein), no change in saturation was observed. Therefore, according to the indirect Fick principle, in the absence of demonstrable change in myocardial metabolic demand, reduction in oxygen saturation of blood draining the anterior myocardial wall implies a sudden reduction in regional myocardial perfusion. This decrease precedes the onset of signs of acute myocardial ischemia, regardless of the direction of the ST-segment or T-wave changes.[30]

Coronary Arteriographic Studies (Figure 6-3)

Another of our objectives was to locate coronary vasospasm and evaluate it in relation to coronary atherosclerosis and transient ECG changes. We therefore performed systematically repeated coronary injections in over 50 patients during anginal episodes, spontaneous or induced by intravenous infusion of ergonovine maleate.[31,32] These investigations

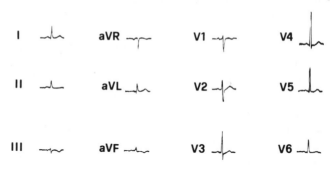

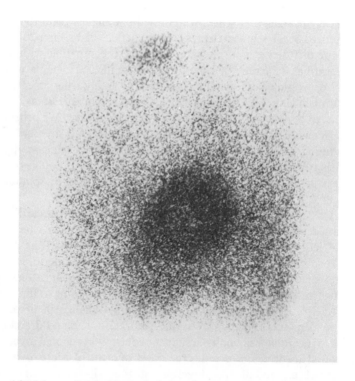

Figure 6-2A Myocardial thallium scintigrams in 45° left anterior oblique projection with corresponding 12-lead electrocardiogram obtained in the absence of symptoms (**A**) and during an anginal episode induced by ergonovine (**B**). Coronary arteriography performed during a similar episode showed an occlusive spasm of the midportion of the left anterior descending and circumflex arteries. The elevation of the S-T segment in the anterior and inferior leads is associated with a massive deficit of tracer uptake in the inferior and anterior heart walls. (Maseri et al. *Am J Cardiol.* 42:1019–1035, 1978. Reproduced with permission.)

documented coronary vasospasm in episodes with ST-segment elevation, depression, and normalization of negative T wave.[5,9,33,34,35] Coronary spasm associated with ST depression has also been documented in other institutions.[36,37]

The vasospasm was observed in vessels that were angiographically normal, in vessels with wall irregularities, and in vessels with stenosis ranging from 50% occlusive to subocclusive. Vasospasm was usually proximal and, when the distal vessel was visible, also distal to the stenosis. Vasospasm was

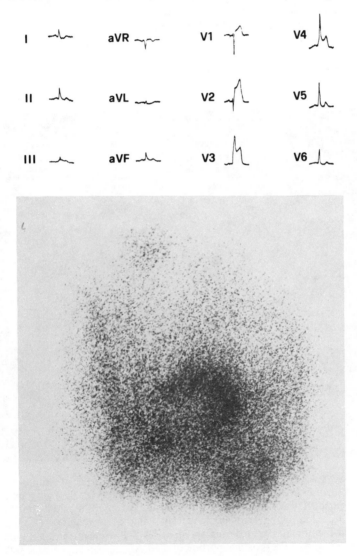

Figure 6-2B

also noted in vessels perfused by collaterals distal to an old occlusion. Contrast injections performed during an anginal attack failed to show detectable coronary changes only in a very small minority of patients. It is possible that a small decrease in caliber at the level of a critical stenosis caused a reduction of perfusion sufficient to produce ischemia without resulting in appreciable changes at angiography. Other causes of angina besides vasospasm and excessive increase of demands may be postulated.

The growing number of observations of spasm during episodes of ST-segment elevation can be attributed to the interest in this ECG pattern stimulated by the Prinzmetal hypothesis and to the more dramatic changes in caliber of main coronary branches usually associated with this pattern.

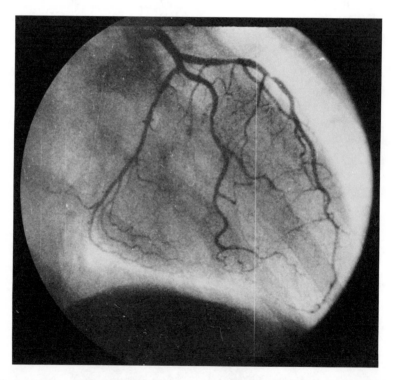

Figure 6-3A Angiogram of the left coronary artery in absence of symptoms showing two stenoses in the left anterior descending branch (LAD). **B** Angiogram during asymptomatic T-wave elevation in V_4: occlusive spasm at the middle third of the LAD. Occlusion disappeared spontaneously within a few minutes. **C** Angiogram obtained five minutes later during spontaneous S-T segment elevation and pain: occlusive spasm of the proximal portion of the LAD. Spasm disappeared following intracoronary isosorbide dinitrate. (Maseri, Thomas Lewis Lecture. *Br Heart J.* 1979. [in press]. Reproduced with permission.)

DIAGNOSTIC IMPLICATIONS

Angina pectoris appears to represent only one of the possible manifestations of acute transient myocardial ischemia that may result from different pathogenic mechanisms and may be associated with variable electrocardiographic changes. Indeed, acute transient myocardial ischemia occurring spontaneously at rest or during stress tests may be completely asymptomatic (always associated with evidence of impairment of left ventricular function, with or without arrhythmias), or it may manifest itself clinically with sudden cardiac dyspnea or with severe rhythm disturbances.

Angina pectoris remains the most easily recognizable form of transient acute myocardial ischemia on a clinical basis because of the characteristics of the pain whether it occurs at rest, on exertion, or both. On the basis of the changing views on the pathogenic mechanisms of transient myocardial ischemia, clinical diagnosis of this problem needs to be further refined with the following in mind:

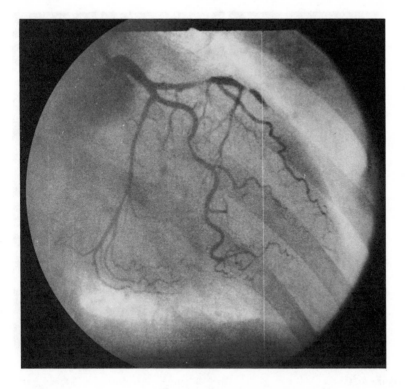

Figure 6-3B

88

- Stress testing can no longer be considered the only "gold standard" for the objective demonstration of acute myocardial ischemia.
- Continuous electrocardiographic ambulatory monitoring represents a tool of great practical importance for evaluating patients with typical or atypical chest pain, regardless of whether it occurs only at rest or only on exertion or both.
- Provocative tests of coronary vasoconstriction also need to be further developed and evaluated.

Since it has now been proved that acute transient myocardial ischemia, apart from traditional extracoronary causes such as anemia or aortic stenosis, can occur in the absence of critical coronary lesions, and since it is known that critical lesions may be compatible with normal submaximal or maximal exercise stress testing, the concept of sensitivity and specificity of diagnostic stress tests should be updated. These tests will need to be compared to a "gold standard" yet to be developed.

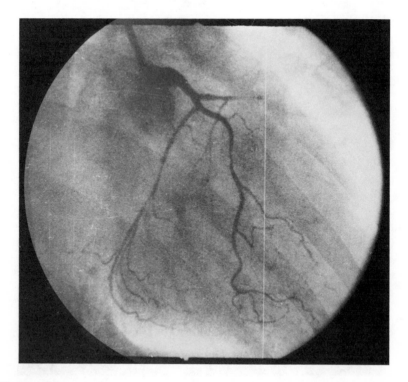

Figure 6-3C

A PRACTICAL PATHOGENIC CLASSIFICATION
OF THE ACUTE MYOCARDIAL ISCHEMIA

The current clinical classification of patients into "stable" and "unstable" angina pectoris groups has only a diagnostic meaning and can be taken to suggest how carefully and intensively the patient should be managed rather than what type of management he should receive. Thus, we would like to propose the following provisional pathogenic classification:

- Traditional angina, or acute transient myocardial ischemia "secondary" to coronary atherosclerotic stenosis (according to now prevailing theory) and brought out in response to increased myocardial demand beyond the fixed limitations of the available blood supply.
- "Primary" angina, or acute myocardial ischemia caused by other mechanisms such as vasospasm.[38,39] The term "primary," borrowed from other fields of medicine, is meant to indicate our present ignorance about the causes of acute transient myocardial ischemia.

This provisional distinction would simply serve the practical purpose of an immediate and clear-cut separation of the traditionally accepted mechanism of "secondary" angina, for which diagnostic and therapeutic approaches are already reasonably well-defined, from all other causes that still require appropriate and specific research and management.

As in the case of classification schemes for systemic hypertension, this pathogenic classification of angina pectoris will become more precise as the causes of primary angina are identified in the future.

The goal should be to identify whether a patient presents: a) only primary, b) only secondary acute transient myocardial ischemic episodes, or c) predominantly attacks of primary or of secondary ischemia (with or without pain and/or demonstrated transient electrocardiographic changes). The mechanisms of primary ischemia and the degree of limitation of the coronary blood flow in secondary ischemia should also be specified.

For primary angina pectoris the only reasonably well-documented cause so far is coronary vasospasm. This is possibly because it was more extensively search for than other postulated causes, such as platelet aggregation,[40] small vessel disease,[41] transient myocardial metabolic abnormalities,[42] and inadequate vasodilatation.[43]

In secondary angina pectoris the severity of impairment of coronary blood flow should be evaluated on the basis of a careful history and of a consistently positive electrocardiographic stress test for similar levels of cardiac work. The level of exertion that the patient can never exceed without the occurrence of symptoms or signs of acute myocardial ischemia should be used to identify the degree of impairment of coronary blood flow.[39] The diagnosis of secondary angina should be confirmed by the demonstrated presence of critical coronary stenosis.

THE CLINICAL PROBLEM

The hypothesis of a primary cause of angina appears reasonable for most patients with angina at rest. Common clinical experience indicates that these attacks usually occur unheralded, with no cause that is recognizable by the patient or by the physician. Most patients report that they can carry out their daily activities, involving effort of variable intensity, without experiencing symptoms. A secondary origin of spontaneous angina at rest implies the reduction of coronary flow reserve to such a low level that even the slightest increase of myocardial metabolic demand above basal values cannot be met and acute myocardial ischemia ensues. Patients with this low degree of cardiac reserve usually have progressive limitation of exercise tolerance in which they can walk a mile at first, then perhaps 100 yards, until finally they cannot walk more than the length of a corridor without developing angina. Relatively few patients with angina at rest have such a history. On the basis of our experience a vasospastic origin of primary angina can be suspected for most patients with recurrent spontaneous attacks at rest. It should be noted, however, that spasm was recently demonstrated during stress testing[44-46] and that patients with secondary angina also appear to have attacks of primary transient acute myocardial ischemia caused by vasoconstriction during cold exposure[43] or by still unidentified factors during ordinary daily activity.[48]

The hypothesis of a secondary cause of angina appears reasonable for patients with exertional angina. It is certainly valid for those who develop angina any time they exercise beyond a rather fixed level and who have severe coronary stenoses. Primary mechanisms may coexist in those who report exertional angina on superficial questioning but, on specific questioning, admit that the level of exertion triggering their attacks is variable and that they can sometimes perform at higher levels of exertion without discomfort.

The prevalence, natural history, and prognosis of primary transient acute myocardial ischemia remain to be defined because all the information currently available on stable and unstable angina probably represents rather heterogeneous clinical syndromes in terms of pathogenic mechanisms. Certainly it is no longer justifiable to attribute, without proof, the frequently observed variability of the threshold of exertional angina only to variable degrees of increase in myocardial demand.

Primary and secondary forms of angina and of asymptomatic myocardial ischemic attacks often coexist in the same patient or occur during successive phases of coronary disease, as frequently ascertained by a careful history of the patient's symptoms. The vast majority of patients we see in our practice fall within the third category and have attacks of both primary and secondary angina. A minority fall into the second category of having only attacks of secondary angina.

THERAPEUTIC IMPLICATIONS

We now recognize the existence of modulatory factors, such as coronary vasospasm, which appear to play a major role in the clinical manifestations of ischemic heart disease. Therefore, our attack on the problem, in terms of therapy and prevention, ought not to be directed solely at treating coronary atherosclerosis but also at identifying these modulatory factors. We need to know what is causing coronary spasm. We need to know whether or not causes other than spasm, can cause angina or acute myocardial ischemia. Such other causes are likely to exist, but if we do not look for them, we may not find them.

A better understanding of the causes of myocardial ischemia will lead to the development and use of an appropriate pharmacology and to intervention measures to prevent the clinical manifestations of ischemic heart disease. Therapy for patients in whom spasm seems to be the main cause of myocardial ischemia is empiric and difficult to evaluate, because long-term study of these patients shows that there is a natural waxing and waning of the disease.

Thus, treatment of primary angina and of coronary vasospasm remains symptomatic. In our experience, patients with vasospastic myocardial ischemia are quite sensitive to psychologic factors. This observation has relevant implications both in terms of management and interpretation of the results of treatment. We believe that in such patients evaluation of the efficacy of a drug in reducing the frequency of attacks can be accomplished only by repeated crossover trials rather than by the usual double-blind group studies.

Crossover trials just completed in our institution have demonstrated a consistent, remarkable effect of intravenous isosorbide dinitrate infusion[49] and of verapamil.[50] Nifedipine, another calcium antagonist drug, also appears to be effective in patients with vasospastic angina.[51]

Beta-blockers, the most widely used antianginal drugs, do not have the same rational indications in primary angina as they do in secondary angina. They were found to be effective in some patients only at doses much higher than those sufficient to produce complete beta blockade.[52]

Further investigations are needed to shed light on the pathogenesis and etiology of vasospasm and other forms of primary acute transient myocardial ischemia and on the mechanisms that control their reversibility or irreversibility.[10] This knowledge is essential to the development of rational therapeutic and preventive interventions. Undoubtedly, the effects of these modulatory factors, such as coronary vasomotor activity, responsible for some of the clinical manifestations of ischemic heart disease, will be more devastating in the presence of severe coronary atherosclerosis. Therefore, coronary bypass surgery may represent a rational form of associated preventive treatment for the patients in whom it has been proven more effective in improving prognosis than an appropriate specific medical therapy.

REFERENCES

1. Friedberg, C.K. *Diseases of the Heart.* Philadelphia: W.B. Saunders, 1966, p 700.

2. Arteriosclerosis. A Report by the National Heart and Lung Institute Task Force on Arteriosclerosis, Vol I, June 1971. U.S. Department of Health, Education, and Welfare, Public Health Service, National Institutes of Health, DHEW Publ. No. (NIH) 72-137, p. 36.

3. Arteriosclerosis. The Report of the 1977 Working Group to Review the 1971 Report by the National Heart and Lung Institute Task Force on Arteriosclerosis, December, 1977. U.S. Department of Health, Education, and Welfare, Public Health Service, National Institutes of Health, DHEW Publ. No. (NIH) 78-1526, p 36.

4. Prinzmetal, M., Kennamer, R., Merliss, R. et al. Angina pectoris. I. A variant form of angina pectoris. *Am J Med.* 27:375–388, 1959.

5. Maseri, A., Mimmo, R., Chierchia, S. et al. Coronary artery spasm as a cause of acute myocardial ischemia in man. *Chest* 68:625–633, 1975.

6. Maseri, A., Parodi, O., Severi, S. et al. Transient transmural reduction of myocardial blood flow, demonstrated by thallium-201 scintigraphy, as a cause of variant angina. *Circulation* 56:280–288, 1976.

7. Meller, J., Pichard, A., and Dack, S. Coronary arterial spasm in Prinzmetal's angina: a proved hypothesis. *Am J Cardiol.* 37:938–940, 1976.

8. Maseri, A., L'Abbate, A., Pesola, A. et al. Coronary vasospasm in angina pectoris. *Lancet* 1:713–717, 1977.

9. Maseri, A., Severi, S., De Nes, M. et al. "Variant" angina: one aspect of a continuous spectrum of vasospastic myocardial ischemia. Pathogenetic mechanisms, estimated incidence, clinical and coronary angiographic findings in 138 patients. *Am J Cardiol.* 42:1019–1035, 1978.

10. Maseri, A., L'Abbate, A., Baroldi, G. et al. Coronary vasospasm as a possible cause of myocardial infarction. A conclusion derived from the study of "preinfarction" angina. *N Engl J Med.* 299:1271–1277, 1978.

11. Hillis, L.D., and Braunwald, E. Coronary-artery spasm. *N Engl J Med.* 299:695–702, 1978.

12. Enos, W.E., Holmes, R.H., and Beyer, J.C. Coronary disease among United States soldiers in action in Korea. *JAMA.* 152:1090–1093, 1953.

13. Baroldi, G. Coronary stenosis: ischemic or non-ischemic factors? *Am Heart J.* 96:139–143, 1978.

14. Friesinger, G.C., Smith, G.F. Correlation of electrocardiographic studies and arteriographic findings with angina pectoris. *Circulation* 46:1173–1184, 1972.

15. Gorlin, R. Angiographic coronary artery findings in patients with typical angina relative to those with myocardial infarction and those with suspect disease only. Edited by A. Maseri, G.A. Klassen, and M. Lesch. In *Primary and Secondary Pectoris*. New York: Grune & Stratton, Inc., 1978, pp 71–79.

16. Neill, W.A., Ritzmann, L.W., and Selden, R. The pathophysiologic basis of acute coronary insufficiency. Observations favoring the hypothesis of intermittent reversible coronary obstruction. *Am Heart J.* 94:439–444, 1977.

17. Fuster, V., Frye, R.L., Connolly, D.C. et al. Arteriographic patterns early in the onset of the coronary syndromes. *Br Heart J.* 37:1250–1255, 1975.

18. Bertolasi, C.A., Trongé, J.E., Carreño, C.A. et al. Unstable angina. Prospective and randomized study of its evolution, with and without surgery. *Am J Cardiol.* 33:201–208, 1974.

19. Conti, C.R. Unstable angina pectoris: National Cooperative Study Group to Compare Medical and Surgical Therapy. I. Report of protocol and patient population. *Am J Cardiol.* 37:896–902, 1976.

20. Chierchia, S., Marchesi, C., and Maseri, A. Evidence of angina not caused by increased myocardial metabolic demand and patterns of electrocardiographic and hemodynamic alterations during "primary" angina. Edited by A. Maseri, G.A. Klassen, and M. Lesch. In *Primary and Secondary Angina Pectoris*. New York: Grune & Stratton, Inc., 1978, pp 145–155.

21. Guazzi, M., Polese, A., Fiorentini, C. et al. Left ventricular performance and related haemodynamic changes in Prinzmetal's variant angina pectoris. *Br Heart J.* 33:84–94, 1971.

22. Chierchia, S., Maseri, A., Simonetti, I. et al. O_2 myocardial extraction in angina at rest. Evidence of a primary reduction of blood supply. (Abstract). *Circulation* 55–56(suppl III):135, 1977.

23. Guazzi, M., Polese, A., Fiorentini, C. et al. Left and right heart hemodynamics during spontaneous angina pectoris. Comparison between angina with S-T segment depression and angina with S-T segment elevation. *Br Heart J.* 37:401–413, 1975.

24. Roughgarden, J.W., and Newman, E.V. Circulatory changes during the pain of angina pectoris. 1772–1965. A critical review. *Am J Med.* 41:935–946, 1966.

25. Robinson, B.F. Relation of heart rate and systolic pressure to the onset of pain and angina pectoris. *Circulation* 35:1073–1083, 1967.

26. Berman, N.D., McLaughlin, P.R., and Huckell, V.F. et al. Prinzmetal's angina with coronary artery spasm. Angiographic, pharmacologic, metabolic and radionuclide perfusion studies. *Am J Med.* 60:727–732, 1976.

27. Ricci, D.R., Orlick, A.E., Dohertu, P.W. et al. Reduction of coronary blood flow during coronary artery spasm occurring spontaneously and after provocation by ergonovine maleate. *Circulation* 57:392–395, 1978.

28. Parodi, O., Severi, S., Uthurralt, N. et al. Angina pectoris at rest: regional myocardial perfusion during S-T segment elevation or depression (abstract). *Circulation* 55–56(suppl III):229, 1977.

29. Uthurralt, N., Parodi, O., Maseri, A. et al. Myocardial scintigraphy in patients with angina at rest. Studies during spontaneous and exercise induced attacks. Presented at the 1st Joint Meeting of the Working Groups of the European Society of Cardiology, Brighton, UK, June 1978 (abstract).

30. Chierchia, S., Maseri, A., Simontti, I. et al. O_2 myocardial extraction in angina at rest. Evidence of a primary reduction of blood supply. (abstract). *Circulation* 55–56(suppl III):135, 1977.

94

31. Curry, R.C., Pepine, C.J., Sabom, M.B. et al. Effects of ergonovine in patients with or without coronary artery disease. *Circulation* 56:803–809, 1977.

32. Schroeder, J.S., Bolen, J.L., Quint, R.A. et al. Provocation of coronary spasm with ergonovine maleate. *Am J Cardiol.* 40:487–491, 1977.

33. Maseri, A., L'Abbate, A., Pesola, A. et al. Coronary vasospasm in angina pectoris. *Lancet* 1:713–717, 1977.

34. Marzilli, M., L'Abbate, A., Ballestra, A.M. et al. Coronary angiography findings during angina at rest with ST depression (abstract). *Circulation* 56(suppl III):83, 1977.

35. Maseri, A., Severi, S., Chierchia, S. et al. Characteristics and pathogenetic mechanism of "primary" angina at rest. Edited by A. Maseri, G.A. Klassen, and M. Lesch. In *Primary and Secondary Angina Pectoris.* New York: Grune & Stratton, 1978, pp. 265–273.

36. Wiener, L., Kasparian, H., Duca, P.R. et al. Spectrum of coronary arterial spasm. Clinical angiographic and myocardial metabolic experience in 29 cases. *Am J Cardiol.* 38:945–955, 1976.

37. Tavazzi, L., Salerno, J.A., Ray, M. et al. Acute myocardial ischemia induced by ergonovine maleate in patients with "primary" angina. In *Primary and Secondary Angina Pectoris.* Edited by A. Maseri, G.A. Klassen, and M. Lesch. New York: Grune & Stratton, 1978, pp. 247–263.

38. Maseri, A. Preface. Edited by A. Maseri, G.A. Klassen, and M. Lesch. In *Primary and Secondary Angina Pectoris.* New York: Grune & Stratton, 1978, pp. xiii–xiv.

39. Maseri, A. Pathogenetic mechanisms of angina pectoris: expanding views. Thomas Lewis Lecture, London, 24th November 1977. *Br Heart J.* (In press).

40. Mustard, J.F. Reversible platelet aggregation and myocardial ischemia. *Circulation* 29(suppl III):30, 1964.

41. James, T.N. Pathology of small coronary arteris. *Am J Cardiol.* 20:679–691, 1967.

42. Richardson, P.J., Jackson, G., Olsen, E.C.J. et al. Angina pectoris with normal coronary arteriograms. A metabolic problem? Edited by A. Maseri, G.A. Klassen, and M. Lesch. In *Primary and Secondary Angina Pectoris.* New York: Grune & Stratton, 1978, pp. 297–301.

43. Kübler, W., Opherk, D., Mehmel, H. et al. Significance of coronary reserve in patients with different forms of "ischemic heart disease." VIII World Congress of Cardiology, Tokyo. Abstract 1:124:0155, 1978.

44. Montemartini, C., Angoli, L., Marinoni, G.P. et al. Coronary spasm during effort test. Presented at the 3rd Congress of the European Society of Cardiovascular Radiology, Florence, May 15–17, 1978.

45. Yasue, H., Omote, S., Takizawa, A. et al. Coronary arterial spasm as a cause of exertional angina pectoris. VIII World Congress of Cardiology, Tokyo, Abstract 1:174:0348, 1978.

46. Falcone, C., De Servi, S., Specchia, G. et al. La prova da sforzo nell'angina variante de Prinzmetal. XXXIX Congress of the Italian Society of Cardiology. Milan. Abstract Book 1978, p 131.

47. Mudge, G.M., Jr., Grossman, W., Millis, R. et al. Reflex increase in coronary vascular resistance in patients with ischemic heart disease. *N Engl J Med.* 295:1333–1337, 1976.

48. Schang, S.J., Jr., and Pepine, C.J. Transient asymptomatic S-T segment depression during daily activity. *Am J Cardiol.* 38:396–401, 1977.

49. Distante, A., Maseri, A., Severi, S. et al. Management of vasospastic "crescendo" angina by continuous infusion of isosorbide dinitrate. (In press).

50. Parodi, O., Maseri, A., and Simonetti, I. Management of unstable angina at rest by verapamil. A double-blind cross-over study in CCU. *Br Heart J.* 41:167-174, 1979.

51. Muller, J.E., and Gunther, S.J. Nifedipine therapy for Prinzmetal's angina. *Circulation* 57:137-139, 1978.

52. Guazzi, M., Fiorentini, C., Polese, A. et al. Use of beta-receptor antagonists in spontaneous angina pectoris. Edited by A. Maseri, G.A. Klassen, and M. Lesch. In *Pathogenetic Mechanisms of Angina Pectoris 1976*. New York: Grune & Stratton, 1978, pp. 373-382.

7 Myocardial Imaging of Patients with Unstable Angina

Peter R. McLaughlin, MD, and
John E. Morch, MD

In recent years a number of isotope imaging techniques have been developed that are clinically useful in the assessment of coronary disease.[1] Some of these techniques are applicable to patients with unstable angina and may be classified as follows:

Imaging with infarct-avid agents such as technetium-99m pyrophosphate

Imaging with potassium-analogue agents such as thallium-20

Radionuclide ventricular angiography

TECHNETIUM-99M PYROPHOSPHATE IMAGING

Technetium-99m pyrophosphate has been used for several years as an infarct-avid agent for acutely infarcted myocardium.[2-5] The mechanism of its uptake in infarcted tissue appears to be concentration of the

97

pyrophosphate chelated with the intracellular calcium precipitations that accumulate in injured myocardial cells.[6,7] Imaging approximately 60 minutes after injection of 15 to 20 mCi. of technetium-99m pyrophosphate permits visualization of the infarct as a "hot spot" from 1 to 7 days after time of infarction. As recently reviewed by Wynne et al,[8] a number of conditions such as breast tumors, rib fractures, and valvular calcification have been reported to cause "false positive" studies. These conditions can often be excluded on clinical grounds. Thus, discrete localized uptake of ^{99m}Tc pyrophosphate using established criteria[4,9] in the absence of conditions known to produce false positive studies is strongly suggestive of recently injured myocardial tissue.

A number of studies have demonstrated uptake of ^{99m}Tc pyrophosphate in patients with unstable angina without enzymatic or electrocardiographic evidence of infarction.[10-12] These data suggest that many patients with unstable angina may be experiencing subclinical infarction, likely in subendocardial areas. Willerson and co-workers found that 35% of their patients with unstable angina had positive scintigrams identical to those seen after acute subendocardial infarction.[4] In the author's own experience 5 to 11 studies in patients with unstable angina without enzymatic or electrocardiographic evidence of infarction had positive images.

Newer imaging techniques with the 7-pinhole collimator give tomographic cuts through the myocardium[13] and may improve the ability to detect, localize, and quantitate the amount of injured tissue in this group of patients. Further studies will be required to answer this question.

A limitation of the method is the uncertainty as to whether a "hot spot" with technetium-99m pyrophosphate in these patients without enzymatic or ECG evidence of infarction represents irreversibly or reversibly injured tissue. One may speculate that the patients with definite abnormal uptake of technetium-99m pyrophosphate and normal enzymes are a subgroup of patients with small areas of infarction who are at higher risk for more extensive infarction without surgery, and perhaps also at a higher surgical risk. The natural and surgical history of these patients will require more detailed follow-up studies.

THALLIUM-201 IMAGING

Imaging with thallium-201 displays myocardial perfusion and theoretically, should be useful in the patient with unstable angina to distinguish the difference between ischemia and necrosis. In the special circumstances of Prinzmetal's angina, thallium-201 administered during painful episodes showed prominent perfusion defects.[14] In order to distinguish between necrosis and ischemia, wash-in imaging was repeated three to four hours postinjection. However, a serious drawback to the technique was the necessity of injecting the isotope during the episode of pain and performing the imaging promptly with delayed wash-in imaging. Wackers et al[15] studied a large number of patients with unstable angina using similar imaging techniques except the injections of isotope were made during the pain-free period. Some patients displayed persistent defects (up to six hours) due to delay in uptake of the isotope in the absence of ECG or enzyme changes of myocardial infarction. The authors raised the question as to whether imaging revealed effects of ischemia long after the clinical and ECG parameters were normal or did this delayed uptake display clinically unrecognizable myocardial damage? The authors further went on to comment that in the presence of previous myocardial infarction, it may be difficult to determine further increases in the perfusion defect due to ischemia. These authors concluded that the patients with the most markedly delayed uptake after the injection of isotope had the most unfavorable clinical course.

In summary, it would appear that although thallium-201 myocardial imaging, which displays myocardial perfusion, theoretically would be useful in unstable angina, there are a number of practical limitations and problems in interpretation of the significance of the delayed uptake in patients without clinically recognizable myocardial damage. Further studies will be necessary to define the applicability of this technique to the management of patients with unstable angina.

RADIONUCLIDE ANGIOGRAPHY

Few data are available on transient changes in ventricular function in the patient with recurrent angina being monitored in the intensive care unit. The newly developed multiple-gated and single-pass isotope angiographic techniques[16,17] will permit serial studies of ventricular function of these patients "in situ." Radionuclide angiography has demonstrated marked reduction in left ventricular performance during exercise- induced ischemia in patients with stable angina.[18] Similar changes might be expected in patients with recurrent spontaneous rest pain. This technique has promise not only in properly defining risk groups in patients with unstable angina but also in assessing the immediate effects on ventricular function of different medical and surgical treatment programs in the acutely ill patient.

REFERENCES

1. McLaughlin, P. Radionuclide imaging in cardiovascular disease. *JAMA.* 236:2439, 1976.

2. Parkey, R.W., Bonte, F.J., Meyer, S.L. et al. A new method for radionuclide imaging of acute myocardial infarction in humans. *Circulation* 50:540, 1974.

3. McLaughlin, P., Coates, G., Wood, D. et al. Detection of acute myocardial infarction by technetium-99m pyrophosphate. *Am J Cardiol.* 35:390, 1975.

4. Willerson, J.T., Parkey, R.W., Bonte, F.J. et al. Technetium stannous pyrophosphate myocardial scintigrams in patients with chest pain of varying etiology. *Circulation* 51:1046, 1975.

5. Willerson, J.T., Parkey, R.W., Bonte, F.J. et al. Acute subendocardial myocardial infarction in patients. *Circulation* 51:436, 1975.

6. Buja, L.M., Parkey, R.W., Dees, J.H. et al. Morphologic correlates of technetium-99m stannouspyrophosphate imaging of acute myocardial infarcts in dogs. *Circulation* 52:596, 1975.

7. Poliner, L.R., Buja, L.M., Parkey, R.W. et al. Clinicopathologic findings in 52 patients studied by technetium-99m stannous pyrophosphate myocardial scintigraphy. *Circulation* 59:257, 1979.

8. Wynne, J., Holman, B.L., and Lesk, M. Myocardial scintigraphy by infarct-avid radiotraurs. *Prog Cardiovasc Dis.* 20:243, 1978.

9. Berman, D.S., Amsterdam, E.A., Hines, H.H. et al. New approach to interpretation of technetium-99m pyrophosphate scintigraphy in detection of acute myocardial infarction. *Am J Cardiol.* 39:341, 1977.

10. Donsky, M.S., Curry, G.C., Parkey, R.W. et al. Unstable angina pectoris. Clinical, angiographic and myocardial scintigraphic observations. *Br Heart J.* 38:257, 1976.

11. Abdulla, A.M., Carredo, M.I., Cortez, B.C. et al. Detection of unstable angina by 99m technetium pyrophosphate myocardial scintigraphy. *Chest* 69:168, 1976.

12. Perez, L.A., Hayt, D.B., and Freeman, L.M. Localization of myocardial disorders other than infarction with 99 Tc-labelled pyrophosphate agents. *J Nucl Med.* 17:241, 1976.

13. Vogel, R.A., Kirch, D.L., LeFree, M.T. et al. Thallium-201 myocardial perfusion scintigraphy: Results of standard and multi-pinhole tomographic techniques. *Am J Cardiol.* 43:787, 1979.

14. Maseri, A., Parodi, O., Severi, S. et al. Transient transmural reduction of myocardial blood flow, demonstrated by thallium-201 scintigraphy, as a cause of variant angina. *Circulation* 54:2; 280, 1976.

15. Wackers, F.J., Lie, K.I., Liem, K.L. et al. Thallium-201 scintigraphy in unstable angina pectoris. *Circulation* 57:4; 738, 1978.

16. Burrow, R.D., Strauss, W., and Singleton, R. Analysis of left ventricular function from multiple gated acquisition (MUGA) cardiac blood pool imaging: comparison to contrast angiography. *Circulation* 56:1024, 1977.

17. Steele, P., Van Dyke, R.S., Trow, R.S. et al. A simple and safe bedside method for serial measurement of left ventricular ejection fraction, cardiac output, and pulmonary blood volume. *Br Heart J.* 36:122, 1974.

18. Borer, J.S., Bacharach, S.L., Green, M.V. et al. Real time radionuclide cineangiography in the non-invasive evaluation of global and regional left ventricular function at rest and during exercise in patients with coronary artery disease. *N Engl J Med.* 296:839, 1977.

SECTION III

Medical Therapy for Unstable Angina

8 Therapeutic Decisions in the Management of Unstable Angina

Ronald S. Baigrie, MD

The editors of this monograph have defined unstable angina pectoris to include the following clinical syndromes: new onset angina, crescendo angina, acute coronary insufficiency, and angina following soon after acute myocardial infarction. New onset angina is defined as the initial appearance of angina within two months of its diagnosis in a patient with no previous history of myocardial ischemic pain or infarction. Crescendo angina implies an increase in the severity or duration of preexistent angina or the occurrence of angina with less provocation.[1] Acute coronary insufficiency is defined as prolonged myocardial ischemic pain, usually greater than 15 minutes in duration and occurring either spontaneously at rest, without obvious provocation, or following exertion. Angina pectoris occurring early or remotely, but arbitrarily within two months of acute myocardial infarction is felt to represent the fourth syndrome within the unstable angina pectoris group. Implicit in the above definitions of the clinical subgroups within the unstable angina pectoris population is that every patient with angina was, at one time, unstable. It must also be recognized that these terms and definitions and subsequent classifications are convenient ones based on the patient's own clinical description of the pattern of occurrence of his chest pain. The use of the designation "unstable" implies an unpredictable early clinical outcome and long-term prognosis.

The majority of patients with unstable angina pectoris have significant coronary atherosclerosis.[2] Assuming that patients with coronary atherosclerosis present with a spectrum of myocardial ischemic syndromes, it is generally felt that unstable angina lies between stable exertional angina pectoris at one end of the spectrum and acute myocardial infarction at the other. This concept has traditionally been very useful with regard to classification as well as therapeutic intervention and prognostication. Heberden[3] described the clinical picture of angina pectoris in 1772 but it was not until 1912 that Herrick[4] recorded the clinical features of acute myocardial infarction. Although the clinical syndrome of unstable angina pectoris was reported in 1937,[5,6] it is only in the past decade that it has become important to distinguish various unstable angina subgroups. The reason is: multiple therapeutic alternatives coupled with an expanding cognizance of the pathophysiology. It is the purpose of this chapter to discuss the various therapeutic decisions in the acute phase of treatment of patients with unstable angina. Before attempting to outline the triage of management of unstable angina pectoric, it is necessary to review some of the traditional and more contemporary concepts regarding this syndrome.

HISTORICAL RESUMÉ

It has been appreciated for many years that several ischemic pain syndromes appear to have a worse clinical course and poorer prognosis than typical exertional angina pectoris and yet not so ominous, perhaps, as does the syndrome of acute myocardial infarction. This intermediate form of pain, presently referred to as unstable angina pectoris was initially mentioned by Osler[7] and Herrick[4] in their descriptions of patients with acute myocardial infarction. This intermediate pain was not appreciated generally as a separate clinical syndrome until reported as such by Sampson and Eliaser[5] and Feil.[6] Since these descriptions, numerous attempts at defining the population of patients who present with these intermediate pain syndromes have led to an extensive and confusing nomenclature. The names given to these syndromes vary according to their content of clinical description and prognostication. For example, the original description of this clinical entity by Sampson and Eliaser[5] termed the syndrome "impending coronary occlusion" since all of their 29 patients eventually developed myocardial infarctions. For similar reasons, Reeves and Harrison[8] used "preinfarction angina" to describe similar intermediate pain syndromes. Both of these names imply a knowledge that myocardial infarction is imminent. Other names of this syndrome emphasize the important feature, intermediate pain, without implying prognosis. Blumgart[9] described a group of patients with intermediate pain under the heading "coronary failure." Although not implied in this name, it was felt that this was prodromal to myocardial infarction. Graybiel[10] used "intermediate coronary syndrome." Master[11] used "acute coronary insufficiency" and, more recently, Fowler[12] coined the term "unstable angina pectoris," a term that is most suitable given current understanding of prognosis and pathophysiologic mechanisms.

A few of the terms given to this important syndrome of myocardial ischemic pain since its original clinical description are: unstable angina,[12] preinfarction angina,[8] acute coronary insufficiency,[11] impending myocardial infarction,[13] intermediate coronary syndrome,[10] status anginosus,[14] accelerated angina,[15] slight coronary attacks,[16] coronary failure,[9] acute fatal coronary insufficiency,[17] impending acute coronary artery occlusion,[5] preliminary pain in coronary thrombosis,[6] and premonitory period.[10] In fact, 29 different names for this clinical syndrome were found during the preparation of this manuscript. Chahine,[18] in a recent editorial, concluded that this abundant terminology likely reflects a lack of clear understanding of these myocardial ischemic syndromes. It is important to note that although the term unstable angina pectoris is now widely accepted because it reflects our inability to predict ultimate prognosis, unstable angina pectoris oversimplifies a broad spectrum of acute myocardial ischemic syndromes that are now grouped under one, perhaps superficial, title.

CLINICAL IMPLICATION AND PROGNOSIS

Two important historical concepts must be considered in order to understand current enthusiasm about unstable angina pectoris as a separate clinical syndrome worthy of urgent or emergent medical or surgical intervention. These are: 1) the revelation that many patients with acute myocardial infarction give histories of prodromal pain patterns compatible with unstable angina pectoris, and 2) the early natural history studies of unstable angina pectoris, which described a poor medium- and long-term prognosis.

Prodromal Pain of Acute Myocardial Infarction

It was not long after the early description of the clinical syndrome of acute myocardial infarction that reports appeared describing a variable incidence of premonitory symptoms in these patients. Anginal pain was the most common of these prodromes, but also described were dyspnea, fatigue, and palpitations. Herrick[4] in his original communication noted a case history in which a premonitory attack of severe unusual angina pain occurred three days prior to acute myocardial infarction. Sampson[5] reported a 48% incidence of prolonged anginal attacks in patients who developed acute myocardial infarction with an average of 7.1 days between the onset of this new symptom and the occurrence of acute myocardial infarction. The incidence of acute myocardial infarction preceded by symptoms presently accepted as compatible with unstable angina pectoris has varied widely; there are recent figures of 19%, 43%, and 63%.[19-21] The duration of the unstable angina symptoms preceding admission for acute myocardial infarction has also varied widely, with mean time of two and three and a half weeks[18,22] being common but with many patients having these complaints for several weeks or months.[21] In addition, the occurrence of rest pain preceding acute myocardial infarction is reported as high as 55%.[20]

These studies and others indicate that prior to acute myocardial infarction, a history of prolonged chest pain, not infrequently occurring at rest, with a duration of several days or weeks is common. In the absence of chest pain, other prodromes, eg, fatigue and dyspnea, have occurred in from 7% to 18% of patients.[18] This rather high incidence of prior unstable angina among patients with fresh acute myocardial infarction should not be interpreted as meaning that all unstable angina patients subsequently suffer acute myocardial infarction. Indeed, natural history studies as well as studies concerned with the therapeutic alternatives in unstable angina pectoris patients have demonstrated that acute myocardial infarction does not invariably follow unstable angina pectoris.

Natural History Studies

The earlier natural history studies, prior to 1970, reported the results of treatment utilizing only nitroglycerin without the benefit of beta-blockers, anticoagulants, or long-acting nitrates.[21,23,24] Subsequent studies, after 1970, included patients receiving various regimens of long-acting nitrates, anticoagulants, and beta-blockers.[25-27] As pointed out by Cairns,[28] infarction and death were more frequent in the earlier compared to the later studies; 21% to 80% infarction and 1% to 60% mortality versus the later figures of 7% to 15% and 1% to 2%, respectively.[2,25] Unfortunately, the great variety of patient populations studied and the diverse medical therapies utilized in these reports makes interpretation somewhat difficult, particularly in the subgroups of unstable angina patients. For example, Duncan[29] reported a 12.7% incidence of acute myocardial infarction and a 3.6% mortality at six months in a prospective analysis of 251 male patients with new onset, recurrent, or crescendo angina pectoris. Gazes[25] reported on 140 patients with either new onset, crescendo, or prolonged rest pain (> 15 min), and found 1-, 2-, 3-, 5-, and 10-year mortality rates of 18%, 25%, 31%, 39%, and 52%, respectively. A high-risk sub-group, those with continuing pain in-hospital had a very poor prognosis, with mortality rates of 43%, 53%, 63%, 73%, and 81%, respectively. Overall, 21% of patients developed acute myocardial infarction within eight months of the clinical diagnosis of preinfarction angina. This figure was 35% at three months for the high-risk subgroup. In Krauss's[26] series of 100 patients with acute coronary insufficiency, defined as prolonged pain greater than 30 minutes at rest, the mortality and infarction rates were 22% and 14% at an average follow-up of 20 months; at six months' follow-up the figures were 8% and 10%. The patients described by Vakel,[24] which included mostly patients with prolonged pain (> 15 min), had a 37% incidence of acute myocardial infarction within a three-month period of follow-up.

A complete discussion of long-term prognosis will not be presented here. It is, however, important to recognize that in Duncan's series 73% of the patients who did not suffer acute myocardial infarction or death had stable angina pectoris at six months' follow-up. Gazes[25] found that at one year, 74% of the survivors had less angina. Krauss[26] found that at 20 months, 52% of the patients had stable angina pectoris or were pain-free, and only 8% had suffered recent acute coronary insufficiency.

In most studies in which beta-blocking agents have been used in-hospital, morbidity and mortality has remained relatively low, ranging from 0% to 13% mortality and 0% to 25% acute myocardial infarction.[26,27,29-31] Recently, the National Cooperative Study Group to compare medical and surgical therapy for unstable angina pectoris reported a 3% mortality and an 8% incidence of acute myocardial infarction in-hospital among 147 patients randomized to medical therapy including beta-blockers.[2] It is important, however, to recognize that although this study included patients with crescendo angina and new onset angina as well as those having angina at rest in the hospital, all patients were pain-free (after receiving medical therapy) prior to randomization. However, even patients with prolonged rest pain in-hospital have responded to aggressive medical therapy (including propranolol) with low short-term morbidity and mortality.[27,32] It is now generally assumed that if patients continue to have spontaneous angina at rest despite aggressive medical therapy that the incidence of subsequent infarction and death in-hospital is far greater.[25] Perhaps more important is the outcome of patients who persist with recurrent spontaneous prolonged pain despite maximal pharmacologic therapy; the debate regarding optimal treatment of these patients continues.

The therapeutic implications of these reports are obvious. Aggressive medical therapy is indicated at the time of first diagnosis, and subsequent urgent or emergent surgical intervention can safely await knowledge of the patients' response to such medical treatment.

CLINICALLY RECOGNIZABLE UNSTABLE ANGINA PECTORIS SUBGROUPS: ATTEMPTS AT CLASSIFICATION

Several investigators have attempted to classify unstable angina pectoris into subgroups with differing prognoses. Gazes[25] found that patients who continued to complain of rest pain during hospitalization had a greater incidence of acute myocardial infarction and death than did patients whose pain subsided on traditional medical therapy. Earlier, Littmann[33] attempted to subclassify 207 consecutive patients admitted to the hospital with "acute atypical coronary artery insufficiency," a term used to describe the group of patients with pain more severe than angina pectoris but who failed to satisfy criteria for acute myocardial infarction. These subgroups were: 1) coronary failure—prolonged pain at rest with transient ECG changes and no relief with nitroglycerin, 2) subendocardial necrosis—prolonged pain with transient ST depression with or without T-wave inversion and slight fever or leukocytosis, and 3) atypical acute myocardial infarction—prolonged pain, symmetric T-wave inversion, and slight fever with leukocytosis. The subendocardial necrosis group had the greatest incidence of acute myocardial infarction and death. Armstrong[34] reported four subgroups of unstable angina pectoris based on ECG and creatine kinase (CK) determinations. If both ECG and CK were normal, the subsequent occurrence of acute coronary insufficiency was 14%, and there was no infarction or mortality. If both ECG and CK were abnormal, there was an 8% infarction rate and 15% mortality at 12 months follow-up. Bertolasi's[35] study of 142 patients with unstable angina pectoris included 20 patients with intermediate syndrome and 20 patients with progressive angina who were treated medically. The mortality rates for patients with intermediate syndrome were 35% and 5% for those with progressive angina at an average follow-up period of 8.3 months. Kraus[26] also noted an increased rate of acute myocardial infarction and mortality in his patients with acute coronary insufficiency who continued to have angina in the hospital. Thirty-six percent of his patients fell into this subgroup with a 17% rate of acute myocardial infarction during the first hospitalization. In the National Cooperative Study Group trial[2] of unstable angina pectoris, a greater in-hospital mortality rate was found among patients with single-vessel disease compared to triple-vessel disease (6% versus 0%). Conversely, there was a greater in-hospital rate of acute myocardial infarction among patients with three-vessel disease compared to single-vessel disease (12% versus 6%). Wiles[36] investigated a number of preoperative risk factors for operative mortality in 124 consecutive patients undergoing coronary bypass surgery for unstable angina pectoris. Factors that significantly increased operative mortality were failure of in-hospital maximal medical treatment, hypertension, and triple-vessel disease. Mortality of patients with all three of these independent risk factors was 41.7%; if only two were present 1.9%, and no mortality occurred if only one or no risk factor was present.

In a recent retrospective study by Weisel et al,[37] 471 patients who underwent aortocoronary saphenous vein bypass grafting for unstable angina pectoris were analyzed. Among 348 patients with brief pain in the form of crescendo angina, the perioperative infarction rate, mortality, and incidence of low output syndrome were 5%, 4%, and 14%, respectively. Those patients with unstable angina pectoris with acute coronary insufficiency in the form of prolonged rest pain but with reversible ischemic ECG changes had a 4%, 4%, and 18% incidence, respectively. Patients with irreversible new ischemic changes on their resting ECG but no enzyme elevations had a 22%, 10%, and 21% incidence. Among those patients felt to have had a subendocardial myocardial infarction with fixed ECG changes and enzyme elevation less than three times normal, the figures were 20%, 7%, and 13%, respectively. Retrospectively then, it would appear that the ECG taken in consideration with serum enzyme determination can be predictive for postoperative morbidity and mortality. Whether such criteria can be applied to a prospectively analyzed group of medical and surgical patients is currently under study.

These important efforts attempting to categorize subgroups of unstable angina pectoris patients are clearly identifying patients at greater or lesser risk. Further investigation will undoubtedly expose subgroups whose prognosis and treatment can be individualized on the basis of more than empirical reasoning.

APPLIED NEWER DIAGNOSTIC TECHNIQUES

The application of newer diagnostic techniques has expanded the understanding of anatomical and functional abnormalities that may occur in patients with unstable angina pectoris. The results have been revealing. Notably, among these newer techniques are those of hemodynamic monitoring, echocardiography, and myocardial nuclear imaging and nuclear angiography. A brief discussion of each will serve to identify potential usefulness and contribution to the understanding of unstable angina pectoris.

Hemodynamics

The first report of clinical observations of circulatory changes during spontaneous anginal attacks was made by T.L. Brunton in 1867.[38] Roughgarden[39] critically reviewed the literature on circulatory changes during angina pectoris and subsequently reported his own observations on hemodynamic changes in 15 patients.[40] He concluded that spontaneous angina was associated with elevation of systemic and pulmonary artery pressures, which preceded the onset of pain in 86% of the cases. Increases in pulse rates were much less striking prior to the onset of pain. M. Guazzi[41] reported hemodynamic changes during spontaneous pain in four patients with Prinzmetal's angina. Typical findings in 38 recorded episodes were progressive reduction in arterial pressure, fall in cardiac output, increase in peripheral resistance and right atrial pressure, prolongation of left ventricular isovolumic contraction time, reduction in mean rate of isovolumic pressure development, and decrease in mean systolic ejection rate. Hemodynamic changes always occurred at the same time as ECG changes. He concluded that this form of angina was unlikely secondary to circulatory changes that acutely increase cardiac oxygen consumption. He later documented disappearance of both the ECG and hemodynamic changes using propranolol.[42]

Cannon et al[43] reported hemodynamic changes occurring at the onset of 56 episodes of spontaneous angina in 26 patients with unstable angina. Three distinctive hemodynamic subsets were defined: increase in heart rate only, increase in systemic arterial pressure and heart rate, and increases in systemic arterial and pulmonary arterial diastolic pressures with minimal changes in heart rate. They were unable to correlate the type of hemodynamic alteration with the location or severity of coronary artery disease, the presence or absence of left ventricular contraction abnormalities or the number of previous myocardial infarctions. Also, the type of hemodynamic abnormality associated with resting angina was not helpful in identifying the high-risk patient for early myocardial infarction.

Scheidt et al[1] hemodynamically studied 54 episodes of spontaneous angina at rest in 17 patients. Heart rate, systolic and diastolic arterial pressures, and left ventricular filling pressure increased usually before the conscious perception of pain. They concluded that spontaneous angina at rest is preceded by hemodynamic changes that increase cardiac work and, by inference, myocardial oxygen consumption.

Maseri et al[44] hemodynamically studied 38 patients with angina at rest. No consistent increase in heart rate, blood pressure, or first derivative of left ventricular pressure was observed in any patient before the onset of ischemic ECG changes. Increases in heart rate and blood pressure were often observed after the onset of ischemic repolarization changes. They concluded that the episodes of acute myocardial ischemia in their patients could not be ascribed to an increase in myocardial oxygen demand.

Figueras et al[45] studied 23 patients with angina at rest. Anginal episodes were always preceded by ischemic ECG changes and increases in pulmonary artery systolic pressure as well as reduction in stroke index. Mean aortic pressure either increased, decreased, or remained unaltered. The double product (heart rate × systolic arterial pressure) before the onset of pain was unchanged or increased slightly. They concluded that the absence of significant alterations in the major determinants of myocardial oxygen consumption at the onset of the ischemic episode raises the possibility of a spontaneous reduction in myocardial perfusion as a primary mechanism of rest angina.

The occurrence of ischemic ECG changes prior to the appearance of hemodynamic alterations that would cause an increase in cardiac work (myocardial oxygen consumption) apparently contradicts traditional thinking regarding the pathophysiology of anginal pain at rest. Although the determinants of myocardial oxygen consumption[46] may be operative in pain occurring with exertion, there are other potential mechanisms that may precipitate ischemia.[47] A few of the alternative entities implicated in myocardial ischemia production when coronary angiography is normal are: coronary artery spasm, small-vessel coronary disease, oxyhemoglobin dissociation defects, misinterpretation of coronary arteriograms, cardiomyopathy, misdiagnosed chest pain, psychosomatic factors, and hypercoagulability.

Echocardiography

Although there are no studies reporting the use of echocardiography (ECHO) in unstable angina pectoris patients, there is much known about ECHO findings in patients with coronary artery disease with or without recent or remote myocardial infarction.[48] The ECHO changes found with myocardial infarction include wall motion abnormalities (segmental dyskinesia), compensatory hyperactivity of nonischemic myocardium, wall thinning, decreased systolic velocity and wall excursion, aneurysmal bulging, and abnormal systolic wall thickening. In coronary artery disease, the pattern of abnormal wall motion has been correlated with the location of occlusive coronary atherosclerosis.[49] Corya[50] has found a 36% incidence of abnormal interventricular septal motion and an 18% incidence of decreased systolic septal thickening in 28 patients without evidence of previous acute myocardial infarction.

Ventricular asynergy during anginal pain provoked by exercise has been reported by Fogelman.[51] Arnett[52] has shown in patients with coronary artery disease utilizing two-dimensional ECHO that the percent of left ventricular wall thickening in wall segments supplied by diseased vessels is significantly less than in wall segments supplied by normal coronary arteries.

The further application of ECHO, particularly multidimensional ECHO techniques, to the study of patients with unstable angina pectoris will undoubtedly add much to knowledge of this syndrome. Perhaps patients could be subgrouped on the basis of presence or absence of wall motion abnormality or the extent and type of dyssynergy. Certain prognostic information may also be forthcoming. The use of this noninvasive modality during both quiescent and painful periods in patients with unstable angina pectoris may prove useful in identifying patients with reversible ischemic dysfunction versus those with biochemically obscure myocardial 'infarction.'

Nuclear Imaging

Notable among the newer techniques that have been applied to the assessment of patients with unstable angina pectoris is nuclear cardiology; specifically, myocardial imaging and gated nuclear angiography. Using cold-spot imaging, Wackers et al[53] found a 39% incidence of definitely positive thallium-201 scintigrams in 98 patients with unstable angina pectoris. When a high-risk subgroup was identified, ie, those who developed acute myocardial infarction as well as those who continued to have angina despite optimal medical therapy, a 76% incidence of positive scintigrams was found. This was in contrast to a 32% incidence of positive scintigrams in patients who subsequently had an uncomplicated course. Abdulla et al[54] found a 71% incidence of positive technetium-99 pyrophosphate scintigrams in patients with unstable angina pectoris. Willerson et al[55] previously described seven patients with positive myocardial scintigrams who were admitted with a diagnosis of unstable angina pectoris.

Nichols et al[56] have recently demonstrated an improvement in left ventricular wall motion abnormality among patients with unstable angina during active intraaortic balloon counterpulsation utilizing technetium-99-labelled human serum albumin multigated cardiac blood pool imaging. Similar improvement in regional contraction was not observed in patients with acute myocardial infarction. Donsky et al[57] have also recently demonstrated positive technetium-99 pyrophosphate scintigrams in one-third of patients with unstable angina pectoris without diagnostic electrocardiographic or enzyme changes suggestive of myocardial infarction. Their findings also suggested that when technetium-99 pyrophosphate scintigrams are the only evidence of profound myocardial ischemia in patients with unstable angina, this does not have prognostic significance in terms of longevity or response to therapy.

The fact that thallium-201 scintigrams are positive in a number of patients with unstable angina pectoris who are not having anginal pain at the time of the study raises questions of prolonged or subclinical myocardial ischemia in their population. The interesting finding of positive technetium-99 pyrophosphate scintigrams in patients with unstable angina pectoris has been postulated as indicating either the occurrence of small areas of myocardial necrosis, which is not detectable by traditional investigation, or that severely ischemic myocardium can take up technetium in the absence of overt myocardial necrosis.

The application of these newer diagnostic techniques to the study of patients with unstable angina pectoris is adding to our knowledge of the pathophysiology of this disease. With this additional information, however, come a number of important questions that will only be answered with further investigation. What is the significance of large versus small areas of wall motion abnormality that occur during spontaneous angina? What is the significance of large versus small defects found by myocardial imaging techniques during spontaneous angina pectoris? Are there subgroups of patients with unstable angina pectoris who can be identified by these newer techniques, in conjunction with traditional assessments, who will benefit from more objective and specific therapeutic intervention? Will the timing of medical or surgical intervention be clarified in subgroups of patients with unstable angina pectoris?

MEDICAL AND SURGICAL TREATMENT

Since this topic is extensively reviewed elsewhere in this book, only some generalizations will be mentioned here. There are many factors that dictate the early and eventual definitive treatment of patients with unstable angina pectoris. Among these are age, sex, general state of health, complicating illnesses, the state of left ventricular function, as well as the coronary pathoanatomy. Prior to the availability of direct myocardial revascularization, the therapeutic options were limited to various medical regimens or indirect myocardial revascularization. Medical therapy has continued to be directed at reducing myocardial oxygen requirements and/or improving coronary blood flow.

Urgent and emergency coronary artery bypass grafting has proved useful in this syndrome since its introduction in 1971.[58] Newer pharmacologic agents, such as verapamil and nifedepine are being investigated, particularly since the suggestion that coronary spasm may be active as a precipitant in unstable angina pectoris.

Patients with exertional brief pain in the setting of new onset or crescendo anginal patterns probably can safely be treated initially at home with limited activity and long-acting nitrates and/or beta-blockers. Subsequent definitive investigation and treatment may be done on an elective or semielective basis. However, patients suffering spontaneous pain, particularly when prolonged, should be hospitalized preferably in a coronary care unit in order to exclude acute myocardial infarction and ischemia-related arrhythmias and to quickly obtain a pain-free status. Bedrest, oxygen, sedation, and perhaps anticoagulants have been traditional measures. The use of nitrates of various types, doses, and modes of administration has a sound physiologic basis.[59] Beta-blockers (propranolol) are useful to control heart rate and blood pressure and hence myocardial oxygen consumption.[60] On these regimens, the majority of patients become free of at least acute pain in the hospital. Some patients continue to have spontaneous pain and represent a previously described high-risk group for acute myocardial infarction.[25] Intravenous nitroglycerin has proved useful in controlling some of these otherwise refractory patients.[61]

Urgent or emergency coronary artery bypass grafting has been advocated prior to a trial of aggressive medical therapy. If this line of treatment is pursued, it is inevitable that inappropriate patients will undergo major cardiac surgery. Typical examples are patients who are operated on in the fact of evolving myocardial infarction. Without the opportunity to rule out significant coexistent medical disease, the risk of emergency surgery in patients with problems such as unrecognized bleeding disorders or diabetes mellitus, are obvious. As well, the risks of perioperative acute myocardial infarction and death in patients with unstable angina pectoris are greater than surgery for stable angina pectoris,[15,62] particularly if ischemic ECG changes persist and slight enzyme elevation is present.[37]

Several studies have shown that stabilization of patients with aggressive medical treatment followed by direct myocardial revascularization on an elective or semielective basis is not associated with excessive morbidity or mortality.[2,63-65] Whether or not elective myocardial revascularization should be performed in patients who are stabilized with aggressive medical therapy remains controversial. The use of coronary angiography is advocated by many in order to identify potentially high-risk subgroups as well as inoperable patients and those with normal coronary arteries.

For those patients who continue to have spontaneous pain in the hospital on aggressive medical treatment, selective coronary angiography with a view to bypass graft surgery for uncontrolled symptoms is indicated. There is a possibility that these patients may be offered newer pharmacologic preparations for the preoperative stabilization of their anginal pain. Further stabilization by use of mechanical intraaortic balloon counterpulsation has been shown to be beneficial.[66,67]

CLINICAL PRESENTATION AND ROUTINE INVESTIGATION

The majority of patients presenting with unstable angina pectoris and admitted to the coronary ICU at the Toronto General Hospital have suffered at least one episode of acute coronary insufficiency. This is defined as prolonged myocardial ischemic pain, usually greater than 15 minutes. Although their initial pain may have been either new onset angina or crescendo angina, they are admitted primarily to rule out myocardial infarction because of a history of prolonged pain usually with, but occasionally without, electrocardiographic abnormalities. The majority of patients show ECG changes in either the ST segment or the T wave. These changes are transient in some and persistent in others. ST-segment elevation of the Prinzmetal type does occur but is less common than ST-segment depression. Elevation of serum enzymes beyond the accepted normal values does occur, but this is usually minimal (less than 50% above normal) and in fact is used to rule out the diagnosis of acute myocardial infarction. This degree of enzyme elevation likely indicates subendocardial necrosis.

It is not unusual, however, for enzymes to rise within the range of normal values. This likely has significance equal in type but not extent to enzyme elevation and decline outside of the normal range. Appearance of the myocardial band (MB) of creatine kinase in the presence of normal traditional enzyme values is not uncommon. It often accompanies an elevation of traditional enzymes, but within the normal range.

Occasionally patients with unstable angina pectoris present with a completely normal ECG even during an episode of angina; definitive diagnosis may require repeated ECGs during recurrent episodes of pain or other diagnostic tests, eg, thallium-201 myocardial imaging. Further subclassification of these patients is necessary to identify subgroups of patients with unstable angina according to historical, electrocardiographic, and enzyme criteria.[34,37] Figures 8-1, 8-2, and 8-3 are examples of 12-lead electrocardiograms taken from patients presenting with acute coronary insufficiency. Another patient — a 40-year-old police officer with type A personality and history of cigarette smoking — presented with atypical anginal pain at rest. All ECGs and enzymes were normal. A submaximal exercise stress test was normal. Two days later he returned with a transmural anterior wall myocardial infarction.

As described earlier, patients with unstable angina pectoris can have other complaints in the absence of (or more apparent than) ischemic pain. The so-called "anginal equivalents" of dyspnea, syncope, ashen gray color with diaphoresis and severe fatigue are difficult to evaluate but likely are equally important prognostically and yet have not been included in the definition of unstable angina pectoris. These symptoms should perhaps be placed in a separate subgroup.

MANAGEMENT TRIAGE

Unstable angina pectoris is a common enough disorder that apparently trivial adjustments in the philosophy of treatment can have a major impact on available health-care resources. The overall management of patients with this syndrome has both qualitative and temporal dimensions and should be approached from the point of view of early or urgent and definitive or elective forms of therapeutic intervention. In order to implement an effective triage of management for any disease entity, a number of

116

factors concerning the disorder must be appreciated. Among these are the natural history of the disease, the results of the various therapeutic interventions, and the local circumstances dictating the availability of contemporary resources. The management triage (introduced in March 1977) utilized at the Toronto General Hospital invokes a rational approach to the temporal sequence of therapeutic intervention in this clinical syndrome. Prior to this date emergency coronary angiography and bypass graft surgery was commonly employed. Important recent studies of unstable angina pectoris have not specifically addressed the temporal dimension in the overall care of patients with unstable anginal pain.

The wide variety of clinical presentations and the creation of an unwieldy descriptive nomenclature is aggravated even more if one assumes that all patients suffering angina pectoris were at one time unstable by definition. Urgent coronary angiography and aortocoronary saphenous vein bypass graft surgery is advocated by some groups. Others have reported that the short-term morbidity is not excessive if it is assumed that an aggressive trial of contemporary medical treatment is the initial therapeutic endeavor.[1,27,32,39,63] Since March 1977, it has been accepted that unstable angina pectoris requires urgent medical intervention and is not a surgical emergency. Patients with at least one episode of prolonged myocardial ischemic pain (acute coronary insufficiency) are admitted to the coronary intensive care unit. Electrocardiograms are done on admission and daily and at any time if the patient experiences an episode of chest pain. Routine cardiac enzymes as well as CK-MB are performed daily. The patient is treated as though he has suffered a myocardial infarction. Oxygen is administered if pain is persistent. Blood is taken for grouping and the serum is reserved for later cross-match if necessary. The patient is started on beta-blocker therapy in the form of propranolol, beginning with 20 mg every six hours and increasing each successive dose by 20 mg. Metoprolol is preferred in asthmatics and diabetics. Nitrates are also begun in the form of topical nitroglycerin or oral isosorbide dinitrate (beginning with 20 mg every six hours). About 48 hours after admission to the hospital, the patient is classified according to his therapeutic response. Figure 8-4 shows the three locally used classifications of patients according to therapeutic response. Group I patients are completely free of anginal pain on medical therapy. Group II patients have a partial response to pharmacologic therapy in that they may have occasional episodes of brief pain with mild exertion, but these are quickly relieved by rest or sublingual nitroglycerin. Group III patients have shown an inadequate response to aggressive medical therapy and continue to have either brief pain at rest, which is quickly relieved with sublingual nitroglycerin (group IIIA) or prolonged pain at rest that does not respond well to sublingual nitroglycerin (group IIIB). In this triage, it is assumed that patients in group I and group II become predictable, at least in the short term, and they are discharged to the medical ward and ambulated provided no arrhythmia is identified. Figure 8-4 also outlines eventual therapeutic options in group I and group II patients. Elective cardiac catheterization may or may not be performed depending on the individual patient and his cardiologist. Selective coronary angiography may be performed during the initial hospitalization and surgical consultation obtained at that time, or coronary angiography may be delayed until such time as the patient proves refractory to increasing medical therapy.

Group III patients taking sufficient propranolol to suppress the heart rate to 50 to 60 beats/min during an episode of pain, receiving large doses of oral or topical nitrates, and persisting with recurrent chest pain are started on intravenous nitroglycerin in increasing doses from 0.4 to 4.0 mg/hr by continuous infusion. These patients generally undergo selective coronary angiography during their initial admission to the coronary ICU. The use of intraaortic balloon counterpulsation in this group of patients prior to angiography was at one time common but recently has declined. Those patients in this category who demonstrate operable coronary atherosclerosis generally undergo either urgent revascularization surgery or temporary intraaortic balloon counterpulsation in order to stabilize them

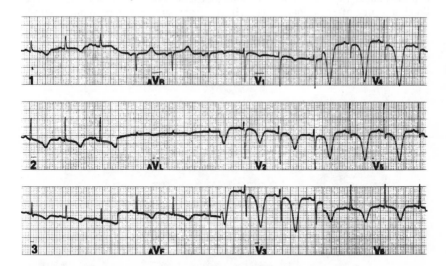

Figure 8-1 Example of a 12-lead ECG of a 39-year-old woman who presented with one prolonged episode of typical angina pectoris at rest. There was no history of hypertension or drug ingestion. No electrolyte disturbance or enzyme elevation was detected. CK-MB was normal. The ECG was persistently abnormal until discharge. Coronary angiography revealed an isolated, very proximal 90% lesion in the left anterior descending coronary artery. Ventricular function was normal. Intravenous ergonovine maleate failed to produce coronary arterial spasm. Her symptoms subsided on propranolol 60 mg four times a day and isosorbide dinitrate 20 mg four times daily.

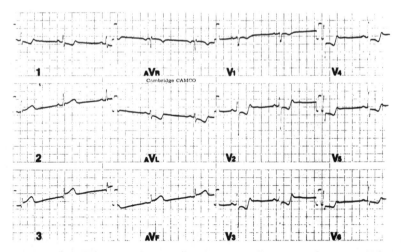

Figure 8-2 Example of a 12-lead ECG of a 50-year-old man who presented with crescendo angina and one episode of prolonged rest pain. The ECG returned to normal after 12 hours and there were no enzyme elevations including CK-MB. At coronary angiography an isolated 90% stenotic lesion was present proximally in the dominant circumflex coronary artery. His symptoms subsided on propranolol 40 mg four times a day and isosorbide dinitrate 60 mg four times daily.

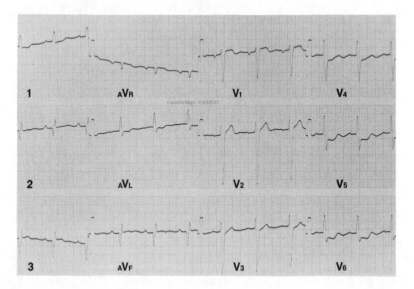

Figure 8-3 Example of a 12-lead ECG of a 65-year-old black man with acute coronary insufficiency. There is an old inferior wall infarct. The anterior and apical ischemic repolarization changes did not resolve following relief of chest pain and no enzyme elevation occurred.

while awaiting semielective bypass grafting. Group III patients who are deemed technically or otherwise inoperable are considered as candidates for newer antianginal therapy in the form of such drugs as verapamil.

This management triage has allowed identification of patients on the basis of their response to aggressive medical therapy. The majority of patients do in fact respond to pharmacologic intervention as has been noted by others.[2] Group I and group II patients then enter into the debate as to whether surgical or medical therapy is most appropriate. Myocardial infarction has been ruled out and they are stabilized on medical therapy. Group III patients, on the other hand, do not enter into this debate since they are having either persistent or recurrent myocardial ischemic pain at rest, and therefore an attempt at revascularization surgery is indicated because of these persistent symptoms. This triage has allowed standardization of the overall approach to these patients within the first 48 hours of their admission to the hospital. Pharmacologic therapy has been standardized in the form of increasing doses of propranolol and nitrates. Since the majority of these patients become pain-free on the aggressive medical regimen, urgent or emergent surgical intervention becomes less common.

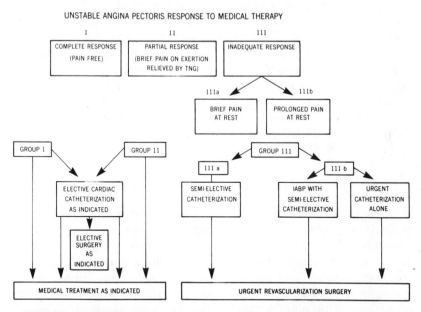

Figure 8-4 The classification of unstable angina pectoris patients based on response to medical therapy introduced at Toronto General Hospital, March 1977. Group I patients are completely pain-free on medical treatment. Group II patients have only exertional pain, which responds well to supplemental nitrates. Group III patients continue to have spontaneous or rest pain that is either brief (IIIa) or prolonged (IIIb) and does not respond well to supplemental nitrates. Further management proceeds electively or urgently, depending upon this therapeutic response, as shown.

More time is allowed for informative communication with the patient and his family and sufficient time is present to rule out the existence of subendocardial myocardial infarction or nonmyocardial ischemic pain syndromes and coexistent medical problems.

It should be obvious that this triage of unstable angina pectoris management makes a number of assumptions: 1) temporal sequence of medical and surgical intervention can safely be guided by symptoms, 2) coronary and myocardial anatomy does not alter appreciably during the period of medical treatment, 3) early morbidity and mortality with optimal medical therapy alone is minimal, and 4) a pain-free state is in fact a stable state for the myocardium. These assumptions may not be entirely true. It is conceivable that medical therapy may mask some forms of myocardial ischemia. It is not known if coronary or myocardial anatomy deteriorates under the guise of a medically stable pain-free state. The newer investigative techniques capable of easily measuring ventricular function may yet answer these questions.

Why bother to medically stabilize patients with unstable angina pectoris? As pointed out, the "cooling off" period allows time for optimal patient selection and classification as well as communication between patient and family and the medical/surgical team. The functional integrity of the catheterization laboratory and surgical team may be threatened by excessive "emergency" procedures. In areas or institutions where surgical intervention is not possible, it is important to protect the patient from unnecessary transfer in an unstable state. It is also important to protect elective catheterization and surgical schedules. It is not the purpose of this communication to discuss the important economic factors associated with excessive use of emergency surgical procedures.

SUMMARY

The assumption that a clinical spectrum exists in which myocardial ischemia presents at one end in the form of stable (predictable) exertional angina to acute myocardial infarction at the other is a reasonable one. However, the assumption that the more severe the anginal pain in terms of frequency, severity, and duration should not necessarily imply that the pathophysiologic mechanism is similar but more profound. The majority of patients with unstable angina pectoris have significant coronary atherosclerosis that is of the same order of magnitude as patients with stable angina. Another unknown factor, therefore, must be implicated to explain the clinical differences between the two. Vasospastic coronary artery disease is one of the possibilities.[68] This other factor must be capable of causing sufficient ischemia to explain acute myocardial infarction in the absence of total vascular occlusion as well as spontaneous episodes of brief or prolonged anginal pain without evidence of detectable myocardial necrosis by traditional laboratory tests.

The current therapeutic approach to patients with unstable angina pectoris is oversimplified for two reasons: 1) our lack of understanding of the pathophysiologic mechanisms in any particular instance, and 2) our lack of specific pharmacologic therapy. The tendency has been to approach the problem on the basis of the supply/demand relationship for myocardial oxygen utilization. Historically and currently, the attack centers on the demand side of the equation. More recent revelations,[43] and future approaches to unstable angina pectoris, particularly forms of spontaneous pain, will likely concentrate more on the supply side of the equation. There should be an attempt to explain and treat the nonatherosclerotic factors involved in the generation of unprovoked myocardial ischemic pain. This may be similar to the factors evoked in the explanation of acute myocardial infarction in the presence of normal coronary arteriograms.[69]

New concepts involving the production, extent, and endogenous control of pain have opened newer challenges to the explanation and treatment of discomfort.[70] Very little is known about the psychologic factors involved in myocardial ischemic pain, but placebo relief has long been appreciated.[71]

Until a more comprehensive understanding of pathophysiologic events is forthcoming, the current management presented here is empirically and practically reasonable. In the short term, the question is not: which of the therapeutic alternatives should be chosen? It is, more rationally: what is the most appropriate temporal sequence of therapeutic intervention in each of the subgroups of unstable angina pectoris?

The author wishes to thank Mrs. Lucy Rapp and Miss Heather Hurst for their careful typing of the manuscript and Drs. Goldman and A. Adelman for their editorial comments and suggestions.

REFERENCES

1. Scheidt, S., Wolk, M., and Killip, T. Unstable angina pectoris: natural history, hemodynamics, uncertainties of treatment and the ethics of clinical study. *Am J Med.* 60:409–417, 1976.

2. Unstable Angina Pectoris: National Co-Operative Study Group to compare medical and surgical therapy. *Am J Cardiol.* 42:839–848, 1978.

3. Heberden, W. Some account of a disorder of the breast. *J R Coll Physicians Lond.* 2:59, 1772.

4. Herrick, J.B. Clinical features of sudden obstruction of the coronary arteries. *JAMA.* 59:2015–2021, 1912.

5. Sampson, J.J., and Eliaser, M. Jr. The diagnosis of impending acute coronary artery occlusion. *Am Heart J.* 13:675–686, 1937.

6. Feil, H. Preliminary pain in coronary thrombosis. *Am J Med Sci.* 193:42–48, 1937.

7. Osler, W. Angina pectoris. *Lancet* 1:839–844, 1910.

8. Reeves, T.J., and Harrison, T.R. Cardiac pain. *J Chronic Dis.* 4:340–349, 1956.

9. Blumgart, H.L., Schlesinger, M.J., and Zoll, P.M. Angina pectoris, coronary failure and acute myocardial infarction. The role of coronary occlusions and collateral circulation. *JAMA.* 116:91–97, 1941.

10. Graybiel, A. The intermediate coronary syndrome. *US Armed Forces Med J.* 6:1, 1955.

11. Master, A.M., Jaffe, H.L., Field, L.E. et al. Acute coronary insufficiency: its differential diagnosis and treatment. *Ann Intern Med.* 45:561–581, 1957.

12. Fowler, N.O. Pre-infarctional angina. *Circulation* 44:755–758, 1971.

13. Waitzkin, L. Impending myocardial infarction. *Ann Intern Med.* 21:421–430, 1944.

14. Papp, C., and Smith, S. Status anginosus. *Br Heart J.* 22:259–273, 1960.

15. Scanlon, P.J., Nemickas, R., Moran, J.F. et al. Accelerated angina pectoris. Clinical, hemodynamic, arteriographic and therapeutic experience in 85 patients. *Circulation* 47:19–26, 1973.

16. Riseman, J.E.F., Altman, G.E., and Koretsky, S. Nitroglycerin and other nitrates in the treatment of angina pectoris. *Circulation* 17:22–39, 1958.

17. Levy, R.L., and Bruenn, M.G. Acute fatal coronary insufficiency. *JAMA.* 106:1080–1085, 1936.

18. Chahine, R.A. Unstable angina. The problem of definition. *Br Heart J.* 37:1246–1249, 1975.

19. Hochberg, H.M. Characteristics & significance of prodromes of coronary care unit patients. *Chest* 59:10–14, 1971.

20. Solomon, H.A., Edwards, A.L., and Killip, T. Prodromata in acute myocardial infarction. *Circulation* 50:463–471, 1969.

21. Wood, P. Acute & subacute coronary insufficiency. *Br Med J.* 1:1179–1182, 1961.

22. Mounsey, R. Prodromal symptoms in myocardial infarction. *Br Heart J.* 13:215–226, 1951.

23. Beamish, R.E., and Storrie, V.M. Impending myocardial infarction: recognition and management. *Circulation* 21:1107–1115, 1960.

24. Vakil, R.J. Intermediate coronary syndrome. *Circulation* 24:557–5571, 1961.

25. Gazes, P.C., Mobley, E.M., Faris, H.M. et al. Preinfarction (unstable) angina—a prospective study—10 year follow-up. *Circulation* 48:131–337, 1973.

26. Kraus, K.R., Hutter, A., and Desanctis, R.W. Acute coronary insufficiency. *Arch Intern Med.* 129:808–813, 1972.

27. Heng, M.K., Norris, R.M., Singh, B.N. et al. Prognosis in unstable angina. *Br Heart J.* 38:921–925, 1976.

28. Cairns, J.A., Fantus, I.G., and Klassen, G.A. Unstable angina pectoris. *Am Heart J.* 92:373–386, 1976.

29. Duncan, B., Fulton, M., Morrison, S.L. et al. Prognosis of new and worsening angina pectoris. *Br Med J.* 1:981–985, 1976.

30. Levy, H. The natural history of changing patterns of angina pectoris. *Ann Intern Med.* 44:1123–1135, 1956.

31. Fulton, M., Lutz, W., Donald, K.W. et al. Natural history of unstable angina. *Lancet* 1:860–865, 1972.

32. Fischl, S., Herman, M.V., and Gorlin, R. The intermediate coronary syndrome: clinical, angiographic and therapeutic aspects. *N Engl J Med.* 288:1193–1199, 1973.

33. Littmann, D., and Barr, J.H. Acute atypical coronary artery insufficiency. *Circulation* 5:189–200, 1952.

34. Armstrong, P.W., Chiong, M.A., and Parker, J.O. The spectrum of unstable angina. *Ann R Coll Phys Surg Can.* 12:28, 1979.

35. Bertolasi, C.A., Tronge, J.E., Carreno, C.A. et al. Unstable angina — prospective and randomized study of its evolution, with and without surgery. *Am J Cardiol.* 33:201–208, 1974.

36. Wiles, J.C., Peduzzi, P.N., Hammond, G.L. et al. Preoperative predictors of operative mortality for coronary bypass grafting in patients with unstable angina pectoris. *Am J Cardiol.* 39:939–943, 1977.

37. Weisel, R.D., Goldman, B.S., Teasdale, S. et al. Surgery for unstable angina and impending infarction. *Ann R Coll Phys Surg.* 12:28, 1979.

38. Brunton, T.L. On the use of nitrate of amyl in angina pectoris. *Lancet* 2:97, 1867.

39. Roughgarden, J.W. Circulatory changes during the pain of angina pectoris. *Am J Med.* 41:935–946, 1966.

40. Roughgarden, J.W., and Newman, E.V. Circulatory changes associated with spontaneous angina pectoris. *Am J Med.* 41:947–961, 1966.

41. Guazzi, M., Polese, A., Fiorentini, C. et al. Left ventricular performance and related hemodynamic changes in Prinzmetal's variant angina pectoris. *Br Heart J.* 33:84–94, 1971.

42. Guazzi, M., Magrini, F., Fiorentini, C. et al. Clinical, electrocardiographic, and hemodynamic effects of long term use of propranolol in Prinzmetal's variant angina pectoris. *Br Heart J.* 33:889–894, 1971.

43. Cannon, D.S., Harrison, D.C., and Schroeder, J.S. Hemodynamic observations in patients with unstable angina pectoris. *Am J cardiol.* 33:17–22, 1974.

44. Maseri, A., Severi, S., De Nes, M. et al. "Variant" angina: one aspect of a continuous spectrum of vasospastic myocardial ischemia. *Am J Cardiol.* 42:1019–1035, 1978.

45. Figueras, J., Singh, B.N., Ganz, W. et al. Mechanism of rest and nocturnal angina: observations during continuous hemodynamic and electrocardiographic monitoring. *Circulation* 59:955–968, 1979.

46. Sonnenblick, E.H., and Skelton, C.L. Myocardial energetics: basic principles and clinical implications. *N Engl J Med.* 285:668–675, 1971.

47. Herman, M.V., Cohn, P.F., and Gorlin, R. Angina-like chest pain without identifiable cause. *Ann Intern Med.* 79:445–447, 1973.

48. Kerber, R.E., and Marcus, M.L. Evaluation of regional myocardial function in ischemic heart disease by echocardiography. *Prog Cardiovasc Dis.* 20:441–450, 1978.

49. Joffe, C.D., Brik, H., Teichholz, L.E. et al. Echocardiographic diagnosis of left anterior descending coronary artery disease. *Am J Cardiol.* 40:16, 1977.

50. Corya, B.C., Rasmussen, S., Feigenbaum, H. et al. Systolic thickening & thinning of the septum and posterior wall in patients with coronary artery disease, congestive cardiomyopathy and atrial septal defect. *Circulation* 55:109–114, 1977.

51. Fogelman, A.M., Abbasi, A.S., Pearse, M.L. et al. Echocardiographic study of abnormal motion of the posterior left ventricular wall during angina pectoris. *Circulation* 46:905–913, 1972.

124

52. Arnett, E.N., Weiss, J.L., Garrison, J.B. et al. Quantitative evaluation of regional left ventricular thickening in man by two dimensional echocardiography. (abstract) *Am J Cardiol*. 43:377, 1979.

53. Wackers, F., Lie, K.I., Liem, K.L. et al. Thallium 201 scintigraphy in unstable angina pectoris. *Circulation* 57:738–742, 1978.

54. Abdulla, A.M., Canedo, M.I., and Cortez, B.C. Detection of unstable angina by 99m technetium pyrophosphate myocardial scintigraphy. *Chest* 69:168–173, 1976.

55. Willerson, J.T., Parkey, R.W., Bonte, F.J. et al. Technetium stannous pyrophosphate myocardial scintigrams in patients with chest pain of varying etiology. *Circulation* 51:1046–1052, 1975.

56. Nichols, A.B., Pohost, G.H., Gold, H.K. et al. Left ventricular function during intraaortic balloon pumping assessed by multirated cardiac blood pool imaging. *Circulation* 58(suppl 1):176–183, 1978.

57. Donsky, M.S., Curry, C.C., Parkey, R.W. et al. Unstable angina pectoris: clinical, angiographic and myocardial scintigraphic observations. *Br Heart J*. 18:257–263, 1976.

58. Hill, J.D., Kerth, W.J., and Kelly, J.J. Emergency aortocoronary bypass for impending or extending myocardial infarction. *Circulation* 43(suppl 1):105, 1971.

59. Aronow, W.S. Management of stable angina. *N Engl J Med*. 289:516–520, 1973.

60. Thadani, U., Davidson, C., Chir, B. et al. Comparison of the immediate effects of five beta-adrenoceptor-blocking drugs with different ancillary properties in angina pectoris. *N Engl J Med*. 300:750–755, 1979.

61. Dauwe, F., Affaki, G., Waters, D.D. et al. Control of refractory and unstable angina with intravenous nitroglycerin. *Ann R Coll Phys Surg Can*. 12:28, 1979.

62. McIntosh, H.D., and Garcia, J.A. The first decade of aortocoronary bypass grafting — 1967–1977 — a review. *Circulation* 57:405–431, 1978.

63. Huret, J.F., Agier, B., Rosier, S.P. et al. Delayed semi-elective coronary bypass surgery for unstable angina pectoris. *J Thorac Cardiovasc Surg*. 75:476–482, 1978.

64. Selden, R., Neill, W.A., Ritzmann, L.W. et al. Medical versus surgical therapy for acute coronary insufficiency. *N Engl J Med*. 293:1329–1333, 1975.

65. Berndt, T.B., Miller, D.C., Silderman, J.F. et al. Coronary bypass surgery for unstable angina pectoris. *Am J Med*. 58:171–176, 1975.

66. Scully, H.E., Gunstensen, J., Williams, W.G. et al. Surgical management of complicated acute coronary insufficiency. *Surgery* 80:437–442, 1976.

67. Aroesty, J.M., Weintraub, R.M., Paulin, S. et al. Medically refractory unstable angina pectoris: 11 hemodynamic and angiographic effects of intra-aortic balloon counterpulsation. *Am J Cardiol*. 43:883–888, 1979.

68. Hillis, L.D., and Braunwald, E., Coronary artery spasm. *N Engl J Med*. 299:695–702, 1978.

69. Kahn, A.H., and Maywood, L.J. Myocardial infarction in nine patients with radiologically patent coronary arteries. *N Engl J Med*. 291:427–431, 1974.

70. Levine, J.D., Gordon, N.C., and Fields, H.L. The mechanism of placebo analgesia. *Lancet* 2:654–656, 1978.

71. Benson, H., and McCallie, D.P. Angina pectoris and the placebo effect. *N Engl J Med*. 300:1424–1429, 1979.

9 The Medical Treatment of Unstable Angina

Henry F. Mizgala, MD

The existence of clinical syndromes of intermediate severity between chronic stable angina and acute myocardial infarction has been recognized for many years. In the earlier literature, terms such as acute coronary insufficiency,[1] intermediate coronary syndrome,[2] preinfarction angina,[3] and impending myocardial infarction[4] were used to describe patients with ischemic chest pain of longer than usual duration accompanied by transient ST-T wave abnormalities on the electrocardiogram and no laboratory evidence of acute myocardial infarction. In later years, angina of recent onset[5] and progressive angina (crescendo angina)[6] were included in this broad category probably because it became quite clear that in a substantial proportion of patients dying suddenly or admitted to hospital with acute myocardial infarction, clinically recognizable prodromata were present during the few weeks preceding the acute event. The term unstable angina, advocated by Conti et al[7] is now used to include all such clinical syndromes.

DEFINITIONS

Because of the variability of symptoms in individual patients it is difficult to be precise in defining unstable angina. However, four broad categories are recognized.

Recent onset angina   Included in this category are previously asymptomatic patients in whom there has been onset of effort angina during the preceding 3 to 6 weeks.

Progressive angina includes patients with or without a previous history of stable angina in whom there has been a recent progression of symptoms. This may take the form of increasing severity and/or frequency of anginal attacks so that over a period of days or weeks, there is worsening of symptoms.

Prolonged chest pain is characterized by one or more attacks of ischemic chest pain at rest, lasting 15 to 30 minutes, accompanied by electrocardiographic changes limited to the ST-T segments and without enzymatic elevations diagnostic of myocardial infarction.

Postinfarction unstable angina   This category includes patients with transient recurrent typical ischemic pains at rest occurring within a few days to a few weeks following an acute myocardial infarction. The ischemic pains are spontaneous, unprovoked, and may be progressive.

For all categories of unstable angina, possible precipitating factors such as anemia, arrhythmia, hyperthyroidism, and congestive cardiac failure should be excluded. It has also been suggested that transient ST-T segment changes should be documented in all categories of unstable angina.

NATURAL HISTORY

Proper evaluation of a medical or surgical treatment presupposes knowledge of the natural history of the disease under consideration. Unfortunately, little is known of the natural history of unstable angina and the quoted incidence of subsequent acute myocardial infarction and mortality is extremely variable. Thus, in early studies of acute coronary insufficiency, impending myocardial infarction and preinfarction angina (prolonged chest pain), the incidence of myocardial infarction occurring within one to three months of onset was reported at 22%[1] to 80%[4] with mortality of 16% to 60%. A long-term study of unstable angina has been reported by Gazes et al[3] and has been quoted extensively in the literature on unstable angina. At three months, 20.7% of their 140 patients had sustained a myocardial infarction and 10% had died; 10% were dead at the end of one year, 39% at the end of five years, and 52% at 10 years. In a later study, Krauss et al[8] reported a 7% incidence of myocardial infarction and a 1% mortality within one month; at one year, there was a 20% incidence of acute myocardial infarction and a

15% mortality. While the first of these studies was prospective and the latter was retrospective, management as well as follow-up was unstructured, and treatment was not standardized in either. The extreme variability in the results is understandable. It can be explained by differences in terminology and methodology within the various protocols as well as by the extreme variability in the management of patients within individual studies. The data resulting from these reports, therefore, were more a reflection of current therapy than of the natural history of these syndromes.

RATIONALE OF EMERGENCY SURGERY

It is on the basis of such statistics and because of the widespread availability of selective coronary arteriography that the emergency surgical treatment of unstable angina became popular. The former implies a horrendous prognosis and the latter demonstrates very graphically the high-grade obstructive coronary artery lesions often found in patients with unstable angina. It was therefore quite logical to proceed to the next step and attempt direct coronary artery revascularization on an emergency basis. The rationale of emergency surgery was based on three logical but unproven hypotheses: 1) that unstable angina was followed by a high incidence of subsequent myocardial infarction and a high mortality; 2) that high-grade coronary artery lesions detected angiographically were "critical," the concept of "critical lesion" implying that the more stenotic the lesion, the more urgently it should be acted upon to prevent myocardial infarction or death, and 3) that emergency direct coronary artery revascularization would prevent myocardial infarction, preserve myocardium, and thus prolong life.

No proof exists at present in support of any of these hypotheses. The true natural outcome of unstable angina remains uncertain, and more recent studies have not confirmed the alarmingly high mortality and morbidity reported in the early studies. Visualization of high-grade proximal stenotic lesions in the coronary arteries naturally conjures up images of massive myocardial infarction and, thus, becomes an almost irresistible stimulus to early intervention. Is such a reflex justified? It certainly appears to be logical, but very little is known about the sequence of events triggering a myocardial infarction. Indeed, similar critical lesions are seen with equal frequency in stable angina, and there is evidence to suggest that the evolution of symptoms as seen in unstable angina may occur for reasons other than the sudden progression of obstructive coronary artery lesions.[9] It also appears logical that bypassing severe coronary artery lesions with vein grafts would prevent the impending infarction, preserve myocardium, and prevent death. Indeed, several early uncontrolled studies of emergency surgical treatment were very encouraging.[10,11] The reported incidence of early infarction and mortality was quite impressive when compared to results quoted in the early studies of medical management, and it rapidly became the practice in many centers to perform coronary angiography in patients with unstable angina soon after admission and proceed on an emergency basis to aortocoronary bypass surgery. However, not only did the logistics of such an approach soon become unmanageable, but as early experience accumulated, it became evident that the majority of patients could be rendered asymptomatic with adequate rest and medical treatment. Results of a recent controlled National Cooperative Study moreover confirmed that there was little to gain from an urgent approach, and that the in-hospital incidence of acute myocardial infarction and the early and late mortalities were not significantly different in the surgical and the medical groups.[12]

BETA-ADRENERGIC BLOCKADE

Early Reports

It has become almost universal practice to treat unstable angina with beta-adrenergic blockers. In North America, propranolol has been used almost exclusively because until recently it was the only beta-blocking agent generally available. Its introduction as a valid therapeutic measure for unstable angina was slow and cautious. There was, first of all, a general reluctance in principle to administer a drug with potent negative chronotropic and inotropic properties to patients with an unstable clinical state. Second, and more specifically, there was widespread concern that the myocardial depressant effect of propranolol would have an adverse influence on the outcome of myocardial infarction in patients receiving therapeutic doses of propranolol.

Earliest reports on the use of propranolol in unstable angina concerned small series of patients with the syndrome of acute coronary insufficiency (type 3 in our classification) who in spite of bedrest, sedation, and nitrates continued to have ischemic pain at rest. In one report,[13] propranolol was given to 15 hospitalized patients whose rest pain had persisted for an average period of 14 days in spite of conventional treatment. Propranolol was administered orally in increasing doses until symptoms subsided, or to a total daily dose of 400 mg/day. After a 16-month follow-up, the only acute event was sudden death in one patient. In another report, six of seven patients with refractory acute coronary insufficiency became asymptomatic after 60 to 80 mg/day of propranolol, and the seventh patient responded to a daily dose of 160 mg/day.[14] Later studies confirmed the safety and efficacy of propranolol in unstable angina. Thus, Fischl[15] reported control of symptoms at rest in 17 of 20 patients with refractory

"intermediate coronary syndrome" within 24 hours of initiating propranolol therapy. Recurrent pain in seven of these patients responded to an
increased dose.[15] Similarly, Conti reported ten patients with acute coronary
insufficiency treated with propranolol for a period of ten months at a mean
dose of 160 mg/day. One suffered a fatal myocardial infarction in the
hospital, and another had an uncomplicated myocardial infarction.[7] These
studies, therefore, indicated that propranolol rather consistently relieved
recurrent ischemic rest pain. Though the series were small, they also tended
to suggest that the subsequent incidence of myocardial infarction and death
was not as high as suggested in earlier reports.

Controlled Studies

Very few prospective controlled studies of propranolol in unstable
angina have been reported. Yet, propranolol is used very extensively in the
treatment of the various forms of this disorder. For this reason and as a
rational explanation for the treatment we advocate, two studies are outlined in some detail. In the first study,[16] 72 patients with unstable angina
were randomized in a double-blind fashion for treatment with propranolol
and placebo and followed prospectively for an average period of 19
months. Three patients on placebo and one receiving propranolol were
refractory to medical treatment and underwent early aortocoronary bypass
surgery. Of the remaining 68, there were 21 patients with recent onset or
recently progressive angina (group A), 23 patients with prolonged chest
pain and no infarction (group C) and 24 patients with postinfarction
unstable angina (group M). Propranolol was given in oral doses ranging
from 80 to 480 mg/day. Mean daily dose was 420 mg. Patients also received
digitalis or diuretics, or both, when indicated. Over a subsequent follow-up
period in the 33 patients allocated to placebo, eight were readmitted with
recurrent unstable angina, four sustained acute myocardial infarction, and
two died. However, in the 35 patients in the propranolol group, four had
recurrent unstable angina, one sustained myocardial infarction, and there
were no deaths (Table 9-1). The difference in the total acute events in the
two treatment groups was statistically significant in favor of propranolol
($p < 0.05$). A valid criticism of this study was the small proportion of patients (18%) who underwent coronary angiography. However, at the time
the study was carried out, it was not considered appropriate and ethically
acceptable to perform coronary angiography unless it was for the purpose
of proceeding with surgical treatment in suitable cases. Nevertheless, the
study did confirm that propranolol could safely be administered to patients
with unstable angina, that it was of immediate symptomatic benefit, and
that it appeared to reduce the subsequent incidence of acute coronary
events.

Table 9-1
Comparative Incidence of Acute Coronary Events Following Onset
of Unstable Angina in Patients Receiving Propranolol and Placebo,
(Follow-up, 19 months)

	Propranolol (n = 35)	Placebo (n = 33)
Recurrent unstable angina	4	8
Acute myocardial infarction	1	4
Death	0	2
	5	14
	$p < 0.05$	

A later study was carried out to compare the short-term results of therapy with propranolol and perhexiline maleate to a control group receiving sublingual isosorbide dinitrate alone. This study was also to determine the efficiency of these agents in preventing recurrent unstable angina, myocardial infarction, and death during an initial follow-up period of three months.[7] Criteria for the diagnosis of unstable angina were identical to those in the previous study. All patients were admitted to the hospital and treated in the coronary care unit. Concurrent medical treatment included sublingual nitroglycerin or, if necessary, intravenous morphine for chest pain as well as mild sedation, digitalis, and diuretics when necessary. A total of 61 patients were randomly allocated to treatment with propranolol in doses of 80 to 400 mg/day (21 patients), perhexiline maleate 400 to 600 mg/day (19 patients), and sublingual isosorbide dinitrate in doses of 5 mg every six hours (21 patients). All patients were reevaluated 72 hours after initiating treatment. Patients who responded to treatment with a total disappearance of their ischemic pain were continued on the same treatment. Patients with persisting or recurrent ischemic pain were crossed over to propranolol treatment if they had previously been in the perhexiline or the control group. If symptoms persisted after another 48 hours, coronary angiography was performed and followed by aortocoronary bypass surgery when feasible. Patients who responded to drug therapy continued on the same medication throughout their hospitalization and were followed at regular intervals as outpatients during the following three months. At 12 to 14 weeks after discharge, patients were readmitted for coronary angiography and left ventriculography was obtained in 48 of the 61 patients (77%). Of the 61 patients entered into the study, six were excluded from analysis because subsequent angiography revealed normal coronary arteries. Results were therefore analyzed in 55 patients. In Figure 9-1, the symptomatic response 72 hours after beginning treatment is compared in the three groups. In the propranolol-treated group, 19 of 20 patients (95%)

experienced complete relief of myocardial ischemic pain, compared to nineof 15 patients (60%) in the perhexiline-treated group and 10 of 20 (50%) in the control group. The difference in immediate response between the propranolol group and each of the other two groups was statistically significant—$p < 0.05$ compared to the perhexiline group and $p < 0.005$ compared to the control. Acute myocardial infarction or other serious complications occurred in no patients during this early phase.

Following the initial 72 hours, the 16 nonresponders in the control group and perhexiline groups were crossed over to the propranolol group. Fourteen of these 16 patients became asymptomatic. The remaining two patients as well as the one patient from the original propranolol group who remained symptomatic after the initial phase of treatment underwent early coronary angiography and aortocoronary bypass surgery.

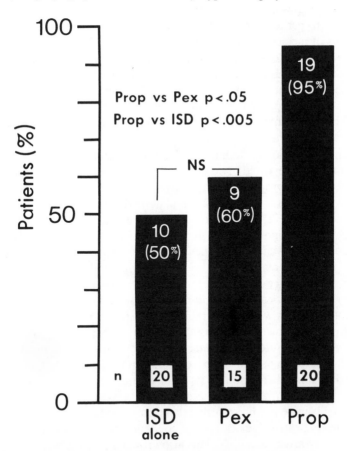

Figure 9-1 Comparison of the early response to treatment with isosorbide dinitrate (ISD), prehexiline maleate (Pex), and propranolol (Prop) in patients with unstable angina (% of patients becoming asymptomatic within 72 hours).

Thus, 52 medically treated patients began the latter phase of treatment, 33 receiving propranolol in mean daily doses of 220 mg (80 to 400 mg/day), nine perhexiline maleate in daily doses of 400 to 600 mg, and 10 controls who continued receiving isosorbide dinitrate 5 mg sublingually every six hours. The acute events in each of the three treatment groups during the subsequent 12-week follow-up are illustrated in Figure 9-2. In the control group, five of 10 patients (50%) developed recurrent unstable angina. In the nine patients at risk in the perhexiline group, four acute myocardial infarctions and one episode of recurrent unstable angina occurred, a rate of total coronary events similar to the control group. However, in the propranolol group, only one myocardial infarction and one episode of recurrent unstable angina occurred in the 33 patients receiving this drug. Thus, the 6% frequency of coronary events in the propranolol group was significantly lower than in either the control group ($p < 0.025$) or the perhexiline group ($p < 0.01$). It should also be noted that after 12 weeks of medical treatment, 14 of 52 patients (27%) had resumed their usual activities and were considered to be in New York Heart Association functional class I or II. Because of unmanageable symptoms or the presence of left main stem disease, 17 of 52 patients (33%) underwent late aortocoronary bypass surgery with no mortality. The 21 remaining patients (40%) continued medical treatment, of whom nine (17%) were considered technically inoperable.

The angiographic findings of the patients entered in this study were similar to those reported in other studies of unstable angina and were comparable to angiographic findings in patients with other coronary artery disease syndromes.[7-15] Thus, 12% had normal coronary arteries, 19% had one-vessel disease, 27% had two-vessel disease, and three-vessel disease was present in 44%. Significant left main stem lesions were present in 12%, and 50% had normal ventricular function. Careful analysis of the angiographic data in these patients also revealed the following findings. The incidence of significant coronary obstructive lesions in one, two or three vessels, and the incidence of significant left main stem disease and of ventricular contraction abnormalities were comparable in the three treatment groups, as well as in the three categories of unstable angina. No significant angiographic differences were noted in patients who responded to initial medical treatment compared to patients who were nonresponders. Similarly, there were no angiographic differences in patients with or without subsequent acute events. In addition, during the ensuing 12 to 14 weeks of medical treatment acute events were not necessarily related to the extent and severity of coronary artery obstructive disease and could not be predicted on the basis of the coronary artery anatomy. This also included patients who were subsequently found to have significant left main stem lesions at angiography done 12 to 14 weeks after the onset of unstable angina.

Several comments are appropriate. Symptoms of unstable angina sub-side in 50% of patients within 72 hours of admission to the coronary care unit with sublingual nitrates alone. The addition of propranolol in ade-quate doses is not only safe but provides rapid symptomatic relief to a ma-jority of such patients and, in the short term at least, appears to reduce the subsequent incidence of acute coronary events. The coronary anatomy in patients with unstable angina is identical to that found in patients with other coronary syndromes, and no specific pattern of obstructive lesions appears to be predictive of subsequent events. It is also of interest that while there is a general urgency to perform early coronary angiography, the course of patients in the second study did not appear to be adversely in-fluenced by postponing this procedure to a later date. Indeed, at 12 weeks after onset, 27% of these patients were virtually asymptomatic and able to resume their usual activities.

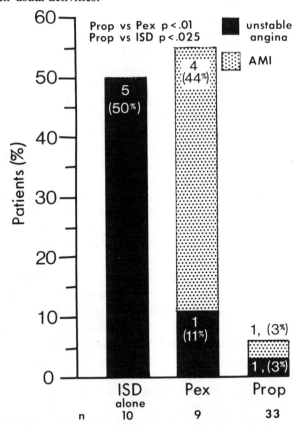

Figure 9-2 Comparison of the incidence of acute coronary events during medical treatment with isosorbide dinitrate (ISD), prehexiline maleate (Pex), and pro-pranolol (Prop) during the 12 weeks following onset of unstable angina.

THERAPEUTIC APPROACH

Principles of Therapy

Medical and surgical treatment in unstable angina should not be considered mutually exclusive, but rather as complementary during the course of what is usually a long-standing disease with exacerbations and remissions. The ultimate aim of treatment must remain the patient's return to a full and productive life, while at the same time initiating and continuing a lifelong program of secondary prevention. Based on the results of the above studies, our approach to the treatment of unstable angina is one of early optimal medical treatment. Unstable angina is an acute coronary event requiring admission to the hospital, preferably in a coronary care unit. Initial medical treatment should be prompt and vigorous with administration of oral and sublingual nitrates and adequate doses of beta-adrenergic blocking drugs. Unstable angina need not be a surgical emergency. Since a significant proportion of patients with unstable angina are found to have either normal coronary arteries or significant left main stem disease, it is our belief that all patients should at some time undergo selective coronary angiography, which provides the physician with valuable information in his ultimate decision to continue medical treatment or recommend surgery. Whatever mode of treatment is chosen, adequate follow-up must be provided, particularly during the first year, to ensure compliance with medical treatment and with the principles of secondary prevention.

Current approaches to the management of unstable angina are outlined in Figure 9-3. While unstable angina is still considered a surgical emergency by some, the practice of initiating early vigorous medical treatment to calm the unstable state and control recurrent ischemic chest pain is rapidly gaining acceptance in most centers. Following successful initial medical treatment for 5 to 10 days, there are, we believe, two options: coronary angiography followed by aortocoronary bypass surgery when technically feasible, or continued medical therapy with angiography postponed to a later date. The choice of options is guided by one's current thinking on the potential long-term benefits of aortocoronary bypass surgery and its effect on the prevention of subsequent myocardial infarction and death.

At present, these issues remain unsettled and controversial in spite of controlled studies done on the subject. Thus, if one believes in the long-term prophylactic value of aortocoronary bypass surgery and if significant obstructive coronary artery lesions are visualized at angiography done immediately after the acute phase, a logical option emerges and surgery is performed prior to discharge from the hospital. One obvious advantage to this option is that a final and ultimate solution can be proposed and executed during the patient's first hospital admission. If, on the other hand, one's philosophy is to consider aortocoronary bypass surgery as merely of symptomatic benefit and having no influence on ultimate prognosis, medical treatment can be continued during the remainder of the hospitalization as well as during convalescence provided that instability does not recur and the patient remains asymptomatic. We personally favor this more conservative approach for several reasons. It is virtually impossible to predict at five to ten days after admission a patient's eventual symptomatic status at three months. Moreover, early angiography usually demonstrates very graphically the presence of significant and sometimes severe lesions, which, of themselves, are an irresistible stimulus to immediate intervention. Our previous studies have shown that there is no increased risk in postponing coronary angiography since the incidence of acute coronary events during the convalescent phase does not exceed the incidence of perioperative infarction and mortality. Also, at three months, nearly 30% of our patients with unstable angina are virtually asymptomatic. Based on the premise that bypass surgery should only be done in symptomatic patients or in individuals with significant left main stem lesions, our tendency is to postpone coronary angiography to 12 to 14 weeks after the onset of unstable angina. At this time, patients are readmitted to the hospital for three to four days and assessed on the basis of symptoms, performance on a treadmill test, and results of coronary angiography. However, if at any time after the first admission symptoms become unmanageable, or there is a recurrence of unstable angina, coronary angiography is carried out and followed by surgical treatment.

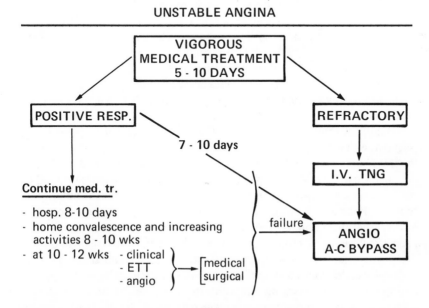

Figure 9-3 Schematic representation of current management of unstable angina.

Acute Phase

Unstable angina should be treated as an acute coronary event. Patients are admitted to a coronary care unit for complete rest and electrocardiographic monitoring. Twelve-lead electrocardiograms should be recorded during chest pain to document transient electrical changes. Patients remain in the hospital for a total of 15 to 20 days and should be told at the outset that they are not expected to return to work for a period of 12 to 14 weeks. Attacks of chest pain are treated with sublingual nitroglycerin or longer acting nitrates such as sublingual isosorbide dinitrate in doses of 5 mg every two to four hours. Nitrates in the form of oral isosorbide dinitrate in doses of 15 to 60 mg every six hours may also be added, as well as nitroglycerin ointment applied topically every four to six hours. Unless there are contraindications, treatment with beta-adrenergic blockers is begun immediately after admission. While several new beta-blockers are now available, we know of no studies confirming their efficacy in unstable angina. For this reason we still favor propranolol although we have utilized metoprolol in a number of patients with unstable angina with good results. Propranolol is begun in initial doses of 20 mg orally and increased progressively in increments of 20 mg six-hourly to a total daily dose necessary to ensure a pulse rate consistently under 60 beats/min, until symptoms subside or to a total dose of 480 mg/day. Intravenous heparin is utilized during the first few days while patients remain on bedrest to prevent thromboembolic complications. Patients with cardiac enlargement or clinical evidence of left ventricular failure are given digitalis and, if necessary, diuretics. Mild sedation is employed as necessary. Possible precipitating factors such as undiscovered anemia, cardiac arrhythmias, congestive heart failure, and, in rare cases, hyperthyroidism should be sought early and corrected. Similarly, risk factors should be identified within the first few days and corrective measures instituted. Thus, appropriate support and motivation for tobacco withdrawal should be provided, systemic hypertension treated, and hyperlipidemia identified, classified, and managed in the appropriate way.

The vast majority of patients with unstable angina respond to this regimen, and within three to five days become asymptomatic. Activities are then gradually increased during the next few days so that by day 12 to 20, patients are up and about, have climbed stairs under supervision, and are ready to be discharged home for continued convalescence if still asymptomatic. Prior to discharge, patients should be advised about continued medical treatment and risk factor correction. The type of medication given, proper dosage, and the appropriate use of sublingual nitroglycerin must be carefully explained. As well, patients should be given adequate guidance with respect to continued gradual increase in their daily activities. The importance of early warning symptoms must be stressed, and they must be advised to report to the emergency department in the event of recurrent chest pain.

The Convalescent and Chronic Phase

After hospital discharge, follow-up is of the utmost importance and should be systematic and structured. This ensures compliance with medical treatment, permits the adjustment of dosages, and provides the necessary support and guidance in the control of risk factors. Patients should be seen frequently during the first few months. It is our practice to set appointments two weeks after hospital discharge, then at four, eight, and twelve weeks. At each visit, the anginal status should be evaluated, patients should be examined, and a 12-lead electrocardiogram recorded. Advice as to physical activities can be given and questions answered.

At 12 to 14 weeks after discharge, patients are electively readmitted to the hospital for three days for a complete assessment including evaluation of symptoms, objective assessment of exercise tolerance, and coronary angiography. Patients who in spite of medical treatment continue to have symptoms precluding a return to their former activities, whose exercise tolerance tests reveal marked ST-segment depression at a low level of activity, and whose coronary arteriograms reveal multiple high-grade obstructive lesions, are offered surgical treatment. Surgery is also proposed whenever significant left main stem disease is discovered. On the other hand, patients who have become virtually asymptomatic or whose anginal attacks occur only with unusual exertion, and whose exercise tolerance tests confirm an acceptable exercise capacity, can be permitted to continue on medical treatment. The decision in regard to ultimate treatment for patients falling between these two extremes is made on an individual basis and the following factors should be considered: age, occupation, degree of adaptability to a life-style of reduced activity, number of coronary arteries involved, and ventricular function. In terms of the patient's ability to adapt to disease, it is interesting to note how widely this can vary. At one extreme one sees patients with minimal symptoms and good exercise tolerance on the treadmill who cannot bear the thought of any disability necessitating the use of medication. At the other extreme there are patients who in spite of a low treadmill tolerance nevertheless are able to carry on with their everyday activities with a minimal number of daily anginal attacks. Such individuals have learned to adapt to a slower pace without having to give up any essential activities.

The decision to continue medical therapy does not preclude eventual surgical treatment should this become necessary. Patients on long-term medical treatment must be followed at intervals of three to six months or oftener if necessary. Biyearly treadmill tests are a useful and objective guide to a patient's anginal threshold and functional capacity. Any significant decrease of this parameter or sudden worsening of the anginal status should alert the physician to a possible progression of the underlying disease or to the occurrence of other precipitating factors or circumstances that are temporary or correctable. When the severity of the anginal syndrome is such that it interferes with a patient's usual life-style, surgical treatment should be reconsidered and, if technically possible, carried out.

Intolerance to nitrates manifests itself early in the form of headaches and can be overcome by increasing the doses gradually. Propranolol is generally well tolerated. The most frequent side effects, usually noted early during therapy, consist of cold extremities, fatigue, and mild gastrointestinal disturbances, which rarely necessitate discontinuing the drug. In most instances these adverse effects disappear after the first few weeks of treatment. Rarely, we have encountered patients in whom propranolol has had to be discontinued because of adverse effects. Substitution with other beta-blockers such as metoprolol or timolol was achieved with no untoward incidents. Because of the negative inotropic effect of beta-adrenergic drugs, patients with preexisting impairment of left ventricular function should be monitored carefully for signs of congestive cardiac failure. The same precautions should be applied to patients with preexisting cardiac enlargement. Indeed, in some patients receiving chronic oral therapy, the first sign of cardiac decompensation may be the occurrence of nocturnal or early morning angina. Careful clinical examination usually reveals signs of fluid retention. Administration of a daily diuretic and, if necessary, digitalis is effective in eliminating such symptoms without the necessity of discontinuing the beta-adrenergic blocker.

There are no data available to indicate how long optimal medical treatment should be continued, and our approach has been empirical. In general, however, it has been our experience that after the initial period of unstable angina has been controlled, longer-term maintenance can be achieved with lower doses of both nitrates and propranolol. It is our practice to discharge patients with doses necessary to achieve symptomatic control. In patients initially requiring very high doses of nitrates and propranolol, the dose may sometimes be reduced at subsequent follow-up visits if patients remain symptom-free. Otherwise, full treatment is continued at least until readmission at 12 to 14 weeks. At this time, oral nitrates are first reduced or discontinued over a period of 7 to 10 days in patients who are asymptomatic or have minimal symptoms. Also (and particularly in patients receiving doses of propranolol in excess of 400 mg/day), this drug is gradually reduced to levels that will ensure a resting heart rate of more than 60 beats/min. While in most patients long-acting nitrates can be discontinued completely, we have empirically continued beta-adrenergic blockers even in asymptomatic patients for a period of a year. The beta-blocker is then gradually discontinued over a period of ten days. In symptomatic patients, treatment with beta-blockers and, if necessary, long-acting nitrates is continued as long as patients have effort angina.

Medically Refractory Patients

If at anytime during initial medical therapy "breakthrough rest angina" recurs, and the patient remains clinically unstable in spite of optimal medical therapy, immediate angiography has been recommended, followed, when appropriate, with bypass surgery. This was our practice until recently. However, carrying out these procedures at a time when the patient remains in an unstable clinical state in spite of full therapy was of some concern. Other than the problems associated with scheduling emergency bypass procedures, the incidence of complications of emergency angiography during the unstable phase is higher and there is evidence to indicate that the complications of aortocoronary bypass surgery are less frequent when the procedure can be carried out in stable patients.[12] While the use of intraaortic balloon pumping has been widely advocated to treat such refractory patients and as a protective measure during coronary angiography, it is not without its hazards.[18]

It must also be stressed that few patients with unstable angina are refractory when medical treatment is adequate. In our experience, the incidence has been on the order of 10%. When encountered, it is now our practice to treat these patients with intravenous nitroglycerin. We have found this to be a safe, effective, and well-tolerated form of treatment.[19] Rest angina is greatly reduced or completely suppressed. In an initial series of 14 patients so treated, of which 12 were hemodynamically monitored throughout treatment, intravenous nitroglycerin was infused for three to six days with virtual suppression of anginal attacks (Figure 9-4), thus stabilizing the patient's clinical status and permitting sufficient time to schedule angiography and surgery on a nonurgent basis. In our initial study, nitroglycerin was infused at a rate of 10 to 180 μg/min with a mean dose of 47 μg/min. Four of the 14 patients complained of dose-related transient headaches, but there were no other adverse effects. During treatment, there were no prolonged bouts of chest pain, no serious arrhythmias, and no myocardial infarction. The infusion was continued during coronary angiography, and there were no complications during this procedure. If chest pain recurred during angiography it was rapidly relieved by additional 100 to 300 μg bolus injections of intravenous nitroglycerin. Of the initial 14 patients so treated, 12 underwent subsequent aortocoronary bypass procedures on an nonurgent basis. The remaining two patients were found to be inoperable, and it is of interest to note that over the next six days both were weaned off intravenous nitroglycerin onto continued medical treatment with no untoward effects. Hemodynamic parameters were measured during infusion at 6, 12, 18, 24, and 48 hours. While there was an overall slight increase in heart rate, pulmonary capillary wedge pressure, systemic arterial pressure, cardiac index, and pressure rate product decreased slightly. These changes were minimal and not statistically significant. We have since employed this mode of treatment in 50 additional patients without hemodynamic monitoring with similarly satisfactory results.

Intravenous nitroglycerin is prepared in the hospital pharmacy in 15-ml vials containing 15 mg of nitroglycerin. A solution containing 30 mg of nitroglycerin (two vials) is added to 470 ml of 5% glucose and water. The

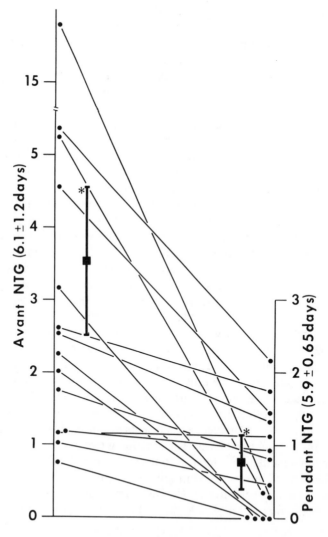

Figure 9-4 Mean daily episodes of rest angina before and during treatment with intravenous nitroglycerin in 14 consecutive patients.

infusion is begun at a rate of 5 μg/min and increased in increments of 5 to 10μg every hour until anginal pains subside or headache develops. With each increase in dose, vital signs are carefully monitored particularly during the first 30 minutes after the rate of infusion has been increased. The infusion is continued during coronary angiography as well as during the interval between this procedure and bypass surgery.

The use of intravenous nitroglycerin is easy, inexpensive, safe, well-tolerated, and effective in totally abolishing or significantly diminishing medically refractory rest angina. It obviates the necessity of proceeding with emergency coronary angiography and, in our experience, makes this procedure safer. It also permits bypass surgery to be performed on a nonurgent basis.

SUMMARY AND CONCLUSIONS

While the various syndromes of unstable angina alert the physician to the possibility of subsequent acute coronary events, its modern medical therapy has not been associated with the high incidence of acute myocardial infarction and death reported in earlier studies. With early optimal medical management, the majority of patients rapidly become asymptomatic. There is, therefore, no need to consider unstable angina as a surgical emergency.

Since 10% of patients with unstable angina will be found to have normal coronary arteries and another 10% will have significant left main stem lesions, selective coronary angiography should be performed in all patients. In the small proportion of patients refractory to initial medical treatment, this procedure should be carried out after symptoms have been suppressed with a continuous infusion of intravenous nitroglycerin. In patients who have responded to initial medical treatment, the timing of coronary angiography and the subsequent decision to continue medical treatment or to proceed with aortocoronary bypass surgery will depend on one's present bias as to the prophylactic value of this procedure. Firm believers in its ability to reduce subsequent acute coronary events will proceed with immediate surgery if operable lesions are found. However, if bypass surgery is considered of symptomatic benefit alone, it is justifiable to continue medical treatment for a further 3 to 4 months at which time about 30% of patients will be relatively asymptomatic. During this convalescent phase, lifelong measures of secondary prevention are instituted, activities are gradually increased and medical treatment is supervised. At 12 to 14 weeks after onset of unstable angina, patients can be readmitted to the hospital for a complete assessment, which includes symptomatic status, performance on an exercise tolerance test, and coronary arteriography. Based on the results of this assessment, a decision can then be made as to whether the patient should continue medical treatment or be referred for bypass surgery.

REFERENCES

1. Wood, P. Acute and subacute coronary insufficiency. *Br Med J.* 1:1779–1784, 1961.

2. Vakil, R.J. Intermediate coronary syndrome. *Circulation* 24:557–571, 1961.

3. Gazes, P.C., Mobley, E.M., Jr., Fares, H.M., Jr. et al. Preinfarctional (unstable) angina — a prospective study — ten year follow-up. Prognostic significance of electrocardiographic changes. *Circulation* 48:331–337, 1973.

4. Beamish, R.E. and Storrie, V.M. Impending myocardial infarction. Recognition and management. *Circulation* 21:1107–1115, 1960.

5. Fulton, M., Lutz, W., Donald, K.W. et al. Natural history of unstable angina. *Lancet* 1:860–865, 1972.

6. Fowler, N.O. Angina pectoris: Clinical diagnosis. *Circulation* 46:1079–1097, 1972.

7. Conti, C.R., Brawley, R.K., Griffith, L.S.C. et al. Unstable angina pectoris: morbidity and mortality in 57 consecutive patients evaluated angiographically. *Am J Cardiol.* 32:745–750, 1973.

8. Krauss, K.R., Hutter, A.M., Jr., De Sanctis, R.W. Acute coronary insufficiency: course and follow-up. *Circulation* 45(suppl):66–71, 1971.

9. Rafflenbeul, W., Smith, L.R., Rogers, W.J. et al. Quantitative coronary arteriography: coronary anatomy of patients with unstable angina pectoris reexamined 1 year after optimal medical therapy. *Am J Cardiol.* 43:699–707, 1979.

10. Favaloro, R.G., Effler, D.B., Cheanvechai, C. et al. Acute coronary insufficiency (impending myocardial infarction and myocardial infarction) surgical treatment by the saphenous vein graft technique. *Am J Cardiol.* 28:598–607, 1971.

11. Spencer, F.C. Bypass grafting for pre-infarction angina. *Circulation* 45:1314–1318, 1972.

12. Unstable angina pectoris: National Cooperative Study Group to compare surgical and medical therapy. II. In hospital experience and initial follow-up results in patients with one, two and three vessel disease. *Am J Cardiol.* 42:839–848, 1978.

13. Mizgala, H.F., Kahn, A.S. and Davies, R.O. The effect of propranolol in acute coronary insufficiency: a preliminary report (abstract). *Circulation* 39(suppl):138, 1969.

14. Papazoglov, N.M. Use of propranolol in pre-infarction angina. *Circulation* 44:303, 1971.

15. Fischl, S.J., Herman, M.V. and Gorlin, R. The intermediate coronary syndrome. Clinical, angiographic and therapeutic aspects. *N Engl J Med.* 288:1193–1198, 1973.

16. Mizgala, H.F., Tinmouth, A.L., Waters, D.D. et al. Prospective controlled trial of long term propranolol on acute coronary events in patients with unstable coronary artery disease (abstract). *Circulation* 50(suppl):235, 1974.

17. Mizgala, H.F., Théroux, P., Convert, G. et al. Prospective randomized trial of perhexiline maleate, isosorbide dinitrate and propranolol in unstable angina (abstract). *Circulation* 56(suppl):225, 1977.

18. Lefemine, A.A., Kosowski, B., Madoff, I. et al. Results and complications of intra-aortic balloon pumping in surgical and medical patients. *Am J Cardiol.* 40:416–420, 1977.

19. Dauwe, F., Affaki, G., Waters, D.D. et al. Intravenous nitroglycerin in refractory unstable angina (abstract). *Am J Cardiol.* 43:416, 1979.

10 Management of Unstable Angina Pectoris

Rolf Michels, MD,
Paul G. Hugenholtz, MD,
Max Haalebos, MD,
Marcel van den Brand, MD,
Patrick W. Serruys, MD, and
Kulasekaram Balakumaran, MD

> When examining a man for illness in his cordia, he has pain in his arms, in his breast, on the side of his cardia... it is death which approaches him.
>
> The Ebers papyrus, 3000 BC

One will never know whether the ancient Egyptian suffered from acute myocardial infarction or from unstable angina pectoris with impending infarction. One thing is certain, even to date, patients with the symptoms described above represent a problem in deciding whether a myocardial infarction has occurred or may still be averted by timely intervention. In an effort to clarify the dilemma, this chapter relates the experience at the Thoraxcenter, Rotterdam with the syndrome of unstable angina in 118 consecutive patients seen between 1977 and 1979.

DIAGNOSIS

Recent onset angina, increasing (crescendo) angina, and angina at rest, are some of the prodromes occurring in most of the patients who sustain acute myocardial infarction.[1,2] So, when managing unstable angina pectoris and suspecting the onset of a first myocardial infarction, the clinician should be well aware of its prognosis[3]: sudden death may occur in at least 30% of patients not treated at all, at least 10% of patients die despite admission to a coronary care unit, and another 15% will die within the first year after discharge from hospital. So every effort must be made to avoid the occurrence of such an infarction in patients in whom this syndrome threatens and in whom timely intervention still seems possible.

Of the many synonyms for the syndromes between stable angina pectoris on the one hand and acute myocardial infarction on the other hand, unstable angina pectoris suggested by Conti et al[4] and utilized later in this series seems most appropriate for our discussion. These workers distinguished three groups:

1. effort-induced angina of recent onset (ie, within the past four weeks)
2. angina on effort with a changing pattern (crescendo)
3. angina at rest (coronary insufficiency), with one or more episodes of pain, with transient ST- or T-wave changes (which returned to normal within 24 hours) without new Q-wave formation or significant elevation of cardiac enzymes.

In this classification, important subgroups with a significantly worse prognosis are constituted by those patients who have a history of previous angina or of myocardial infarction.

In the Myocardial Infarction Research Unit[5,6] studies, unstable angina was classified as:

1. angina pectoris of new onset occurring on effort or at rest
2. changing pattern of angina (crescendo), occurring on effort or at rest.

In both groups, pain could occur in single episodes, in discrete repetitive episodes, or in multiple episodes throughout the day or night. This classification is distinctly less specific than that by Conti, and both leave out the category of postinfarction unstable angina, which constitutes a major therapeutic challenge, since extension of an infarct may run a clinical course that is worse than the first infarction episode.

The collective diagnosis "unstable angina pectoris," if left unspecified, must, therefore, have great variability in its course and hence in prognosis and its therapeutic considerations.[7-9] Recent-onset effort angina (Conti group 1)[4] frequently can be effectively managed by medical means alone and subsequent prognosis does not differ from that of stable angina pectoris. Patients with intractable angina pectoris at rest (Conti group 3)[4] are at a particularly high risk of sustaining acute myocardial infarction or death.[7] Patients with angina at rest, refractory to medical therapy, require emergency coronary angiography and revascularization, each reportedly associated with a higher mortality and myocardial infarction rate than under stable conditions.[2,4,10] Patients with angina at rest, who can be "cooled off" with medical therapy, deserve consideration of surgical therapy at a later stage, or may avoid this entirely. Let us, therefore, discuss the concepts of surgical treatment and management with drugs first, before entering the detailed discussion of the subgroups in our 118 patients.

MANAGEMENT WITH SURGERY

Management of unstable angina pectoris with surgery aims not only at reduction of symptoms, but also at a diminution of the incidence of subsequent myocardial infarction and of premature death. Efforts to demonstrate the efficacy of this therapy are best reflected by the national cooperative randomized study to compare surgical and medical therapy.[5,6] Its results have clearly demonstrated that, after adequate control of pain by medical means, patients with unstable angina, either of recent onset or as a changing pattern in previously stable angina, with transient ST- or T-wave changes, without Q formation or cardiac enzyme elevation, have no higher early mortality (2% to 3%) with medical therapy than when they undergo surgery. It should be pointed out, however, that in this study patients with obstruction of the left main coronary artery, patients with severe distal obstructions, patients with severe left ventricular dysfunction, and patients not responding to optimal medical therapy were excluded from randomization. While the initial in-hospital myocardial infarction rate was significantly higher in the surgically treated group (17% versus 8%, $p < 0.05$), later, no statistically significant difference could be demonstrated (13% and 10%). Further, it was of great interest that in the follow-up period, disabling angina pectoris (New York Heart Association criteria, class III and IV) was more common in the medically than in surgically treated patients with one-vessel disease (22% versus 3%, $p < 0.05$), two-vessel disease (40% versus 13%, $p < 0.01$), and three-vessel disease (40% versus 15%, $p < 0.01$). For this reason 36% of the patients initially treated with a variety of drugs subsequently underwent surgery. Of these, 3% did so during the original hospitalization, 13% within six months, 19% by one year, and 31% by two years. While no predictive correlation could be demonstrated with the type of angina, the anatomic extent of the disease correlated well with subsequent need for surgery; 20% of the patients with one-vessel disease, 33% of those with two-vessel disease, and 49% of patients with three-vessel disease underwent surgery later for disabling angina pectoris. From these results it may be concluded that, while there is no need for urgent coronary artery surgery in all but those not reacting promptly to medical therapy or those with main stem lesions, the majority of the remainder, while becoming asymptomatic in the short term, will require bypass surgery sooner rather than later, depending on the extent of their coronary artery disease.

Whether or not surgery should be obligatory in single-vessel coronary artery obstruction of the more distal segments of the left anterior descending artery remains unclear at the moment.[3,11] However, in our experience, as well as that of others,[3] single proximal occlusion of the left anterior descending artery is not infrequently encountered in patients with recent onset angina pectoris. Furthermore, a higher five-year cardiac mortality has been reported for nonsurgical patients with single-vessel left anterior descending artery obstruction, when compared with single-vessel obstruction of the right coronary artery.[12] Favaloro has stressed the fact[3] that, in patients with single-vessel left anterior descending artery obstruction, angina often is associated with loss of physical capacity. Since this artery not only feeds a large proportion of the anterior free left ventricular wall but also the greater part of the interventricular septum, anterior myocardial infarctions with atrioventricular nodal or bundle branch conduction disturbances understandably have a bad prognosis. Also, large aneurysms of the left ventricle are often associated with proximal obstructive disease of the left anterior descending artery. In our experience, cardiogenic shock following acute myocardial infarction is more often than not associated with obstruction of the left anterior descending artery. In almost all such patients, extensive involvement of the area supplied by the left anterior descending artery can be found. In over 60 patients with cardiogenic shock reported from this center in the past 3 years,[13] 91% had anterior wall myocardial infarction, often associated with atrioventricular nodal and bundle branch conduction disturbances. Furthermore, cardiogenic shock may be the complication of a first anterior myocardial infarction in a young person without a history of previous coronary artery disease and with the prodrome of recent onset angina. In 30% of the 32 patients surviving (out of 65 total patients) to be catheterized, a single proximal occlusion of the left anterior descending artery was the sole expression of the coronary artery disease. For all these reasons proximal lesions of the left anterior descending artery in patients with unstable angina without a previous anterior myocardial infarction appear to be a special subset where the course of the coronary artery disease may be fulminant. In such individuals with severe one-vessel obstruction and an as yet uncompromised myocardium, early surgery with revascularization appears mandatory. A similar approach has been recommended, with proximal narrowing of a dominant right coronary artery.[3]

In conclusion, we believe a case for urgent surgery should be made in all patients with breakthrough angina despite optimal medical therapy, in all patients with left main stem obstruction, and in patients with single-vessel obstruction of the proximal anterior descending artery. Urgent surgery seems unnecessary for any other category, since elective surgery at a later stage under controlled conditions may offer less risk to these patients.

MANAGEMENT WITH DRUGS

Anticoagulation Although trials before 1964[14-17] indicated the efficacy of anticoagulation, none of these studies meet the statistical criteria currently mandatory for such studies.[18] As coronary thrombosis, instead of preceding myocardial infarction, may well be the consequence of myocardial infarction,[19,20] widespread therapeutic nihilism with these drugs for this indication has occurred. Furthermore, to date no well-designed studies are available to support the use of anticoagulants in unstable angina pectoris. Although, recently, much interest has been focused on the use of platelet-aggregation inhibitors, the role of these drugs in unstable angina pectoris also has not yet been established. Even so, short-term anticoagulants are advocated in all patients with prolonged periods of bedrest in an effort to avoid deep vein thrombosis and pulmonary artery thrombosis in patients being monitored with intravascular catheters. Heparin, IV, 5000 units, six times daily appears to be the ideal choice under subsequent laboratory control.

Nitrates Nitroglycerin tablets sublingually relieve most acute attacks of angina pectoris. They may be used in a prophylactic fashion even in the coronary care unit. The direct vasodilating effect on the venous system lowers preload, and thus filling pressure, as well as afterload and therefore wall stress in the left ventricle. An additional dilating effect on the larger arteries possibly lowers afterload further, and may increase coronary flow. However, unwanted side effects do take place.[21] Hypotension and bradyarrhythmias in the clinical situation can be managed by raising the legs to improve venous return and, if not effective, atropine 0.25 to 1.0 mg IV, and plasma infusions can be employed.

Nitroglycerin acts within minutes, but the duration of action is equally short. Longer effects can be obtained by using nitroglycerin ointment for topical application. This mode of application is especially effective for the prevention and treatment of angina pectoris attacks at night. A prolonged effect can also be obtained with isosorbide dinitrate. The 5-mg tablets for sublingual use are effective within minutes with the duration of action extending from one to three hours. Tablets of 20 mg are being used for oral administration, which, if absorption is total, provide a longer lasting effect. Orally administered, isosorbide dinitrate quickly passes through the liver and is transferred by glutathione-S transferase into two metabolites, isosorbide 2- and isosorbide 5-mononitrate. These two mononitrate metabolites were found to persist in the dog for over four hours after intravenous administration,[22] and hemodynamic effects qualitatively similar to those after isosorbide dinitrate have been demonstrated for the two monocomponents.[23] A sustained effect on exercise performance in patients with angina pectoris has been demonstrated both for the IV administered mononitrates[24] and for orally administered isosorbide dinitrate.[25]

When anginal attacks at rest persist despite beta-blocking agents and sublingual nitrates, both isosorbide dinitrate and nitroglycerin infusions may be helpful in managing these patients. Isosorbide dinitrate here has the advantage over nitroglycerin of a greater stability. The intravenous mode of administration is always used prior to the decision to use the intraaortic balloon pump in order to verify the need for this device.

Beta-blocking agents   As myocardial oxygen consumption is determined by contractile state, heart rate, wall tension, and duration of contraction, the use of this group of drugs appears obvious. Indeed, decreased oxygen consumption takes place in the myocardium when beta-blocking agents reduce contractility and heart rate, but they also prolong systolic ejection time[26] and may increase wall tension when cardiac size increases. Usually the initial net effect for the heart, which is not in congestive failure, is a significant reduction in oxygen consumption. To be effective the heart rate must be brought to 60 beats/min or less while not increasing heart size. Beta-blockade has also been reported to redirect the limited blood supply from normally or overperfused healthy areas to ischemic areas.[27] The rationale for the use of these agents, therefore, is to reduce general oxygen demand and to redirect the supply to the underperfused ischemic area, both mechanisms hopefully avoiding cardiac necrosis in cells in marginal conditions.

Other drugs   The calcium antagonist, verapamil,[28,29] has been helpful in suppressing supraventricular tachycardias[30] as well as in the management of angina pectoris. However, the combination of verapamil and beta-blocking agents proved unfavorable as severe left ventricular failure and cardiogenic shock have been observed.

Another calcium antagonist, nifedipine, has recently derived much attention because of its success in the management of Prinzmetal's variant angina.[31,32] Nifedipine effectively inhibits transmembrane calcium influx into muscle fibers. This results in less phosphate-bound energy being transformed into mechanical work by calcium-dependent myofibrillar adenosine triphosphate. This decreases cardiac oxidative metabolism and thus reduces the need for oxygen. Nifedipine also decreases calcium-dependent contractile tone of large extramural coronary stem arteries, thereby increasing flow. An indirect decrease in cardiac oxygen demand may also be reached by diminishing arterial blood pressure and thus ventricular afterload.[33,34]

Nifedipine in our experience is a useful adjuvant when beta-blocking agents and nitrates are not effective. In fact, a randomized study comparing the efficacy of nifedipine versus propranolol is currently underway in our institute. The combination of nifedipine and beta-blockers has not had acute serious untoward effects except in one case. One should be particularly careful in patients with obvious left ventricular failure.

MECHANICAL SUPPORT

Intraaortic balloon pumping   Intraaortic balloon pumping (IABP) offers the combined advantages of afterload reduction and enhancement of coronary perfusion pressure. However, as with all efficacious measures its use is not without risks. Experience with IABP in cardiogenic shock following acute myocardial infarction[13,35,36] and in angina at rest refractory to medical therapy[37] has been increasing in our center over the past few years. So far, over 70 patients in shock and over 65 patients with angina at rest refractory to medical therapy have been treated. In unstable angina, it is our routine to introduce the intraaortic balloon pump when, despite adequate medical therapy over 24 hours, breakthrough angina makes its appearance. The routine prophylactic use of the IABP advocated by some[38,39] does not seem to be justified and may be unnecessarily hazardous. It should be stressed, however, that there are patients that do not yield to any form of medical therapy, and in these special cases the IABP should be introduced without delay.[9]

Left heart catheterization in patients on the intraarotic balloon pump   To demonstrate IABP efficacy, hemodynamic studies were carried out during cardiac catheterization.[40] A Swan-Ganz thermodilution catheter was introduced into the pulmonary artery, and a tip manometer catheter (angio-Millar) was placed in the left ventricular cavity. The effect of a two-minute interruption of IABP on cardiac output, pulmonary capillary wedge pressure, and left ventricular pressures as well as on the isometric parameters (V_{max} total, peak dP/dt, peak V_{ce}) were studied in 23 consecutive patients with refractory unstable angina (Table 10-1). It has been shown that this short interruption induces marked changes in cardiac output, pulmonary capillary wedge pressure, and left ventricular pressures without untoward clinical effects. Since a random study to judge the efficacy of the IABP appeared impossible, it has become routine to validate IABP support in all patients by measuring cardiac output and pulmonary capillary wedge pressure prior to and during a short interruption of IABP. As shown in Table 10-1, in 22 of 23 patients, pain relief after institution of IABP was prompt, and in the one patient not benefiting from IABP, no hemodynamic effects could be demonstrated. These hemodynamic effects constitute the reason why so many patients benefit by the application of the IABP.

Table 10-1
Hemodynamic Effects of IABP Demonstrated by a 2′ Interruption (Paired Student's T Test)

Case No.	C.O. (L/min) on	off	C.I. (L/min/m²) on	off	H.R. (b/min) on	off	pkLVP (mm Hg) on	off	LVEDP (mm Hg) on	off	pkdP/dt (mm Hg/sec) on	off
1	5,2	4,2					188	210	28	24	2025	2180
2							90	100	8	24	1200	1230
3	5,6	4,3	3,1	2,4	80	100	96	105	26	32	1020	890
4	5,7	5,8	3,1	3,1	97	97	120	132	16	12	2414	2460
5	7,5	6,5	4,3	3,7	55	55	147	143	16	23	1710	1562
6	4,6	4.0	2,6	2,2	76	76	129	148	25	33	890	890
7	5,5	5,2	3,0	2,9	66	66					1305	1415
8	4,9	5,7	2,7	3,1	81	81	109	132	6	8	1695	1655
9	4,5	4,2	2,3	2,2	62	65	100	133	11	14	860	1075
10	4,9	4,5	2,5	2,3	74	79	130	178	18	30	1780	1785
11	5,6	4,3	2,7	2,1	62	62	119	132	30	41	1260	1275
12	6,1	6,0	3,2	3,1	70	70	100	130	8	10	1350	1610
13							123	149	10	13	1175	1230
14							140	154	25	25	1480	1590
15							123	141	14	16	1310	1365
16							126	150	26	32	1290	1400
17	4,8	3,1	2,9	1,9	61	67	108	168	16	30	1290	2015
18							90	90	26	28	990	920
19							120	152	15	32	2139	2619
20							115	154	9	12	1960	1990
21	5,3	5,1	2,4	2,3	94	87	113	127	12	13		
22							160	188	14	10		
23							120	130	4	2		
	5,4	4,8	2,9	2,6	73	75	121	143	17	21	1457	1557
	±	±	±	±	±	±	±	±	±	±	±	±
	0,8	1,0	0,5	0,6	13	14	23	28	8	10	433	497
	n = 13		n = 12		n = 12		n = 22		n = 22		n = 20	
	p < 0,01		p < 0,02		NS		p < 0,000001		p < 0.0025		p < 0.04	

Surgical Mortality: 0
Surgical complications: 0

DESCRIPTION OF CURRENT APPROACHES (Figures 10-1 and 10-2)

When a patient with unstable angina with sufficient symptoms for hospitalization is admitted to the coronary care unit, the patient is given bedrest in semi-isolation. The rooms contain all necessary intensive care equipment and are separated from other patients but directly accessible to the nursing staff. Visitors are initially not allowed. Hemodynamic monitoring is done via a Swan-Ganz thermodilution catheter. In cases of hypotension or hypertension an arterial line is inserted in the left radial artery. All

Table 10-1 *(continued)*

pkVCE (sec⁻¹) on	off	Vmax (sec⁻¹) on	off	No. of Vessels Diseased (> 70%) LMCA	LAD	LCX	RCA	No. of bypasses	IABP efficacy (resolution of pain)	Follow-up 3 mos– 2 yrs
27	33	43	45		+			1	+	
28	19	53	34		+		+	2	+	
21	18	27	21		+	+		2	+	
39	49	46	64		+	+		1	+	
38	34	45	40		+			1	+	
18	16	30	25		+	+	+	3	+	
33	33	48	45		+	+		2	+	
45	41	53	52		+	+	+	3	+	
25	24	34	35		+			1	+	
32	23	49	46		+	+	+	3	+	
23	18	48	43		+	+	+	2	+	a.p.NYHA
38	31	46	45		+	+	+	3	+	
33	31	41	37	+			+	3	+	
28	30	45	45		+			1	+	
30	28	44	41		+	+	+	3	+	
23	20	46	40		+			1	+	
29	25	38	40		+	+		1	+	
20	18	38	32		+	+	+	2	–	a.p.NYHA
31	40	43	63		+	+	+	3	+	
37	35	45	47		+		+	2	+	
					+	+	+	3	+	
						+	+	2	+	
					+			1	+	
30 ± 7 n = 20 NS	28 ± 9	43 ± 7 n = 20 NS	42 ± 10	Total No. Vessel Diseased 49				Total No. Bypasses 46		

patients with indwelling catheters receive anticoagulant therapy with intravenous heparin (5000 units, six times daily). The parameters monitored during and after pain include heart rate and rhythm, systemic blood pressure, pulmonary artery pressures, and cardiac output. During and following every attack of pain, a twelve-lead ECG is recorded and, with persisting pain, repeated at 15-minute intervals. Six hours after every attack of pain the cardiac enzymes (CPK, CPK-MB, and α-HBDH) are determined. After an initial sedative, preferably diazepam (5 to 10 mg orally three times a day), isosorbide dinitrate (5 mg sublingually every two hours) is given and the intravenous administration of propranolol (at 1 to 10 mg, $\leqslant$ 1 mg/min) is begun until a heart rate $\leqslant$ 60 beats/min has been reached.

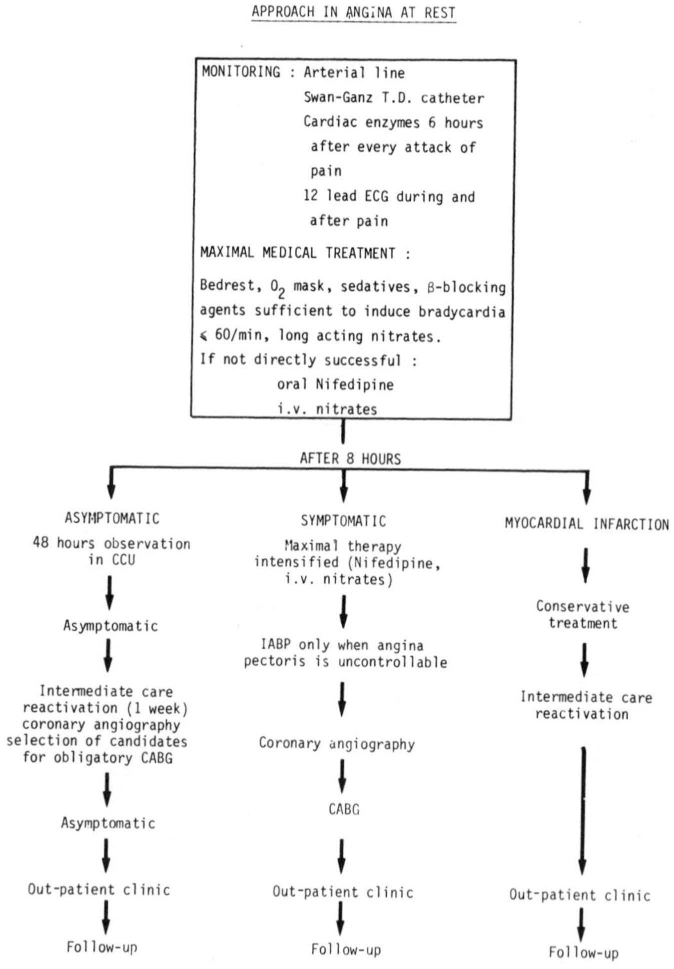

Figure 10-1 Approach in angina at rest.

After this an oral maintenance dosage (400 to 800 mg/24 hr) is instituted. When propranolol is contraindicated, such as in the presence of lung disease, a more selective beta-blocker may be chosen.

Patients who develop an acute myocardial infarction despite optimal therapy with drugs are treated conservatively. Propranolol is discontinued only if cardiac or pulmonary problems arise from its use. For the patient who becomes asymptomatic within eight hours of optimal medical therapy, a 48-hour period of observation in the coronary care unit follows. If the patient is still asymptomatic, he is transferred to the intermediate care unit and mobilized over the course of one week. If the patient is still asymptomatic, discharge from the hospital follows. Upon discharge the patient is instructed to report immediately should symptoms recur. Also, an appointment is made for the outpatient clinic at which time, in the absence of unstable angina pectoris or other contraindications, a symptom-limited bicycle exercise test is performed. At a variable interval, preferably during the initial hospitalization, cardiac catheterization with coronary angiography is carried out, and the decision is made whether or not to operate with bypass surgery.

APPROACH IN ANGINA AT REST

One or more attacks of severe anginal pain
at rest, associated with transient ST- or
T-wave changes, without significant
(> 2 x control value) cardiac enzyme
elevation, or the appearance of new Q-waves.

Bedrest
long acting nitrates
β-blocking agents
sedatives

CORONARY ANGIOGRAPHY

Surgery :
- Left main coronary artery obstruction
- Angina at rest (class IV) despite optimal
  medical therapy for 24 - 48 hours.
- Proximal left anterior descending artery
  obstruction.

Medical therapy :
- Mild stable angina pectoris (NYHA II),
  not violating life style, (even with
  2 - 3 vessel disease)
- Mild coronary obstruction (<50%)
- Surgically unsuitable coronary artery
  disease.
- Untreatable associated disease.

Figure 10-2 Approach in angina at rest. One or more attacks of severe anginal pain at rest, associated with transient ST- or T-wave changes, without significant (> 2 × control value) cardiac enzyme elevation, or the appearance of new Q-waves.

154

When the patient is still symptomatic after eight hours of medical therapy, treatment is considered unsuccessful, and for another 0 to 16 hours intensive medical therapy is given. By and large this course of events indicates that he is a candidate for early coronary angiography and coronary artery bypass grafting (CABG). When, despite further intensive medical therapy including intravenous nitroglycerin over a period up to 16 hours, breakthrough angina makes its appearance, the intraaortic balloon pump is introduced without delay.

CURRENT PATIENT MATERIAL (Figure 10-3)

In the period from January 1977 to January 1979, 118 patients (aged 30 to 69 years; median, 54 years), in whom follow-up of three months to two years was available, were admitted to the coronary care unit of the Thoraxcenter. They showed angina at rest, either of new onset or occurring as a changing pattern of previously stable angina pectoris, with transient ST- or T-wave changes (reverting towards the control pattern after relief of

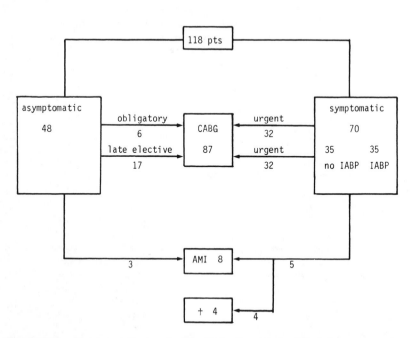

Figure 10-3 Current patient material. Clinical results in 118 patients presenting with unstable angina (AMI = acute myocardial infarction; CABG = coronary artery bypass grafting; IABP = intraaortic balloon pump).

pain), without new Q-wave formation or cardiac enzyme elevation. In 12 of these patients the unstable episode occurred within two weeks after sustaining an acute transmural myocardial infarction (postinfarction unstable angina pectoris). These 12 are discussed in a separate section.

Of the 118 patients, 48 responded favorably to bedrest and medical therapy within eight hours, while 70 patients had breakthrough angina pectoris despite this maximal medical therapy (Figure 10-4). This number of patients refractory to medical therapy has been steadily increasing over the last two years, reflecting the fact that our clinic has become a referral center for unstable angina pectoris.

PATIENTS SYMPTOMATIC AFTER 8 HOURS OF
OPTIMAL MEDICAL THERAPY

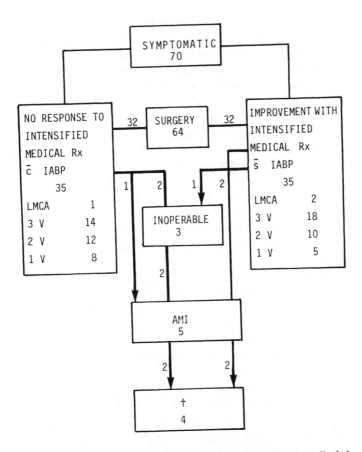

Figure 10-4 Patients symptomatic after eight hours of optimal medical therapy.

Of the 48 patients who became asymptomatic, six later became candidates for obligatory surgery; two patients had a significant (> 50%) narrowing of the left main coronary artery, and four with recent onset angina at rest, but without a previous myocardial infarction, had proximal obstruction (> 75%) of the left anterior descending artery (LAD) before the origin of the first septal branch.

The remaining 42 patients were treated with medical therapy for periods up to six months until elective cardiac catheterization. Sixteen had ≥ 75% narrowing of three vessels, 14 had two-vessel disease, and in 12 only one vessel was affected. Although these patients all initially did well on medical therapy, early recurrence of symptoms resulted in a nonfatal in-hospital myocardial infarction in one patient with three-vessel obstruction. Within three months following discharge, two more patients had nonfatal myocardial infarctions (one patient with three-vessel disease and one patient with a single occlusion of the LAD). Late (ie, six months) elective coronary artery bypass grafting had to be performed in 12 patients for incapacitating angina pectoris (New York Heart Association, class III and IV) and for angina pectoris severe enough to interfere with their usual lifestyle (five patients). Of the patients with three-vessel disease, nine (56%) underwent late CABG, of those with two-vessel disease six (43%), while two patients (17%) with single-vessel narrowing (both of the LAD) underwent CABG at a later stage. Twenty-five patients did not require CABG in the follow-up period of three months to two years. Five patients (three with three-vessel and two with two-vessel disease) now have mild angina pectoris, and 20 patients (four with three-vessel, six with two-vessel, and ten with one-vessel disease [all with 75% or more narrowing of the lumen]) are asymptomatic. Maximal medical therapy did not relieve pain in 70 patients during the initial eight-hour observation period in the coronary care unit (see Figure 10-3). In 35 of these (group A), rapid deterioration necessitated early institution of IABP while thirty-five other patients (group B) gradually improved on prolonged intensive pharmacological therapy and did not require IABP. In group A, a special subgroup was constituted by the 12 patients who had postinfarct unstable angina pectoris (Table 10-2). In the remaining 23 patients, pain relief was prompt in 22 after institution of IABP (see Table 10-1). Cardiac catheterization showed significant obstruction in three vessels or more in nine patients, of two vessels in seven and of one vessel in six, all with proximal occlusion of the LAD. One patient had a significant narrowing of the left main coronary artery. After CABG, 21 patients became asymptomatic, two had mild angina pectoris, none died, and none developed myocardial infarction.

When unstable angina returned in the 12 patients who sustained an acute myocardial infarction one week before (see Table 10-2), pain relief after IABP institution was equally impressive and prompt in 11 patients. All 12 underwent coronary angiography. Three-vessel disease was encountered in five patients, two-vessel disease in five patients and single-

Table 10-2
Postinfarction Unstable Angina Pectoris

No. Vessels Diseased	No. of Patients	IABP Efficacy	Inoperable	Infarction Despite IABP	< 1 mo
1 V	2	2			
2 V	5	5			
3 V	5	4	2	2 (1†)	2
Total	12	11	2	2	2

vessel obstruction in two patients (both of the LAD, both with a good distal run-off). Two patients were considered not operable because of diffuse distal coronary obstructions. Both had a poor left ventricular performance with an ejection fraction less than 30%, and both had a long history of coronary artery disease with several earlier infarctions. One of these two patients suffered an acute myocardial infarction during IABP and died in shock. The other died of an acute myocardial infarction within one month after treatment. One patient had a nonfatal acute myocardial infarction despite IABP, and was not considered a candidate for CABG subsequently. After a varying interval of treatment with the IABP (1 to 14 days, mean of 6), nine patients underwent CABG. Eight of these became asymptomatic, one had mild angina, none died, and none developed an acute myocardial infarction. While this subgroup appears different in terms of the time of occurrence of angina, the course is quite similar to those whose angina was not preceded by infarction.

Since the introduction of the intraaortic balloon pump at the Thoraxcenter (1972) over 65 patients with breakthrough angina despite optimal medical therapy have been treated with it, with consistently good results. Only one patient sustained an infarction while on the IABP. One patient died following surgery, and no serious complications were encountered. The virtual absence of surgical mortality in the subgroup with postinfarction breakthrough angina encourages us to continue this approach. Here the prolonged use of the IABP (in our experience seldom associated with serious side effects)[13,35-37] may enable the surgeon to perform surgery at a well-chosen moment, when all clinical aspects appear to have reduced the risks.

In two of the 35 patients in group B, who could not be cooled off completely, but in whom the IABP did not seem to be indicated urgently, an obstruction of the left main coronary artery was encountered. Eighteen patients had narrowing of three or more vessels, ten patients had two-vessel disease and five patients had single-vessel involvement (four of the LAD and one of the right coronary artery).

The two patients in this group, with extensive coronary artery disease, as well as a significant obstruction of the left main coronary artery, sustained a fatal acute myocardial infarction while in the hospital shortly following coronary angiography. This is considered more than a coincidence. One other patient, with extensive and diffuse distal coronary artery disease, was considered inoperable. To date this patient has chronic stable incapacitating angina pectoris. Of the 32 patients who underwent urgent surgery, six still have mild angina pectoris, but 26 are asymptomatic. None developed an acute myocardial infarction.

EXTENT OF CORONARY ARTERY DISEASE

As evident from Table 10-3, five of 118 patients (4%) had significant narrowing (≥ 50%) of the left main coronary artery, 48 of 118 (41%) had narrowing (≥ 75%) of three vessels, 36 of 118 (31%) had narrowing (≥ 75%) of two vessels, and 29 of 118 (25%) had one narrowed vessel.

It was remarkable that roughly the same distribution in the extent of coronary artery occlusive disease was seen regardless of whether the treatment chosen turned out to be pharmacologic or surgical (see Table 10-3). Only single-vessel obstruction was more frequently (33%) encountered in the group that could be managed by pharmacologic means alone. On the other hand the majority (12/20) of patients with a single proximal occlusion of the LAD remained unstable despite maximal therapy. Of those patients with single proximal occlusions of the LAD that responded to medical therapy, one developed an early myocardial infarction and three were candidates for late elective surgery because of incapacitating angina pectoris.

As outlined earlier, these experiences, as well as those in patients in cardiogenic shock treated with IABP, make patients with proximal LAD obstruction candidates for early obligatory CABG. This was in fact performed in the four remaining patients. As a whole, the 29 patients with single-vessel obstruction were younger (30 to 58 years, median 48 years) and had prodromes of only recent onset without a history of an earlier myocardial infarction. Perhaps they do deserve a different approach, and now this has become a rule at our institute.

MORTALITY AND MORBIDITY

In our experience extending over two years, total mortality was low (4/118 patients, 3%). Three in-hospital deaths occurred: two patients with left main coronary artery obstructions died shortly following angiography, one patient with postinfarction breakthrough angina whose anatomic lesions proved inoperable died during treatment with the IABP. The fourth patient, also considered inoperable, died three months after discharge.

Table 10-3
Extent of Coronary Artery Disease

	Total Group		Medical Therapy Effective in CCU		Medical Therapy Ineffective					
					No IABP 35 Patients		IABP 35 Patients			
							12 Patients Postinfarct.		23 Patients	
	118 Patients		48 Patients							
	nr.	%	nr.	%	nr.	%	nr.	%	nr.	%
LMCA narrowing	5	4	2	4	2	6	-	-	1	4
Triple-vessel narrowing	48	41	16	33	18	51	5	42	9	39
Double-vessel narrowing	36	31	14	29	10	29	5	42	7	30
Single-vessel narrowing	29	25	16	33	5	14	2	17	6	26
LAD	20	17	8	17	4	11	2	17	6	26
LCX	5	4	5	10						
RCA	4	3	3	6	1	3				

No mortality or myocardial infarction was related to the surgical procedure in these series. This absence of surgical mortality does not necessarily reflect the quality of surgical management and may be a chance observation. In a larger group of 499 patients undergoing CABG in our center between 1971 to 1978,[41] the perioperative mortality rate was 3% for patients with unstable angina pectoris refractory to medical therapy, and 1% for the total group. In this same experience the perioperative myocardial infarction rate (as demonstrated by new Q-wave formation on the twelve-lead ECG) was 10%, and the incidence of the perioperative infarctions did not differ for stable or unstable angina pectoris. Mortality related to urgent coronary angiography proved higher in these unstable conditions. Of the 70 patients undergoing urgent catheterization, two (3%) died within 24 hours following the procedure, and both had an obstruction of the left main coronary artery, suggesting a higher risk for patients with unstable angina and left main coronary artery obstructions.

SUGGESTED MANAGEMENT (see Figures 10-1 and 10-2)

Bedrest and aggressive medical therapy (including sedatives, beta-blocking agents and long-acting nitrates) must constitute the initial approach in unstable angina pectoris, when pain and transient ECG changes at rest indicate the threat of an infarction. When the symptoms persist despite this approach, IV nitroglycerin or isosorbide dinitrate may offer benefit in the short term, while nifedipine may be helpful especially when variant forms of angina with spasm are suspected. The IABP should be instituted only when symptoms worsen despite optimal medical therapy. Candidates for early revascularization are those not responding to optimal medical therapy. Early catheterization, preferably during the initial hospitalization, is recommended for all patients. Revascularization is obligatory in patients with significant left main coronary artery obstructions and patients with proximal narrowing of the LAD, who have not yet sustained a massive anterior myocardial infarction. Our experience supports the results reported from the National Cooperative Study Group on Unstable Angina Pectoris.[5,6] A large group (17/42 [40%]) of patients who could be managed by medical means alone later required CABG for incapacitating angina pectoris, especially with three-vessel (56%) and two-vessel disease (43%). Thus the extent of coronary artery disease determines the later recurrence of symptoms and the subsequent need for surgery in patients who initially can be managed by medical means alone. Aggressive medical therapy may save these patients and the clinical and nursing staff, the burden and hazards of emergency procedures. On the other hand, depending on extent of disease, it may fail in the end and expose the patient to a longer period of socioeconomic invalidation. In patients without extensive coronary artery disease, or left main stem narrowings, or proximal narrowings of the LAD, who remain asymptomatic after discharge, elective surgery does not seem to have an advantage over medical therapy. Surgical risk may exceed that of medical management alone. If these patients remain asymptomatic during careful follow-up and do not reveal a seriously diminished physical capacity with early pain with ischemic ECG changes or decreases in arterial pressure during exercise testing, bypass grafting does not appear mandatory. Since, for logistic reasons, it is not always feasible to analyze all patients at an early stage, early angiography could be restricted to symptomatic patients and to those in whom left main obstruction or proximal LAD obstruction is suspected. Both these subsets of coronary artery disease demonstrate a conspicuous loss of physical capacity during exercise testing, which is often associated with lowering of blood pressure. Astute clinical observations with thallium perfusion studies during exercise may prove most helpful in detecting these and other high-risk patients.

REFERENCES

1. Fulton, M., Lutz, W., Donald, K.W. et al. Natural history of unstable angina. *Lancet* 1:860, 1972.

2. Cairns, J.A., Fantus, I.G., and Klassen, G.A. Unstable angina pectoris. *Am Heart J.* 92:373, 1976.

3. Favaloro, R.G. Direct myocardial revascularization: a ten-years journey. *Am J Cardiol.* 43(1):109, 1979.

4. Conti, C.R., Brawley, R.K., Griffith, L.S.C. et al. Unstable angina pectoris: morbidity and mortality in 57 consecutive patients evaluated angiographically. *Am J Cardiol.* 32:745, 1973.

5. Unstable angina pectoris: National Cooperative Study Group to compare medical and surgical therapy. Report of protocol and patient population. *Am J Cardiol.* 37:899, 1976.

6. Unstable angina pectoris: National Cooperative Study Group to compare surgical and medical therapy. II. In hospital experience and initial follow-up results in patients with one, two and three vessel disease. *Am J Cardiol.* 42:839, 1979.

7. Gazes, P.C., Mobley, E.M., Jr., Faris, H.M., Jr. et al. Pre-infarctional (unstable) angina—a prospective study—ten year follow-up. *Circulation* 48:331, 1973.

8. Bertolasi, C.A., Tronge, J.E., Riccitelli, M.A. et al. Natural history of unstable angina with medical or surgical therapy. *Chest* 70:596, 1976.

9. Olinger, G.N., Bonchek, L.I., Keelan, M.H. et al. Unstable angina: the case for operation. *Am J Cardiol.* 42:634, 1978.

10. Scanlon, P.J., Rimgandas, N., Mozan, J.F. et al. Accelerated angina pectoris, clinical, hemodynamic, arteriographic and therapeutic experience in 85 patients. *Circulation* 47(1):19, 1973.

11. Abedin, Z., and Dack, S. Isolated left anterior descending coronary artery disease. *Am J Cardiol.* 40(4):654, 1977.

12. Bruschke, A.V.G., Proudfit, W.L., and Sones, F.M. Progress study of 590 consecutive nonsurgical cases of coronary disease followed 5-9 years. I. Arteriographic correlations. *Circulation* 47(2):1147, 1973.

13. Michels, R., Hugenholtz, P.G. Intraaortic balloon pumping. *Circulation* 59(4):846, 1979.

14. Nichol, E.S., Phillips, W.C., and Gasten, G.G. Virtue of prompt anti-coagulant therapy in impending myocardial infarction. Experience with 318 patients during a 10 year period. *Ann Intern Med.* 50:1158, 1959.

15. Beamish, R.E., and Storrie, V.M. Impending myocardial infarction. Recognition and management. *Circulation* 21:1107, 1960.

16. Wood, P. Acute and subacute coronary insufficiency. *Br Med J.* 1:1779, 1961.

17. Vakil, R.J. Preinfarction syndrome—management and follow-up. *Am J Cardiol.* 14:55, 1964.

18. Gifford, R.H., and Feinstein, A.R. A critique of methodology in studies of anticoagulant therapy for acute myocardial infarction. *N Engl J Med.* 280:351, 1969.

19. Branwood, A.W., and Montgomery, G.L. Observations on the morbid anatomy of coronary disease. *Scott Med J.* 1:367, 1956.

20. Roberts, W.C., and Buja, L.C. The frequency and significance of coronary arterial thrombi and other observations in fatal acute myocardial infarction. *Am J Med.* 52:423, 1972.

21. Come, P.C., and Pitt, B. Nitroglycerin-induced severe hypotension and bradycardia in patients with acute myocardial infarction. *Circulation* 54(4):624, 1976.

22. Sisenwine, S.E., and Rawlins, H.W. Plasma concentrations and urinary excretion of isosorbide dinitrate and its metabolites in the dog. *J Pharmacol Exp Ther.* 176:296, 1971.

23. Wendt, R.L. Systemic and coronary vascular effects of the 2 and 5 mononitrate esters of isosorbide. *J Pharmacol Exp Ther.* 180:732, 1972.

24. Michel, D. Der Einfluss van Metabolieten des Isosorbide Dinitrats auf das Belastungs-EKG bei koronair Insuffisienz. *Herz/Kreisl.* 8(8):444, 1976.

25. Markis, J.E., Gorlin, R., Mills, R.M. et al. Sustained effect of orally administered isosorbide dinitrate on exercise performance of patients with angina pectoris. *Am J Cardiol.* 43(2):265, 1979.

26. Epstein, S.E., Redwood, D.R., Goldstein, R.E. et al. Angina pectoris: pathophysiology, evaluation and treatment. *Ann Intern Med.* 75:263, 1971.

27. Watson, S., and Gorlin, R. Cardiovascular pharmacology of propranolol in man. *Circulation* 40:501, 1969.

28. Ferlinz, J., Easthope, J.L., and Aronow, W.S. Effects of Verapamil on myocardial performance in coronary artery disease. *Circulation* 59(2):313, 1979.

29. Nayler, W.G., and Szeto, J. Effect of Verapamil on contractility, oxygen utilization and calcium exchangeability in mammalian heart muscle. *Cardiovasc Res.* 6:120, 1972.

30. Hagemeijer, F. Verapamil in the management of supraventricular tachyarrhythmias after a recent myocardial infarction. *Circulation* 57:751, 1978.

31. Endo, M., Kanda, I., Hosoda, S. et al. Prinzmetal's variant form of angina pectoris. Re-evaluation of mechanisms. *Circulation* 53:33, 1975.

32. Goldberg, S., Reichek, N., Muller, J. et al. Nifedipine: a useful new agent for the therapy of variant angina. *Circulation* 58(suppl II)(4):101, 1978.

33. Fleckenstein, A., Tritthart, H., Doring, H.J. et al. Bay 0 1040 - ein hochaktiver Ca⁺⁺ antagonistischer Inhibitor der elektromechanischen Koppelungsprozesse in Warmblutter-myokard. *Arzneim Forsch* 22:22, 1972.

34. Gerson, M.C., Noble, R.J., Wann, L.S. et al. Non-invasive documentation of Prinzmetals' angina. *Am J Cardiol.* 43(2):329, 1979.

35. Hagemeijer, F., Laird, J.D., Haalebos, M.M.P. et al. Effectiveness of intraaortic balloon pumping without cardiac surgery for patients with severe heart failure, secondary to a recent myocardial infarction. *Am J Cardiol.* 40:951, 1977.

36. Hagemeijer, F., Michels, H.R., Balakumaran, K. et al. Experience actuelle de l'assistance circulatoire. *Ann Cardiol Angeiol.* 26:463, 1977.

37. Hugenholtz, P.G., Balakumaran, K., Hagemeijer, F. et al. Intraaortic balloon pumping for impending myocardial infarction. *Circulation* 58(suppl II)(4):172, 1978.

38. Gold, H.K., Leinbach, R.C., Buckley, M.J. et al. Refractory angina pectoris: follow-up after intra-aortic balloon pumping and surgery. *Circulation* 54(suppl III):41, 1976.

39. Scully, H.E., Gunstensen, J., Williams, W.G. et al. Surgical management of complicated acute coronary insufficiency. *Surgery* 80:437, 1976.

40. Michels, H.R., Serruys, P.W., van den Brand, M. The hemodynamic response to interruption of intraaortic balloon pumping. *Trans Eur Soc Cardiol.* 1:96 (abst. #374), 1978.

41. van den Brand, M., Serruys, P.W., Bos, E. et al. Coronair chirurgie in het Thoraxcentrum Rotterdam. *Hart Bull.* 9:114, 1978.

11 Unstable Angina Pectoris: Speculations on an Enigma

Kulasekaram Balakumaran, MD, and
Paul G. Hugenholtz, MD

Conceptually, unstable angina pectoris seems to occupy a space between the syndromes of stable angina pectoris and acute myocardial infarction, while at the further extremes of this axis are to be found asymptomatic myocardial ischemia and sudden ischemic cardiac death. Viewed as a spatial arrangement, one is inclined to think that the prognosis for survival in ischemic heart disease worsens as one moves from asymptomatic disease to sudden death. However, whether correct or not, this view is partly unverifiable, for a follow-up of asymptomatic ischemic heart disease would not appear to be feasible. Yet, it is also partly clarified. Thus, although we have learned that the syndrome of sudden ischemic cardiac death is not necessarily fatal,[1,2] the chance of survival, even with prompt and trained assistance, is on the order of 14% to 18%, with a one-year mortality rate in survivors of 30%.[1,3] Acute myocardial infarction shows a somewhat better prognosis, 50% to 60%[4,5] surviving the acute attack, with a further 6% to 10% deaths in the first year thereafter.[5,6] An uncertain aspect in this connection is the phenomenon of unrecognized myocardial infarction.[7] For it seems probable that if one were to consider these cases with those of manifest myocardial infarction, there would be some improvement in the survival figures. As regards angina pectoris, early studies[8-10] demonstrated a yearly mortality ranging from 2.5%[10] to around 12%.[8] The more recent Framingham study showed a 4% annual mortality after a ten-year follow-up.[11] Subsequent studies[12-15] in patients with demonstrated coronary sclerosis yielded an annual mortality varying between 5.5%[14] and 15%.[13] The follow-up in unstable angina pectoris has produced a greater spread in mortality rate. Bertolasi et al[16] had a 20% mortality in 40 patients at eight months, with a 35% mortality in a high-risk group. Conti et al[17] had five deaths in 73 medically treated patients, or 7% in the seven months. Duncan et al[18] had a 4% mortality in 251 patients within six months. Gazes et al[19] in a study of 140 patients found an 18% mortality at one year, and they were able to define a high-risk group of 54 patients with a 43% mortality at the end of the first year.

Viewing the figures, one has to conclude that the criterion of first year mortality does not clearly distinguish between unstable angina pectoris and unselected angina pectoris. This is perhaps partly attributable to the fact that unselected angina pectoris would include a proportion of cases of unstable angina pectoris, thus intermingling the groups. The only proper way to clarify this matter would be to compare the prognosis in a cohort of well defined stable angina pectoris with one of well defined unstable angina pectoris. Such a study, it seems, has not been done. It is not possible to conclude with confidence that unstable angina pectoris represents a more severe form of the disease than stable angina pectoris. However, one does seem to recognize within the group of unstable angina pectoris, a subset at high risk of myocardial infarction and sudden death.[16,19] The identification of this high-risk group seems important, for there is some indication that intensive medical therapy helps in cooling off this emergency and improves the prognosis.[20,21] Furthermore, urgent coronary artery bypass surgery is an attractive therapeutic approach in an effort to modify the somber immediate prognosis. At the very least, one would like to know whether, and to what degree, bypass surgery does alter the outcome in this discouraging situation. The central isssue here is whether these patients are identifiable as a group. Clinically one knows that myocardial infarction and sudden death can announce themselves unequivocally. Crescendo angina, or repeated severe angina at rest ending in infarction or sudden death make a vivid and memorable sequel. But the cases in which the prodromata are as dramatic, but which subsequently cool off without infarction or death, lack theatrical completeness and so tend to be forgotten. Yet they dilute the high-risk group and change the concept of impending infarction/impending sudden death.

Phenomenonologically, the distinguishing feature between stable and unstable angina pectoris is predictability. In stable angina pectoris the attack is predictable in its occurrence, duration, provocation, presentation, and severity. The attack of unstable angina pectoris is unexpected in one or more of these features. Day-to-day variation in the number and severity of anginal attacks by itself does not constitute unstable angina pectoris, when this variation is correlated to, say, the degree of exertion, thus making the variation predictable. However, anginal attacks that appear, for the patient under consideration, in unusual circumstances are excessively prolonged (but not excessively curtailed); arise unprovoked by effort, emotion, cold, meals, or arrhythmia; or are uncommonly severe (but not uncommonly mild) would be considered unstable angina pectoris. Also, angina that, though provoked, arises, for that patient, from milder provocation than before would also come under the concept of unstable angina pectoris. Furthermore, new onset angina and early postinfarction angina are similarly classified, no doubt because newness makes for unpredictability.

Pathophysiologically, this unpredictability in unstable angina pectoris, which implies a lack of clinically identifiable cause for the attack, compounds the problems of ischemic heart disease. Furthermore, unprovoked angina, angina at rest, crescendo angina leading to myocardial infarction and/or sudden death, and all of these "cooling off" and settling down to stable angina or the asymptomatic state give a variety and a depth to the illness that the more easily comprehensible stable angina, infarction, and sudden death do not show. These protean manifestations underscore our lack of understanding of the pathophysiology and have made coronary artery spasm seem likely from Heberden's day to the present,[22,23] spasm for which there is now considerable evidence.[24,25] However, it seems gratuitous to employ the term spasm to bridge all the gaps in the understanding. Perhaps more refined conceptual models will take us some of the way. The discussion that follows will be a speculative effort to construct such a dynamic model for the better understanding of unstable angina pectoris. Hopefully the model will provide, in addition, insight into other aspects of myocardial ischemia. To begin with, the basic tenets of myocardial oxygen demand and oxygen delivery will be briefly considered.

The major determinants of myocardial oxygen demand are[26-28]:

1. Left ventricular wall stress, which is a function of afterload or aortic pressure, of preload or left ventricular end-diastolic pressure, of ventricular volume by the Laplace equation, and of wall thickness.
2. Inotropic state of the myocardium.
3. Heart rate.

Increases in the values of any of these factors lead to increased myocardial oxygen demand.

Oxygen delivery to the myocardium varies with coronary blood flow, which is determined by the perfusion pressure or aortic pressure, and coronary vascular resistance. Coronary blood flow is capable of autoregulation, rising in situations of increasing oxygen demand and falling with reduced demand.[29-31] This adjustment is achieved by means of appropriate alterations in coronary vascular resistance, mainly via humoral factors. Further, as the major part of coronary flow occurs during diastole, tachycardia, which encroaches upon diastole, tends to reduce coronary flow, as does increased left ventricular diastolic pressure, for the perfusion pressure proper of the coronary circulation is the difference between the aortic pressure and the left ventricular diastolic pressure.[32,33]

Myocardial ischemia is essentially a regional phenomenon. If inadequacy of blood flow with respect to the oxygen demand at that moment develops rapidly in some part of the myocardium, acute myocardial ischemia will occur. This could arise from either increased myocardial oxygen demand, as in exercise, emotion, and tachycardia[34,35] or diminished oxygen delivery, as in coronary thrombosis and coronary spasm.[36] Once myocardial ischemia occurs, contractile function of the ischemic cells is rapidly lost,[37] and a state resembling that of cardiac failure tends to follow.[38,39] Or, as is often seen at catheterization, myocardial ischemia leads to regional abnormalities, akinesia or dyskinesia of ventricular contraction, and to elevated left ventricular end-diastolic pressure. If pain occurs, sympathetic stimulation should tend to give rise to tachycardia and a raised blood pressure. Further, in the presence of ischemia, one would expect a fall in coronary vascular resistance and a rise in regional and total coronary flow.

These hemodynamic changes, namely raised left ventricular end-diastolic pressure, raised blood pressure, tachycardia, and increased coronary blood flow, have, in the main, been observed during episodes of myocardial ischemia. Friesinger[40] in a review of the literature on this subject, concluded that a raised left ventricular end-diastolic pressure was usual and a raised blood pressure and tachycardia frequent in spontaneous and provoked angina. Grossman and Mann,[41] by direct measurement in pacing induced angina, found a raised left ventricular end-diastolic pressure, increased coronary flow (despite coronary sclerosis), and a moderate rise in blood pressure. These four changes would, of themselves, tend to produce direct or indirect alterations in myocardial oxygen demand and in oxygen delivery. Thus, increased left ventricular end-diastolic pressure and raised blood pressure (ie, increased preload and afterload) would increase ventricular wall stress and hence increase oxygen demand over the whole ventricle. Elevated left ventricular end-diastolic pressure would have the additional effect of tending to reduce coronary flow, while elevated blood pressure would tend to increase it; tachycardia would augment further the total and regional myocardial oxygen demand, and reduced coronary vascular resistance would help to increase coronary blood flow. Hence, one finds that at the onset of myocardial ischemia there is, as a result of the hemodynamic changes, a rapid nonlinear increase in myocardial oxygen demand over the whole ventricle, and at the same time an increase in coronary blood flow. These two increases, one tending to aggravate the ischemia and the other to overcome it, being multifactorially and relatively independently determined, are not likely to match directly. This leaves the way open for exacerbation of ischemia, on the one hand, or its termination, on the other.

Let us consider a simplified ventricle consisting of three regions: A, B, and C. Suppose region B becomes ischemic, from whatever cause. The myocardial fibers would lose their contractile function, and region B would become akinetic. As a result the ventricular end-diastolic pressure would rise, and hence so would the wall stress in all three regions. (Alterations in aortic pressure and heart rate are being ignored for simplicity.) The oxygen demand of the entire ventricle would rise; region B, already ischemic, suffers a further and inappropriate increase in demand, while regions A and C would experience an increase in oxygen demand solely as a consequence of the change in a neighboring region. Coronary autoregulation is set in motion, coronary vascular resistance tends to fall, and flow to all three regions rises. Should the increase in blood flow to region A be inadequate or sluggish, this region too would become ischemic, the cells would lose their contractile function, region A would become akinetic, and the ventricular end-diastolic pressure would show another incremental rise. Another round of increase in oxygen demand in all three regions would be set in motion. Region C could now become threatened. On the other hand, regions A and B, having become ischemic, the blood supply to region A, after a time lag, perhaps involving opening up of collaterals, catches up with oxygen demand. The cells in region A would recover contractile function and the ventricular end-diastolic pressure would fall, and hence also the oxygen demand of all three regions. This could lead to disappearance of ischemia in region B and result in oxygen demand/supply balance over the entire ventricle. Thus, one sees that while the onset of myocardial ischemia tends to generate a mounting spiral of increasing ischemia, the onset of recovery from ischemia tends to set in motion a spreading wave of recovery; or, to state it in other terms, both the tendency to deterioration and to recovery are subject to multiplier, or cascade, effects. Hence one might expect every attack of myocardial ischemia to find its equilibrium through the interplay of these two tendencies. If the equilibrium is reached with all regions nonischemic, the attack would be one of angina pectoris. If the equilibrium is long in coming, the pain is likely to be prolonged, and the attack would be described as acute coronary insufficiency. If equilibrium is arrived at only with a region of persisting ischemia, a myocardial infarction would result. If equilibrium is not reached before extensive loss of ventricular function, this could be one form of sudden death.[42]

This manner of considering each incident of myocardial ischemia as a search for an equilibrium and hence as an entity capable of development, ie, with the possibilities of worsening, stabilization or recovery, (tendencies that can persist or succeed one another in any combination) permits one to conceive of serious events evolving out of relatively trivial causes. The necessary condition is that the initiating event should generate a situation within which lies the possibility of further aggravation. This condition of dynamism is fulfilled by the model under consideration. The magnification of the effect of a cause by a multiplier or cascade mechanism is of special significance in attempting to grasp a clinical situation where no sufficient cause is evident. Where a sufficient cause exists, the understanding of the situation is problem-free. Thus, in exercise-induced angina and pacing-induced angina, the exercise and the pacing are causes sufficient to explain the angina, which, indeed, in most cases disappears soon after the cessation of exertion or pacing. Then, thrombosis, embolism, and spasm of major coronary arteries are generally recognized as sufficient causes of myocardial infarction and sudden death, although whether they are important or frequent causes is under active dispute.[43] However, when one turns to unstable angina pectoris, which is inherently unpredictable (unpredictable because no sufficient cause directly antedates the attack), mechanisms with some form of multiplier effect would seem essential for it to be comprehended. Part of the increased oxygen demand was due to increased wall stress, but what was the cause of this increase and hence, the cause of the attack? One suspects that the cause was often too trivial to be noticed by the investigators, and thus, it could have produced its effect only by being imperceptibly magnified to, or beyond, some threshold to precipitate the attack. Gorlin,[44] calling "spontaneously occurring acute myocardial ischemia" a misnomer, is satisfied that the alteration in mechanical factors leading to increased oxygen demand is the cause in most cases. One would then like to know whether the "alterations in mechanical factors" were "spontaneous." A mechanism similar in nature to the one being discussed would seem essential to resolve the difficulty and to make unstable, unprovoked angina understandable. The readiness to set such multiplier or cascade mechanisms in motion would determine the degree of instability of the angina. Background factors will, of course, interact with, influence, and often predominate over this mechanism: long-term factors such as increasing coronary stenosis, coronary collateral development, myocardial hypertrophy and degeneration, and increasing impedance via hypertension and aortic sclerosis, and short-term factors such as variation in sympathetic tone, in propensity to coronary artery spasm, in platelet adhesiveness and release of thromboxane A_2, in thyroid stimulation, in level of hematocrit and undoubtedly others. Each of these factors is independently variable in its capacity to aggravate or ameliorate the tendency toward myocardial ischemia. On the interactive model described each would provide a unified concept of sufficient pliancy to make the multiform manifestations of ischemic heart disease comprehensible.

An account of the possible manner in which an attack of unprovoked angina pectoris evolves needs to be given. Coronary autoregulation is a well recognized phenomenon.[29,30] This means that an increase in myocardial oxygen demand tends to produce a fall in coronary vascular resistance and hence, an increase in coronary resistance and a fall in coronary flow. Thus, in conditions of increasing oxygen demand, coronary blood flow increases with, while lagging behind, demand, and in conditions of falling oxygen demand, coronary blood flow also falls, but with a relative excess over demand. That is to say, in rising demand there is relative ischemia; in falling demand there is relative hyperemia. This is a schematic way of appreciating that demand and supply never precisely match for any length of time, that coronary flow constantly fluctuates between small excess and small deficit, minor hyperemia and minor ischemia.

Usually, the excesses soon disappear, and the deficits are easily made up, except in the at-risk heart or the heart with a narrowed limit of deficit. In such a heart the "normal" fluctuation of supply below demand could trigger incipient, localized ischemia, which in turn could be built up by the multiplier mechanism into angina pectoris, or even into infarction or sudden death. As Hood[28] states in a theoretical discussion, minor inadequacies of local coronary flow, especially in a damaged heart, would be sufficient to impair left ventricular function. This then would be sufficient to spark off a multiplier round of disturbances. These minor inadequacies of flow could arise in many ways; for instance, slight and transient increases in blood pressure, or heart rate, trivial increase in coronary vasomotor tone, fleeting platelet aggregates and other minimal events, which, if a multiplier mechanism were not available to them, would be of no significance.

It is necessary to ask whether or not there is any direct evidence for such a multiplier mechanism in angina pectoris. Minimal events and the early rounds of the multiplier would seem too subtle to be detectable, and most observations are of the large events and the more advanced occurrences. However, Maseri et al[45] were able to make detailed electrocardiographic, hemodynamic, and clinical recordings of attacks of spontaneous angina pectoris. The sequence they invariably found was:

electrical ischemia→mechanical dysfunction and
hemodynamic change→symptomatology→further hemodynamic change
followed by a subsidence in the reverse order.

A multiplier of aggravation interacting with a multiplier of improvement would seem an eminently suitable model to explain this sequence. Furthermore, if the multiplier mechanism were of importance in angina pectoris, one would expect a greater preponderance of subclinical ischemic episodes over clinical attacks. Continuous ECG monitoring with respect to ST-segments[46,47] has indeed shown that this is the case. However, this observation would also be compatible with other views of angina.

Unstable angina pectoris could be a long-lasting condition, the tendency to unpredictable and unprovoked angina being persistent over months or years. Impending infarction, however, can be only of short duration. It can mean only the relatively short run up of unstable angina to infarction. Often this short run up cools off into stable angina or the asymptomatic state.[18] What is the nature of this cooling off? How does a brittle disequilibrium in the myocardial oxygen demand/coronary blood supply relationship become less brittle? Or, to use the language of the model described, how does the multiplier mechanism become toned down? Fluctuations in sympathetic tone in the tendency to coronary artery spasm (if it expresses itself as a tendency) and in platelet function, to mention a few factors, could account for the transformation from severe to milder instability. Similarly, beta-blockade, vasodilators, hypotensives, and treatment of incipient heart failure would appear capable of easing instability. Rest, sedation, and admission to hospital would reduce the incidence of the minimal events that invoke the multiplier mechanism, and so produce symptomatic improvement. But why does this improvement often persist? Every episode of ischemia causes some metabolic and mechanical derangement in the myocardium,[48] albeit temporarily. Oxygen and blood and time are needed to recover from this derangement. The more severe the episode of ischemia, the longer, one would expect, the time to full recovery. Prior to full recovery, the ease of activating a multiplier mechanism would appear to be greater, and if ischemia recurs, the myocardial derangement would tend to be more intense. This is to say that every attack of ischemia makes another attack more likely, and more likely to be more severe, a tendency to a repetitive response, a sort of domino effect. Thus, severe unstable angina pectoris could become self-generating and start a vicious circle, which is approximately the form that impending infarction takes. This sequence can be recognized clearly on occasion in the patient who develops unstable angina pectoris following a severe, exercise-induced attack of angina. The converse could also be true; namely, the longer the pain-free interval, the lesser the likelihood of another episode of ischemia, which implies that cooling off can be of long duration. When intensive efforts to cool off impending infarction fail and breakthrough angina occurs, the prognosis, as Gazes et al[19] found, can be expected to be poor, and radical therapy is called for.

It will be appreciated that the above described dynamic model for the oxygen demand/supply interaction of the heart differs importantly from a straightforward equilibrium model. Physiologically, it is the case that demand/supply balance tends to be maintained and that if the balance is disturbed, mechanisms are set in motion to lead to a new balance. However, if the disturbance is too great, or the compensating mechanisms defective, disequilibrium tendencies can appear that further aggravate the disturbance. Eventually equilibrium is reached, or tends to be reached, but it could be at the cost of any degree of symptomatology and/or pathology. The unsophisticated view that coronary thrombosis causes infarction, that effort, by increasing myocardial oxygen demand, causes angina, and that coronary spasm can cause either, is no doubt at least partly true. Yet, following such events, disequilibrium/equilibrium forces become active, and, it is suggested, the ensuing result, which can seem incompatibly large or small with respect to the cause, is determined by the multiplier mechanism.

REFERENCES

Liberthson, R.R., Nagel, E.L., Hirschman, J.C. et al. Pre-hospital ventricular fibrillation. Prognosis and follow-up course. *N Engl J Med.* 291:317, 1974.

2. Baum, R.S., Alaverez, H., and Cobb, L.A. Survival after resuscitation from out-of-hospital ventricular fibrillation. *Circulation* 50:1231, 1974.

3. Schaffer, W.A., and Cobb, L.A. Recurrent ventricular fibrillation and modes of death in survivors of out-of-hospital ventricular fibrillation. *N Engl J Med.* 293:259, 1975.

4. Blackburn, H. Edited by P.N. Yu, and J.F. Goodwin. In *Progress in Cardiology 3.* Philadelphia: Lea and Febiger, 1974.

5. Myocardial Infarction Community Registers. Copenhagen: World Health Organization, 1976.

6. Juergens, J.L., Edwards, J.E., Achor, R.W.P. et al. Prognosis of patients surviving first clinically diagnosed myocardial infarction. *Arch Intern Med.* 105:134, 1960.

7. Medalie, J.H., and Goldbourt, U. Unrecognized myocardial infarction: five-year incidence, mortality and risk factors. *Ann Intern Med.* 84:526, 1976.

8. Sigler, L.H. Prognosis of angina pectoris and coronary occlusion. Follow up of 1,700 cases. *JAMA.* 146:998, 1951.

9. Block, W.J., Jr., Crumpacker, E.L., Dry, T.J. et al. Prognosis of angina pectoris. Observations in 6,882 cases. *JAMA.* 150:259, 1952.

10. Zuckel, W.J., Cohen, B.M., Mattingly, T.W. et al. Survival following first diagnosis of coronary heart disease. *Am Heart J.* 78:159, 1969.

11. Kannel, W.B., and Feinleib, M. Natural history of angina pectoris in the Framingham study. *Am J Cardiol.* 29:154, 1972.

12. Oberman, A., Jones, W.B., Riley, C.P. et al. Natural history of coronary artery disease. *Bull NY Acad Med.* 48:1109, 1972.

13. Slagel, R.C. Natural history of angiographically documented coronary artery disease. (abstract) *Circulation* 45(suppl II):60, 1972.

14. Bruggraf, G.W., and Parker, J.O. Prognosis in coronary artery disease. *Circulation* 51:146, 1975.

15. Bruschke, A.V.G., Prondfit, W.L., and Sones, F.M. Progress study of 590 consecutive nonsurgical cases of coronary disease followed 5-9 years. *Circulation* 47:1147, 1973.

174

16. Bertolasi, C.A., Trongé, J.E., Carreño, C.A. et al. Unstable angina—prospective and randomized study of its evolution with and without surgery. *Am J Cardiol.* 33:201, 1974.

17. Conti, R., Gilbert, J.B., Hodges, M. et al. Unstable angina pectoris: randomized study of surgical vs medical therapy. (abstract) *Am J Cardiol.* 38:201, 1974.

18. Duncan, B., Fulton, M., Morrison, S.L. et al. Prognosis of new and worsening angina pectoris. *Br Med J.* 1:981, 1976.

19. Gazes, P.C., Mobley, E.M., Faris, H.M., Jr. et al. Pre-infarctional (unstable) angina—a prospective study—ten year follow-up. *Circulation* 48:331, 1973.

20. Kraus, K.R., Hutter, A.M., Jr., and De Sanctis, R.W. Acute coronary insufficiency. Course and follow-up. *Circulation* 45(suppl 1):66, 1972.

21. National Cooperative Study Group: Unstable angina pectoris. In-hospital experience and initial follow-up. *Am J Cardiol.* 42:839, 1978.

22. Heberden, W. Commentaries on the history and cure of diseases. Pectoris dolor. Edited by F.A. Willius, and T.E. Keys. In *Cardiac Classics.* New York: Dover Publications, 1802.

23. Hellstrom, H.R. Coronary artery vasospasm: the likely immediate cause of acute myocardial infarction. *Br Heart J.* 41:426, 1979.

24. Oliva, P.B., and Breckinridge, J.C. Arteriographic evidence of coronary arterial spasm in acute myocardial infarction. *Circulation* 56:366, 1977.

25. Maseri, A., L'Abbate, A., Pesola, A. et al. Coronary vasospasm in angina pectoris. *Lancet* 1:713, 1977.

26. Braunwald, E. Control of myocardial oxygen consumption. *Am J Cardiol.* 27:416, 1971.

27. Braunwald, E. Sonnenblick, E.H., and Ross, J.R. Mechanisms of contraction of the normal and failing heart, 2nd Ed. Boston: Little, Brown and Co., 1976.

28. Hood, W.B., Jr. Pathophysiology of ischemic heart disease. *Prog Cardiovasc Dis.* 14:297, 1971.

29. Berne, R.M. Cardiac nucleotides in hypoxia: possible role in regulation of coronary blood flow. *Am J Physiol.* 204:317, 1963.

30. Green, H.D., and Wegira, R. Effects of asphyxia, anoxia and myocardial ischemia on coronary blood flow. *Am J Physiol.* 135:271, 1942.

31. Rubio, R., Berne, R.M., and Katori, M. Release of adenosine in reactive hyperemia of the dog heart. *Am J Physiol.* 216:56, 1969.

32. Brazier, J., Cooper, N., and Buckberg, G.D. The adequacy of subendocardial oxygen delivery: the interaction of determinants of flow, arterial oxygen content and myocardial oxygen need. *Circulation* 49:968, 1974.

33. Hoffman, J.I.E. Determinants and prediction of transmural myocardial perfusion. *Circulation* 58:381, 1978.

34. Robinson, B.F. Relation of heart rate and systolic blood pressure to the onset of pain in angina pectoris. *Circulation* 35:1073, 1967.

35. Sowton, G.E., Balcon, R., Cross, D. et al. Measurement of anginal threshold using arterial pacing: a new technique for the study of angina pectoris. *Cardiovasc Res.* 1:301, 1967.

36. Oliva, P.B., Potts, D.E., and Pluss, R.G. Coronary spasm in Prinzmetal's angina. Documentation by coronary arteriography. *N Engl J Med.* 288:745, 1973.

37. Tyberg, J.V., Parmley, W.W., and Sonnenblick, E.H. In vitro studies of ventricular asynchrony and regional hypoxia. *Circ Res.* 25:569, 1969.

38. Distante, A., Landini, L., Berassi, A. et al. Echocardiographic changes during vasospastic angina. 3rd Sympsoium on Echocardiology, Rotterdam, 1979.

39. Parker, J.O., Ledwich, J.R., West, R.O. et al. Reversible cardiac failure during angina pectoris: hemodynamic effects of atrial pacing in coronary artery disease. *Circulation* 39:745, 1969.

40. Friesinger, G.C. Edited by D.G. Julian. In *Angina Pectoris.* London: Churchill Livingstone, 1977.

41. Grossman, J., and Mann, J.T. Evidence for impaired left ventricular relaxation during acute ischaemia in man. *Eur J Cardiol.* 7(suppl):239, 1978.

42. Raizes, G., Wagner, G.S., and Hackel, D.B. Instantaneous non-arrhythmic cardiac death in acute myocardial infarction. *Am J Cardiol.* 39:1, 1977.

43. Roberts, W.C., and Buja, L.M. The frequency and significance of coronary arterial thrombi and other observations in fatal acute myocardial infarction. *Am J Med.* 34:870, 1972.

44. Gorlin, R. *Coronary artery disease.* Philadelphia: W.B. Saunders Co., 1976.

45. Maseri, A., Mimmo, R., Chierchia, S. et al. Coronary artery spasm as a cause of acute myocardial ischemia in man. *Chest* 68:625, 1975.

46. Schang, S.J., and Pepine, C.J. Transient asymptomatic ST segment depression during daily activity. *Am J Cardiol.* 39:396, 1977.

47. Selwyn, A.P., Fox, K., Eves, M. et al. Myocardial ischaemia in patients with frequent angina pectoris. *Br Med J.* 4:1594, 1978.

48. Jennings, R.B. Early phase of myocardial ischaemic injury and infarction. *Am J Cardiol.* 24:753, 1969.

SECTION IV

Surgical Therapy for Unstable Angina

12 Anesthesia for Patients with Unstable Angina

Sallie J. Teasdale, MD

Anesthesia for the patient with unstable angina presents a real challenge to the anesthesiologist. This class of patient is intermediate between stable angina and acute myocardial infarction, and even without the stress of anesthesia and surgery the incidence of infarction and death during the first year after diagnosis has been reported to vary from 10% to more than 50%.[1]

Studies at our center have shown a significantly higher CPK-MB release and infarction rate associated with revascularization procedures for patients with unstable angina as compared with those for patients with stable angina.[2]

The anesthesiologist concerned with this precarious group of patients must have a complete understanding of the pathophysiology of the potentially ischemic myocardium; he must provide continuous monitoring for prevention or early recognition of myocardial ischemia, and he must use anesthetic agents and techniques least likely to unfavorably upset the delicate balance between myocardial oxygen supply and demand. Imbalance in the myocardial oxygen supply:demand ratio appears to be the essential underlying mechanism of myocardial ischemia and injury. The determinants of each are listed in Table 12-1.

PREOPERATIVE EVALUATION

Preoperative assessment places the patient into one of two major groups: a) unstable angina with good ventricular function, ie, no congestive heart failure, ejection fraction (EF) greater than 0.4, left ventricular end-diastolic pressure (LVEDP) less than 15 mm Hg, and cardiac index (CI) more than 2.5 liters/min/m²; and b) unstable angina with poor left ventricular function, ie, history of multiple myocardial infarctions; signs and symptoms of congestive heart failure; LVEDP more than 18 mm Hg; EF less than 0.4; areas of left ventricular hypokinesia or akinesia; and history of episodic shortness of breath with angina. Adequacy of left ven-

Table 12-1
Determinants of Myocardial Oxygen Supply and Demand

Myocardial Oxygen Supply Myocardial Perfusion	Myocardial Oxygen Demand (MVO_2)
Degree of coronary artery stenosis	Heart rate
Perfusion pressure (aortic diastolic pressure − LVEDP)	Contractile state
Distal coronary artery resistance (vascular tone + blood viscosity)	Wall tension Aortic systolic BP LVEDP
Extracoronary artery bed resistance	Ventricular geometry or synergy Wall thickness
Transmyocardial pressure gradient	
Collateral blood flow	
Diastolic time	
Oxygen Content Hemoglobin	
PaO_2	
pH	
$PaCO_2$	
2,3 DPG	

tricular function influences the whole anesthetic approach and must be recognized. Patients with good ventricular function require suppressive anesthesia to avoid hypertension and tachycardia, while those with poor ventricular function require nondepressant agents to avoid hypotension and elevated LVEDP.

Once the function of the ventricle has been assessed, one may consider vessel involvement. Left main coronary artery stenosis or left main equivalent, proximal left anterior descending coronary artery lesions, and multiple-vessel involvement mean more of the ventricle is at risk and the patient is less able to tolerate ischemia. The severity of the obstruction and the function of collateral flow should be noted, as should the presence or absence of coronary spasm during catheterization. There is growing evidence that angina at rest or angina of a prolonged duration may be indicative of coronary artery spasm either superimposed on a fixed atherosclerotic plaque or involving collateral flow to the ischemic zone. Figueras et al,[3] by providing continuous hemodynamic monitoring of 23 patients with rest pain, were able to demonstrate in some the development of acute left ventricular failure (increasing pulmonary artery diastolic pressure) associated with ischemic ECG changes without significant alterations in major determinants of myocardial oxygen consumption. The results suggest a decrease in myocardial perfusion as the primary mechanism of rest angina in many patients with coronary artery disease. Patients who show very little reduction in frequency or severity of angina with increasing propranolol dosage, or who show characteristic changes of Prinzmetal's angina, may also fall into this subset. These patients respond best to nitrates, and intravenous nitroglycerin should be infused preoperatively, perioperatively and postoperatively.

The patient with unstable angina and established systemic hypertension merits special attention.[4] This is the patient who is most susceptible to surges of blood pressure during laryngoscopy and intubation,[5] has the highest incidence of dysrhythmias (especially ventricular premature beats [VPBs]) and exhibits the greatest hemodynamic instability postoperatively. These patients do better if their antihypertensive drugs (with the exception of monomine oxidase inhibitors) are continued until the day of surgery.[6]

ANESTHETIC MANAGEMENT

Preoperative Sedation

Few operations produce such anxiety in the patient as do heart operations. Added to this is the feeling of doom often associated with severe angina. A calm, unhurried explanation by the anesthesiologist of what to expect in the next few days may help to allay that anxiety.

Patients are premedicated with a combination of diazepam and/or morphine and hyoscine. The dose is varied to produce a well-sedated patient. Slightly smaller doses are required in the patient with compromised ventricular function.

Although coronary artery disease is a regional perfusion deficiency, adequacy of localized perfusion is not easily measured, and medical management as well as anesthetic management is aimed primarily at reduction of global oxygen demand. Propranolol has often been pushed to very high levels to accomplish this in the patient with unstable angina. In order to avoid the rebound effect of discontinuation of propranolol,[7] and recognizing that endogenous catecholamines are elevated in the 24 hours prior to surgery,[8] propranolol therapy should be continued until the time of surgery.

Propranolol therapy decreases the three major determinants of myocardial oxygen consumption (heart rate, contractility, and systolic blood pressure) (see Table 12-1), and has been shown to decrease the extent of acute myocardial infarction.[9,10] As well, oxygen delivery to the tissues may be facilitated by a shift of the oxygen dissociation curve to the right.[11]

Studies done in our hospital have shown that small doses of propranolol (10 to 20 mg four times a day) may well control heart rate at rest but may not produce therapeutic blood levels (30 to 50 ng/ml) sufficient to block tachycardic response to stress. We have found a linear relationship between the oral dose taken chronically and plasma levels two hours after the last oral dose. Propranolol dosage of 60 mg or more four times a day could be discontinued the night before surgery and the patient would usually arrive in the operating room at 8 AM with therapeutic blood levels and adequate beta-blockade effect. Patients with unstable angina on 40 mg or less four times a day usually had inadequate nonprotective blood levels by the following morning and could profit from a repeat dose of 20 to 40 mg by mouth two hours preoperatively, depending on left ventricular function. However, continuing patients on full-dose propranolol therapy until two hours preoperatively and maintaining blood levels with IV infusion of propranolol (1 Mg/hr) did not effect a reduction in incidence of perioperative myocardial injury as measured by ECG changes or CPK-MB release when compared with patients whose propranolol was discontinued the night before.[12] Thus, although some beta blockade is advantageous to control perioperative sympathetic response, we could not show that more was of any greater advantage, and it could add to difficulties of weaning from cardiopulmonary bypass postoperatively. Patients who received beta-blocking drugs postoperatively could not compensate as well for hypovolemia by increasing contractility or heart rate and had to be given replacement volume very carefully.

Nitroglycerin, on the other hand, not only decreases oxygen demand by decreasing preload and wall tension, but may also increase coronary perfusion to the ischemic area by decreasing intramyocardial pressure and causing vasodilatation of coronary vasculature with resultant increase in collateral blood flow.[13] We continue nitroglycerin as a cutaneous paste one hour before induction and by continuous IV infusion in the operating room in the patient who has been on chronic vasodilator therapy, has a high resting LVEDP, gives a history of rest angina, or is known to have coronary artery spasm.

The patient with unstable angina and ECG changes on his resting ECG should be considered for preoperative intraaortic balloon pumping (IABP). If the patient is hemodynamically stable, IABP is not necessary, but significant left ventricular dysfunction with evidence of recent myocardial infarction should make IABP a serious consideration preoperatively.[14]

The patient with chronic or episodic signs of left ventricular failure or with an elevated LVEDP should be partially digitalized before surgery.

Monitoring

When the sedated patient arrives in the operating room he is transferred to the operating table and immediately connected to a seven-lead electrocardiograph (limb leads, augmented limb leads and a precordial lead V_5) with a calibrated write-out. A trace is recorded for future reference. As yet we have no better monitor for early recognition of myocardial ischemia than the ECG. In most cases the location of the ST-segment change correlates with the arteriographic localization of the patient's coronary artery disease,[15] so that the lead showing the most change with angina preoperatively would be the lead to monitor continuously in the operating room. This is usually V_5. Blackburn et al[16] showed that 89% of ST-segment information contained in the conventional 12-lead exercise ECG is found in lead V_5, while Mason et al[17] showed that in 56 patients with ST-segment changes, leads V_4 and V_6 were the most informative.

Under local anesthesia a #20 gauge Teflon needle is inserted into the radial artery after establishing the presence of a collateral ulnar artery circulation using the Allen test to allow continuous readout of arterial pressure and to obtain periodic blood gas, hematocrit, and electrolyte estimations.

Swan-Ganz catheterization is indicated in all patients with unstable angina and compromised left ventricular function. Recent studies have shown that myocardial ischemia is not predictable by monitoring pulmonary capillary wedge pressure (PCWP) in patients with normal left ventricular function, but can be predictive in those with poor ventricular function.[18] Insertion of Swan-Ganz catheters has been shown by one group to be associated with significant increases in arterial pressure and heart rate in the awake premedicated patients,[19] and we usually insert them after induction in the unstable patient believing that undetected increases in PCWP during intubation is the lesser risk except in the severely decompensated patient. Estimations of cardiac output by thermodilution, calculation of systemic and pulmonary vascular resistances, and the establishment of a Starling left ventricular function curve is essential to choose between vasodilators and inotropes in the failing heart.

In patients with normal left (and right) ventricular function a central venous pressure catheter and perioperative left atrial line should suffice.

The most likely times for sympathetic nervous system response stimulating hypertension and tachycardia are during intubation, skin incision, sternotomy, and the first four hours in the recovery room. These periods require special alertness to keep the heart rate below 90 beats/min and the rate-pressure product less than 12,000. These are the oxygen demand limits established by Kaplan and Jones[20] to avoid ischemia in patients under anesthesia undergoing aortocoronary bypass. Hypotension, a threat to coronary perfusion, is more likely to occur during cannulation and manipulation of the heart before bypass (interference with venous return and sinus rhythm) and sometimes coming off bypass after a prolonged period of ischemic arrest. This fall in blood pressure usually responds to restoration of rhythm, increasing blood volume, or, postbypass, the administration of intravenous calcium chloride.

INDUCTION

All patients have a large bore (#14-gauge) intravenous catheter inserted and 300 to 500 ml of crystalloid solution administered, as peripheral vasodilation associated with sedation may exaggerate the hypovolemia found in patients with coronary artery disease.[21] Anesthesia is induced with a loading dose of fentanyl, at least 5 μg/kg, followed by 1 to 2 mg of pancuronium to prevent rigidity, and diazepam in 5-mg increments until consciousness is lost. Fentanyl, a synthetic narcotic 100 times more potent than morphine, exhibits no clinically significant hemodynamic effects in doses up to 50 μg/kg, except a desirable bradycardia.[22] In contrast to morphine, there is no histamine release or dilatation of venous capacitance vessels. It is remarkably effective in blocking the sympathetic response to laryngoscopy and intubation and is the ideal drug in the patient with unstable angina, even in the presence of poor left ventricular function.

Diazepam, a benzodiazepine tranquilizer, is superior to barbiturates for induction because in the small doses used it is associated with only a small reduction in arterial blood pressure (5% to 20%), and slight fall in cardiac output and LVEDP.[23] It may also produce coronary vasodilatation.[24] Certainly, hypnosis is more prolonged and associated with some amnesia.

Pancuronium bromide (0.1 mg/kg) is the muscle relaxant most frequently used and, following a fentanyl reduction, results in a very stable hemodynamic response. Addition of 50% nitrous oxide lowers the anesthesia level and, although it may significantly depress cardiac output in the failing heart, it has very slight depressant effect on a normal left ventricle.

We monitored the endocardial viability ratio (EVR)

$$\frac{\text{Diastolic pressure time index - PCWP}}{\text{Systolic pressure time index}}$$

as a clinical index of epicardial/endocardial blood flow[25] during three different induction techniques and found the fentanyl citrate and diazepam combination to preserve this ratio very well.[26] This comparison is represented graphically in Figure 12-1.

ENDOCARDIAL
VIABILITY RATIO (E.V.R.)

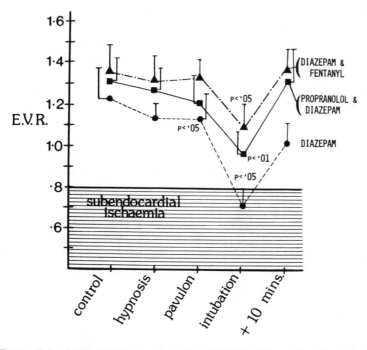

Figure 12-1   Graph showing a comparison of three different induction techniques on endocardial viability ratio. Techniques include: 1) diazepam (0.5 mg/kg) and fentanyl (5.0 μg/kg), 2) diazepam (0.5 mg/kg) and continued full dose oral propranolol, and 3) diazepam (0.5 mg/kg).

The development of tachycardia and hypertension in patients with good ventricular function is controlled with myocardial depressants such as enflurane or halothane, while carefully titrated nitroglycerin infusion is the first line of approach to the control of blood pressure in the patient with poor left ventricular function. Persistent hypertension may require infusion of the more potent vasodilator, nitroprusside. Longer acting narcotics, (ie, morphine 1 mg/kg) are usually used to maintain anesthesia after induction.

Tachyarrhythmias may be managed with incremental doses of intravenous propranolol (0.5–1.0 mg).

ON BYPASS

Anesthesia administration is discontinued as cardiopulmonary bypass is begun. Hypothermia to 24°C to 28°C diminishes the need for any anesthetic agent on bypass as indicated by EEG. The sudden hemodilution and drop in hematocrit produced by initiation of cardiopulmonary bypass results in a sudden fall in total vascular resistance and hypotension, which at normothermia may necessitate the use of an alpha agonist (eg, phenylephrine) to maintain perfusion pressures between 70 and 100 torr. Systemic cooling to 25°C will restore systemic vascular resistance to normal when the hematocrit is 20%.[27] Hematocrits should approach 30% or more when the patient is rewarmed to 37°C. Hematocrits of less than 20% may significantly lower total oxygen transport and make the maintenance of normal PaO_2, $PaCO_2$, and pH critical. Serum potassium levels fluctuate with temperature and cardioplegia and should be in the high normal range (4.5 to 5.0 mEq/liter) at the end of bypass.

Patients with poor left ventricular function may require an inotropic agent to maintain cardiac output with discontinuation of bypass. The appropriate drug will depend upon left atrial pressure, cardiac output estimations, pulmonary and systemic resistance, cardiac rate and rhythm, and urine output. Possible inotropes include calcium chloride, dopamine, dobutamine, isoproterenol, and epinephrine. Nitroprusside may be required to decrease left ventricular wall tension. Continued poor ventricular performance or persistent ST elevation may require insertion of the intraaortic balloon pump.

TRANSPORT

At the conclusion of the operation the patient must be safely moved to the intensive care unit. We do not attempt this transfer until blood pressure and heart rhythm are stable and blood volume replacement, blood gases, and electrolytes are considered optimal for the particular patient. A continuous display of ECG, blood pressure, and LVEDP equivalent is mandatory throughout transfer and is accomplished using a battery-powered three-channel portable oscilloscope. A portable battery-powered defibrillator is included if the patient has demonstrated evidence of ventricular irritability. Ventilation during transport is accomplished by a self-inflating resuscitation bag with supplemental oxygen or a pressure-cycled Bird ventilator. Delivered tidal volume and inspired oxygen concentration is checked before the patient leaves the operating room.

POSTOPERATIVE PERIOD

Unfortunately, the postoperative period can still be a time of major concern. Although the heart has been surgically revascularized beyond the major stenoses, there are frequently diseased peripheral vessels with residual small areas of potential myocardial ischemia. As well, coronary spasm of collateral or diseased vessels is still a possibility. Blood volume redistribution with rewarming and diuresis can produce hemodynamic instability, which could threaten the patency of the aortocoronary graft. The same cardiac risk factors that apply to patients undergoing noncardiac surgery hold some relevance for the aortocoronary bypass patient as well. Recent preoperative myocardial infarction (within six months), preoperative congestive failure, preoperative dysrhythmias, especially premature ventricular contractions, age of more than seventy, preoperative aortic stenosis, or mitral insufficiency and intraoperative hypotension are all factors that may adversely influence the postoperative course.[28] Patients undergoing noncardiac surgery have the highest incidence of perioperative infarctions from the third[29] to the fifth postoperative day.[28]

The aortocoronary bypass patients are at special risk postoperatively because tissue temperature gradients that may persist as a result of inadequate rewarming time cause shivering and arterial hypoxemia and so compromise oxygen-carrying capacity at a time when hematocrits may still be low. Warming blankets and care taken to normalize core temperature before allowing patients to become unparalyzed prevent this complication. Potassium shifts with temperature change and postoperative diuresis require vigilant attention to avoid hypokalemic-induced dysrhythmias. We strive to keep serum potassium between 4.5 and 5.5 mEq/liter postoperatively via routine potassium chloride infusion based on hourly urine volumes.

Systemic hypertension is the main hemodynamic problem. Of 158 aortocoronary bypass patients followed postoperatively, we found a 70% incidence of hypertension (more than 140/90 mm Hg) within one hour postoperatively and a 31% incidence after four hours, in patients without established hypertension preoperatively.

Hypertension can be controlled by nitroglycerin infusion, or, if more persistent, by nitroprusside infusion and usually resolves in four to eight hours without the need of continuing therapy. A more perplexing problem was that of tachycardia. We found about 28% of these patients exhibited a persistent tachycardia (more than 100 beats/min) for more than 24 hours not always responsive to therapy with beta blockade and with no obvious cause or obvious deleterious effect.

Patients with a history of preoperative hypertension invariably require nitroprusside intraoperatively and postoperatively and the early reinstitution of preoperative longer acting vasodilators for smoother blood pressure control.

Immediately postoperatively, myocardial function may be (transiently) depressed by intraoperative manipulations, and right-sided pressures cannot be assumed to be indicative of left-sided pressures. A left atrial line or Swan-Ganz catheter is mandatory.

Patients are usually mechanically ventilated overnight via an endotracheal tube using either intermittent mandatory or assisted ventilation and 5 cm H_2O positive end-expiratory pressure. Extubation in the morning (or sometimes earlier) is indicated in most cases when the patient is awake, the hematocrit is greater than 30%, cardiac performance is adequate with no life-threatening dysrhythmias, vital capacity is greater than 10 cc/kg and inspiratory force is greater than 20 to 25 cm H_2O, and electrolytes and coagulation time are within normal limits. After extubation, all patients require supplemental oxygen for several days, while a very few may require it for one to two weeks.

SUMMARY

Anesthesia for the patient with unstable angina requires careful preoperative assessment of the adequacy of ventricular function and of the critical nature of myocardial oxygen supply in terms of degree of stenosis, vessels affected, collateral supply, and possibility of coronary spasm. All other preexisting pathologic conditions that might have some effect on myocardial demands or anesthesia management must be considered, ie, pulmonary disease, renal or endocrine disease, hypertension, etc. The depression of global oxygen demand as obtained by medical therapy with drugs such as propranolol and the nitrates must be maintained but not to the detriment of myocardial function postbypass. Adequate preoperative sedation combined with intravenous fentanyl and diazepam anesthetizes the patient effectively and blocks sympathetic response to laryngoscopy, but does not significantly depress myocardial function. Potent inhalational agents and long-acting narcotics are used as required to maintain hemodynamic equilibrium after induction. Alert ECG and pressure monitoring as instituted preinduction is continued throughout the operation and into the recovery room phase. A comprehensive understanding of the pathophysiology of the potentially ischemic myocardium and of the pharmacology of all drugs involved is essential to the anesthetic management of this precarious group of patients.

REFERENCES

1. Report of Task Force appointed by the Deputy Ministers of Health. Manifestations and natural history of coronary artery disease: development and evaluation of aortocoronary bypass surgery. *Can Med Assoc J.* 117(5):451–459, 1977.

2. Weisel, R.D., Shardey, G., Teasdale, S.J. et al. Myocardial performance in unstable angina. (abstract) Proceedings of the 30th meeting of the Canadian Cardiovascular Society, Toronto, October 1977.

3. Figueras, J., Singh, B.N., Ganz, W. et al. Mechanism of rest and noctural angina: observations during continuous hemodynamic and electrocardiographic monitoring. *Circulation* 59:955–968, 1979.

4. Prys-Roberts, C., Greene, L.T., Meloche, R. et al. Studies of anesthesia in relation to hypertension. I. Cardiovascular responses of treated and untreated patients. *Br J Anaesth.* 43:122, 1971.

5. Prys-Roberts, C., Greene, L.T., Meloche, R. et al. Studies of anesthesia in relation to hypertension. II. Haemodynamic consequences of induction and endotracheal intubation. *Br J Anaesth.* 43:531, 1971.

6. Edwards, W.T. Letter to the Editor. Preanesthetic management of the hypertensive patient. *N Engl J Med.* 301(3):158, 1979.

7. Miller, R.R., Olson, H.G., Amsterdam, E.A. et al. Propranolol withdrawal rebound phenomenon. *N Engl J Med.* 293:416, 1975.

8. Boudoulas, H., Snyder, G.L., Lewis, R.P. et al. Safety and rationale for continuation of propranolol therapy during coronary bypass operation. *Ann Thorac Surg.* 26:222, 1978.

9. Norris, R.M., Clarke, E.D., Sammel, N.L. et al. Protective effect of propranolol in threatened myocardial infarction. *Lancet* 2:907, 1978.

10. Peter, T., Norris, R.M., Clarke, E.D. et al. Reduction of enzyme level by propranolol after acute myocardial infarction. *Circulation* 57:1091–1095, 1978.

11. Schrumpf, J.D., Sheps, D.S., Wolfson, S. et al. Altered hemoglobin-oxygen affinity with long-term propranolol therapy in patients with coronary artery disease. *Am J Cardiol.* 40:76, 1977.

12. Dosch, E., Teasdale, S. Continued propranolol therapy for myocardial protection during anesthesia for AC bypass surgery. (In press).

13. Logue, R.B., King, S.B., Douglas, J.S. A practical approach to coronary artery disease, with special reference to coronary bypass surgery. Edited by W.P. Harvey. In *Current Problems in Cardiology.* Vol. 1, Chicago: Year Book Medical Publishers, 1976.

14. Jones, E.L., Douglas, J.S., Craver, J.M. et al. Results of coronary revascularization in patients with recent myocardial infarction. *J Thorac Cardiovasc Surg.* 76:545, 1978.

15. Robertson, D., Kostuk, W.T., Ahuja, S.P. The localization of coronary artery stenosis by 12-lead ECG response to graded exercise test. *Am Heart J.* 91:437, 1976.

190

16. Blackburn, H., Taylor, H.L., Okamoto, N. et al. The exercise electrocardiogram: a systematic comparison of chest lead configurations employed for monitoring during exercise. Edited by M. Karlomen. In *Physical Activity and the Heart*. Springfield, Ill.: Charles C Thomas, 1966.

17. Mason, R.E., Likar, I., Biern, R.O. et al. Multiple lead exercise electrocardiography. *Circulation* 36:517, 1967.

18. Lieberman, R.W., Schartz, A.J., Jobes, D.R. et al. Wedge pressure as a predictor of ischemia during CABG. (abstract) *Anesthesiology* 51(suppl 3):S59, 1979.

19. Lunn, J.K., and Stanley, T.H. Arterial blood pressure and pulse rate responses to pulmonary artery catheterization prior to cardiac and major vascular surgery. Abstracts of Scientific Papers, American Society of Anesthesiology Annual Meeting, 1978, pp. 577–578.

20. Kaplan, J.A., and Jones, E. L. Monitoring of myocardial ischemia during coronary artery surgery (abstract) Presented at the Annual Meeting of the American Society of Anesthesiologists, 1977, pp. 507–508.

21. Cohn, L.H., Moore, F.D., and Collins, J.J. Intrinsic plasma volume deficits in patients with coronary artery disease. *Arch Surg.* 108:57, 1974.

22. Stanley, T.H., and Webster, L.R. Anesthetic requirements and cardiovascular effects of fentanyl-oxygen and fentanyl-diazepam-oxygen anesthesia in man. *Anesth Analg.* (Cleve) 57:411–416, 1978.

23. Côté, P., Campeau, L., and Bourassa, M.G. Therapeutic implications of diazepam in patients with elevated left ventricular filling pressure. *Am Heart J.* 91:747, 1976.

24. Ikran, H., Rubin, A.P., and Jewkes, R.F. Effect of diazepam on myocardial blood flow of patients with and without coronary artery disease. *Br Heart J.* 35:626–630, 1973.

25. Philips, P.A., Marty, A.T., and Miyamoto, A.M. A clinical method for detecting subendocardial ischemia after cardiopulmonary bypass. *J Thorac Cardiovasc Surg.* 69:30–36, 1975.

26. Teasdale, S.J., Heiner, M.M., Goldman, B.S. et al. Comparison of induction techniques on cardiac stress and performance in patients for aorto-coronary bypass surgery. *Can Anaesth Soc J.* (In press).

27. Gordon, R.J., Ravin, M.B. Rheology and anesthesia. *Anesth Analg.* 57:252–261, 1978.

28. Goldman, L., Caldera, D.L., Southwick, F.S. et al. Cardiac risk factors and complications in non-cardiac surgery. *Medicine* 57(4):357–370, 1978.

29. Tarhan, S., Moffitt, E.A., Taylor, W.F. et al. Myocardial infarction after general anesthesia. *JAMA.* 220:1451, 1972.

13 Myocardial Protection During Surgery for Unstable Angina

Richard D. Weisel, MD,
Robert J. Cusimano,
Sallie J. Teasdale, MD,
Bernard S. Goldman, MD, and
Ronald J. Baird, MD

The goal of perioperative myocardial protection is to minimize the morbidity and mortality when aortocoronary bypass is performed for unstable angina. The results of surgery for stable angina are dependent on the extent of coronary artery disease and the degree of impairment of left ventricular function. Patients undergoing urgent or semielective surgery, because rest pain is not controlled by medical management, face a higher perioperative risk. In these patients the extent of preoperative ischemic injury appears to influence significantly the results obtained. The technique of intraoperative myocardial protection is more important in patients with unstable than stable angina because preoperative ischemia renders these patients more sensitive to perioperative injury. In addition, the surgical risks appear to correlate with the extent of preoperative ischemia. The uniform decrease in the hospital mortality and incidence of perioperative complications has rendered these clinical indices insensitive to perioperative events. To adequately evaluate the adequacy of perioperative myocardial protection of patients undergoing aortocoronary bypass for unstable angina, they must be subdivided according to the extent of their preoperative ischemia, and more sensitive indices of perioperative injury must be employed.

The report of Adams et al[1] describes an improved perioperative mortality in patients with preinfarction angina when potassium cardioplegia is employed rather than intermittent anoxic arrest. An exact definition of preinfarction angina is necessary in order to determine whether case selection or the technique of myocardial protection significantly influenced the results of surgery.

At the University of Toronto hospitals in the past two years, 1240 patients have undergone elective coronary bypass. There was a 1.8% hospital mortality and a 4.2% incidence of perioperative infarction. This low incidence of morbidity and mortality makes these factors insensitive to changes in perioperative protection. A study group of 165 patients had a similar perioperative morbidity and mortality. However, when CK-MB and the hemodynamic response to volume loading were measured serially following surgery, substantial alterations were discovered in most patients. These alterations can be quantitated, and the results employed to evaluate the type of myocardial protection used.

Fifty-four patients undergoing triple aortocoronary bypass grafting were prospectively evaluated to determine the influence of myocardial protective techniques on the result of aortocoronary bypass surgery. Table 13-1 illustrates the distribution of patients in the study group. Twenty-three patients had stable angina pectoris and were undergoing elective surgery. Thirty-one patients had unstable angina pectoris and underwent elective or semielective (same hospitalization) surgery. Patients with unstable angina had episodes of prolonged rest pain despite medical attention. Eighty-seven percent of these patients had reversible new ischemic electrocardiographic changes; whereas the remaining 13% did not. No patient had elevation of standard enzymes, and the new ischemic changes did not appear to persist after the pain was relieved in the preoperative period.

Table 13-1
Fifty-four Patients Undergoing Triple Aortocoronary Bypass Grafting Divided into Four Groups Dependent on Their Clinical Presentation and the Technique of Intraoperative Myocardial Presentation.

No. of Patients	
	Clinical presentation
23	Stable angina (SA)
31	Unstable angina (UA)
	Myocardial presentation
25	Intermittent anoxic arrest (IAA) 28°C
29	Cold potassium cardioplegia (CPC) 20°C

Two myocardial preservation techniques were employed. In 25 patients distal anastomoses were performed with episodes of intermittent anoxic arrest. Systemic temperature was maintained at 28°C during the performance of the distal anastomoses. In the other 29 patients, distal anastomoses were performed during the single aortic cross-clamp period. A cold potassium cardioplegic solution was infused into the aortic root to induce immediate cardioplegia and produce profound cardiac hypothermia. The technique of cardioplegia had a significant influence on the adequacy of the protection afforded by this method. Interventricular septal myocardial temperature was continuously monitored. Sufficient cardioplegic solution was infused to lower the septal temperature to near 15°C. As illustrated in Figure 13-1, the myocardial temperature tends to rise shortly after the cardioplegic infusion is discontinued. Therefore, multiple infusions are necessary to maintain the temperature below 24°C. To ensure a cold myocardium, the systemic temperature must be lowered to 25°C. The mean myocardial temperature is calculated as the mean of the integral under the temperature-time curve as recorded from the interventricular septal thermistor probe.

The distribution of the 54 patients is outlined in Figure 13-2. There were 13 patients with unstable angina and 12 with stable angina who had an aortocoronary bypass performed using intermittent anoxic arrest. Eighteen

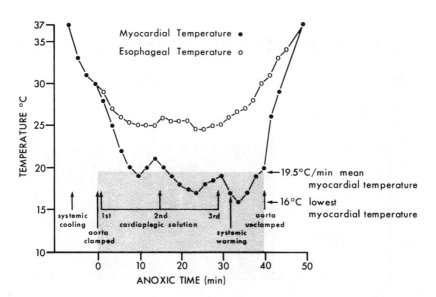

Figure 13-1 The interventricular septal temperature during the use of cold potassium cardioplegia for a triple aortocoronary bypass procedure is illustrated. Three doses of the cardioplegic solution were required to induce a significant fall in septal temperature. The most appropriate temperature during arrest is the mean rather than the lowest myocardial temperature attained.

with unstable and eleven with stable angina had an aortocoronary bypass performed using cold potassium cardioplegia. Since all patients were undergoing triple aortocoronary bypass grafting, the extent of coronary artery disease was found to be the same in all groups. In addition, left ventricular function was not different between groups.

To evaluate the adequacy of the two myocardial protective techniques, serial measurements of a cardiac specific enzyme (CK-MB) were made in the perioperative period. A new antibody inhibition technique was employed to measure postoperative isoenzyme concentrations[2] (Mickle, D.A.G., Washington, G., and Porter, D.J., unpublished data). The patient's serum was exposed to an anti-M antiserum (Merck) in order to block the activity of M subunits of CK. The resultant creatinine phosphokinase activity was felt to reflect the amount of CK-MB present in the original serum.

Postoperatively, all patients were found to have elevations in CK-MB. The highest values were found between one and two hours following anoxic arrest. No patients had CK-MB present 12 hours postoperatively. The peak value was determined for each patient. It is likely that the peak value is representative of the area under the concentration-time curve. We have

PATIENTS UNDERGOING TRIPLE ACB

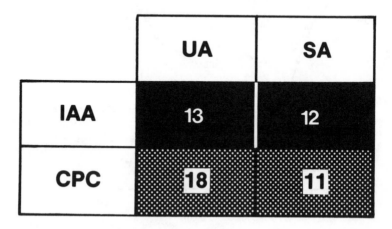

Figure 13-2   The four subgroups of patients undergoing aortocoronary bypass surgery is illustrated. They include patients with stable (SA) or unstable (UA) angina receiving either intermittent anoxic arrest (IAA) or cold potassium cardioplegia (CPC) for intraoperative myocardial protection.

employed the peak value as indicative of the amount of enzyme released from the heart. Previous studies have confirmed this impression (Mickle et al, unpublished data).

Myocardial performance was evaluated in each patient. A Swan-Ganz thermodilution cardiac output catheter was inserted through a central vein preoperatively. Left ventricular filling pressure (LVFP) was measured using either pulmonary artery wedge pressure (PWAP) or left atrial pressure (LAP). Myocardial performance was evaluated by measuring the hemodynamic response to volume loading. Before and immediately after cardiopulmonary bypass, blood was infused from the pump oxygenator to raise the LVFP.

Figure 13-3 demonstrates the response to this volume load. Cardiac output was measured with each 2- to 4-mm increase in LVFP. Cardiac index was then plotted against LVFP. In addition, stroke work index (SWI) was calculated from the primary data and also plotted against LVFP for each volume loading episode.

$$SWI = \frac{(CI)}{P} (MAP - LVFP) \quad (13.6)$$

The curves were then qualitatively compared. Any qualitative differences in the cardiac index (CI) and stroke work index volume loading curves were scrutinized. Any measurements that had more than a 10% change in mean arterial pressure (MAP) or pulse (P) during volume loading were eliminated. The resulting points were then evaluated as illustrated in Figure 13-3. An upslope was calculated using a linear regression analysis. The intercepts of the curve were calculated as: 1) the coordinates of the lowest LVFP and 2) the coordinates of the highest cardiac index and stroke work index attained. This technique permitted a comparison of myocardial performance curves.

A depression of myocardial performance occurred when all the following conditions were discovered (Figure 13-4): 1) a decreased upslope, 2) a lower highest cardiac index or stroke work index attained, and 3) a higher left ventricular filling pressure of the highest cardiac or stroke work index. When two or more measurements were found with a lower cardiac index or stroke work index despite a higher left ventricular filling pressure than the highest cardiac index or stroke work index attained, then a downslope was diagnosed (Figure 13-5). A downslope is an abnormal response to volume loading and is considered indicative (but not diagnostic) of myocardial depression.

Myocardial performance curves were performed prior to the institution of cardiopulmonary bypass, shortly after discontinuance of cardiopulmonary bypass, between two and four hours postoperatively, and again 20 hours postoperatively.

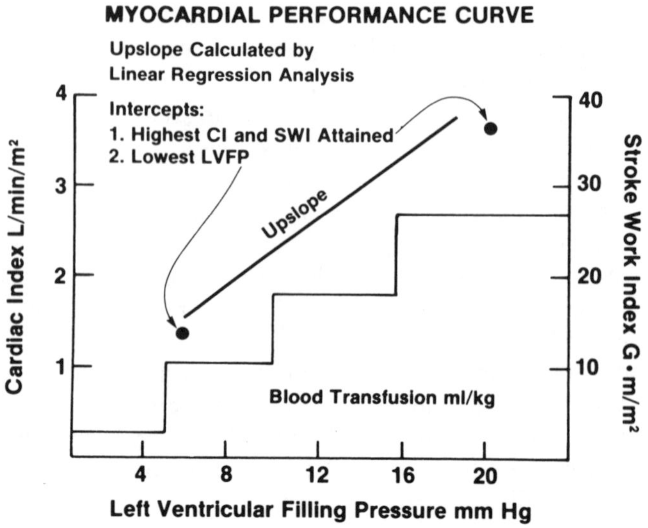

196

MYOCARDIAL PERFORMANCE CURVE

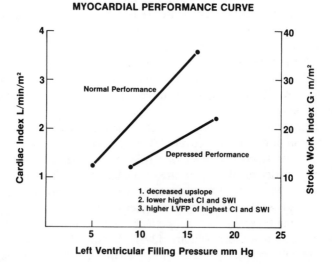

Figure 13-3 An analysis of a myocardial performance curve is illustrated. Volume loading by blood transfusion induces a rise in left ventricular filling pressure (LVFP) and a subsequent increase in cardiac index (CI) and stroke work index (SWI). The rate of rise is calculated by a linear regression analysis and termed the upslope. The position of the curve is determined by calculating the two intercepts: coordinates of the lowest LVFP and the highest CI or SWI attained.

MYOCARDIAL PERFORMANCE CURVE

Figure 13-4 A depression in myocardial performance occurs when there is a decrease in upslope, a decrease in the highest cardiac index (CI) or stroke work index (SWI) attained despite higher levels of left ventricular filling pressure (LVFP) in response to a standard volume load. A diagnosis of depressed performance requires the comparison of a myocardial performance curve to a theoretical normal population or to the same patient at a different time.

RESULTS

Figure 13-6 demonstrates the results of serial CK-MB measurements. The peak values of CK-MB are illustrated in Figure 13-7. Following intermittent anoxic arrest, patients with unstable angina released significantly more CK-MB ($p < 0.01$) than patients with stable angina. Patients protected with cold potassium cardioplegia had similar CK-MB vlaues whether they had stable or unstable angina.

Figure 13-8 demonstrates the myocardial performance curves performed prior to aortocoronary bypass. Patients with stable angina had slightly better performance than patients with unstable angina. However, this trend was not statistically significant. As illustrated in the figure, the highest stroke work attained was lower in unstable than stable angina patients. Figure 13-9 demonstrates the myocardial performance curves 60 minutes after aortocoronary bypass. Unstable angina patients protected by

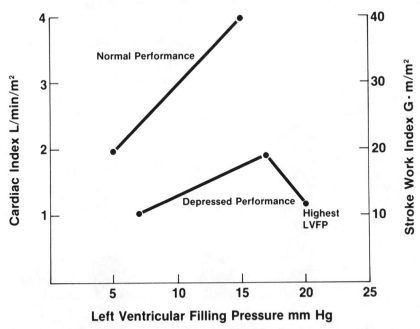

Figure 13-5 The occurrence of decreases in cardiac index (CI) or stroke work index (SWI) despite further increases in left ventricular filling pressure (LVFP) indicates an abnormality of myocardial performance. This abnormality is generally associated with depressed performance.

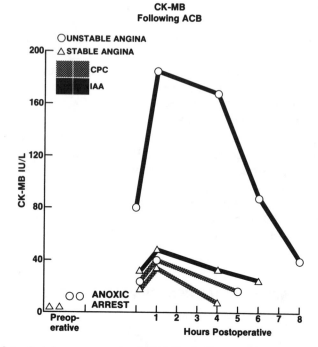

Figure 13-6 Serial measurements of CK-MB are illustrated in the four subgroups.

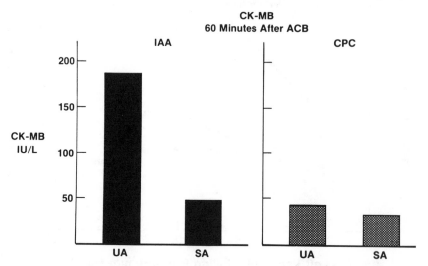

Figure 13-7 The peak postoperative CK-MB values are illustrated. Patients with unstable angina (UA) protected by intermittent anoxic arrest (IAA) released more CK-MB in the postoperative period than patients with stable angina (SA). Patients protected by cold potassium cardioplegia (CPC) show the same amount of postoperative CK-MB whether they had UA or SA.

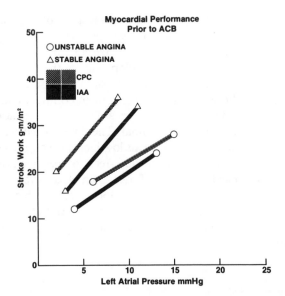

Figure 13-8 The mean values of myocardial performance curves performed preoperatively in the four subgroups of patients is illustrated. Patients with unstable angina tended to have a lower upslope and were unable to attain as high a cardiac index or stroke work index in response to volume loading than patients with stable angina.

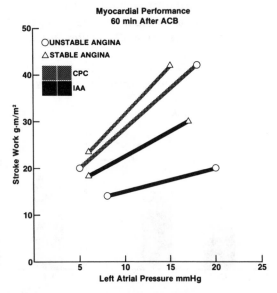

Figure 13-9 The mean values for myocardial performance curves performed following aortocoronary bypass surgery in the four subgroups is illustrated. Patients protected by cold potassium cardioplegia tended to have better performance than patients protected by intermittent anoxic arrest.

intermittent anoxic arrest had a further depression of myocardial performance, whereas unstable angina patients protected by cold potassium cardioplegia showed improvement in postoperative performance. Figure 13-10 demonstrates the difference in upslope among the four groups. The upslope of patients protected by cold potassium cardioplegia was better than the upslope of those patients protected by intermittent anoxic arrest.

The morbidity and mortality for myocardial revascularization among the 54 patients in this group was minimal. There were no deaths and one perioperative myocardial infarction. This low incidence of gross complications is thus relatively insensitive to the effects of perioperative events. Patients with prolonged episodes of rest pain and reversible electrocardiographic abnormalities tolerated an aortocoronary bypass without difficulty, provided preoperative ischemia was limited. Patients with more extensive preoperative ischemic injury have a higher perioperative morbidity and mortality.

High Risk Subgroups

A subsequent study was performed among 52 patients undergoing aortocoronary bypass for unstable angina using either intermittent anoxic arrest or cold potassium cardioplegia. These high-risk patients with unstable angina were evaluated by the pattern and duration of pain and by electrocardiographic abnormalities and enzyme changes. Patients who had short episodes of pain (less than 20 minutes, usually exertional or

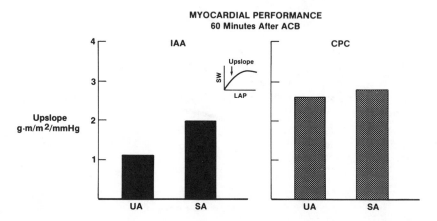

Figure 13-10 The upslope of the myocardial performance curve is lower in unstable angina patients protected by intermittent anoxic arrest (IAA) than in stable angina patients protected by IAA. This difference was not seen in patients protected by cold potassium cardioplegia.

provoked) and no electrocardiographic and enzyme abnormalities had crescendo angina. Patients with prolonged episodes of rest pain without persistent electrocardiographic or enzyme abnormalities had acute coronary insufficiency. The majority of these patients had reversible electrocardiographic changes associated with their pain. Patients who had a persistence of new ischemic electrocardiographic changes but did not have enzyme elevations suggestive of infarction had a probable infarction. Those with persistent ECG changes and slight enzyme elevations (less than 1.5 times normal) had a subendocardial infarction.

This new categorization of high subgroups of patients with rest angina and a crescendo pain pattern does not correspond to the usual differentiation of patients with unstable angina. The National Cooperative Study[3] would have included patients with acute coronary insufficiency since they had prolonged episodes of rest pain and reversible electrocardiographic abnormalities. Surgical results in this group are similar to those reported in the study. However, many patients presenting to the coronary care unit with prolonged episodes of rest pain have persistent electrocardiographic abnormalities or slight enzyme elevations. These patients are frequently felt to have had a small subendocardial infarction. They are considered surgical candidates by many and are therefore included in this classification of unstable angina (probable infarction and subendocardial infarction). Since the surgical risk is higher for patients with more extensive preoperative ischemia, it is important to review the role of myocardial protection when employed for high-risk subgroups.

Serial measurements of CK-MB were performed as previously described. The values 60 minutes following anoxic arrest are illustrated in Figure 13-11. Patients with evidence of more extensive preoperative ischemic injury were found to release more CK-MB in the immediate postoperative period. These high-risk subgroups represent a significant challenge to the surgeon. The use of cold potassium cardioplegia was found to reduce the quantity of CK-MB released in patients at highest risk.

Measurements of myocardial performance were performed postoperatively as previously described. The upslope of the myocardial performance curve was found to be more severely depressed in patients with more significant preoperative ischemic injury. The upslope 60 minutes after surgery is illustrated in Figure 13-12. Again, patients with more extensive preoperative ischemic injury had more depression in myocardial performance. Again, the use of cold potassium cardioplegia was found to provide better postoperative performance than intermittent anoxic arrest in each of the high-risk subgroups.

The results suggested that cold potassium cardioplegia provides better myocardial preservation than intermittent anoxic arrest for patients at high risk for perioperative ischemic injury, ie, those with extensive preoperative ischemia. The use of serial measurements of CK-MB and the evaluation of myocardial performance in the immediate postoperative period are sensitive indices of the adequacy of myocardial preservation. These techniques demonstrate the importance of the extent of preoperative ischemic injury on the postoperative result of surgery. In addition, the use of cold potassium cardioplegia provides an additional incremental benefit for high-risk patients undergoing aortocoronary bypass for unstable angina.

DISCUSSION

The results of aortocoronary bypass surgery in patients with unstable angina are dependent primarily on the preoperative presentation. Patients with extensive preoperative ischemia who require urgent surgery have the highest incidence of perioperative complications. Patients undergoing semielective surgery for persistent symptoms but without evidence of

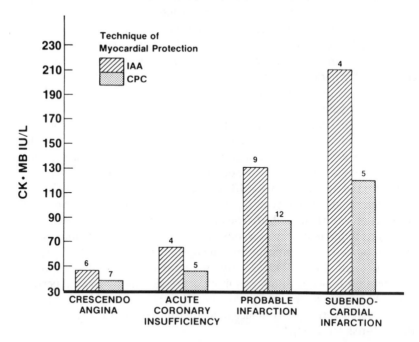

CK·MB RELEASE 60 MINUTES FOLLOWING ACB FOR UA

Figure 13-11 The peak value of CK-MB measured 60 minutes following aortocoronary bypass surgery in each of the subgroups of unstable angina is illustrated. The extent of preoperative ischemic injury had the greatest influence on postoperative CK-MB values. The incremental influence of the type of intraoperative myocardial protection is also demonstrated.

preoperative ischemia undergo revascularization without substantial morbidity or mortality with most types of myocardial preservation. The newer techniques of myocardial preservation should be most beneficial in high-risk patients. However, it is difficult to demonstrate this beneficial effect clinically. We have selected a uniform group of patients with acute coronary insufficiency (prolonged episodes of rest pain, reversible ECG changes without persistent ECG or enzyme elevations). The results in this group have been encouraging. Other studies also have reported improved results using cold potassium cardioplegia in patients with unstable angina.[1,4-6] Sensitive measurements are required to differentiate the effects of the patient's presentation from the technique of intraoperative myocardial protection.

To reduce the release of CK-MB and improve performance following surgery requires the maintenance of cardioplegia and maintenance of profound cardiac cooling during the ischemic period. Severe coronary artery

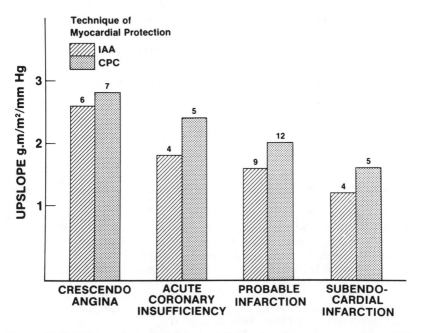

Figure 13-12 The upslope of the myocardial performance curve performed 60 minutes following aortocoronary bypass surgery for unstable angina is illustrated. Patients with greater extent of preoperative ischemic injury had greater depression in postoperative myocardial performance. Patients protected by cold potassium cardioplegia appeared to have the least amount of postoperative myocardial protection within the same group of unstable angina.

disease may limit the distribution of the cardioplegic solution. The use of systemic hypothermia as well as topical hypothermia permits more uniform cardiac cooling. Ventricular venting is necessary when left atrial pressure rises despite adequate drainage from a single right atrial cannula. Reperfusion of the myocardium should be prolonged to allow an adequate repayment of oxygen debt following anoxic arrest. The pressure of reperfusion **should be sufficient to perfuse the subendocardium, yet avoid edema.** Bypass should be discontinued slowly with adequate hemodynamic monitoring. The use of inotropic drugs in the immediate postoperative period may induce further ischemic injury. An additional reperfusion period by **vented bypass is preferable to prolonged inotropic support.** The use of intraaortic balloon pump assistance to support the ischemic myocardium is preferable to large doses of catecholamines.

Myocardial protection for unstable angina begins with the identification of high risk patients. Adequate preoperative preparation includes full beta-blockade and intensive medical management to control symptomatology. The use of the intraaortic balloon pump assistance prior to surgery remains controversial. However, in patients whose symptoms cannot be controlled, this modality can permit aortocoronary bypass under controlled conditions. Intraoperative techniques to preserve myocardial function and integrity must complement preoperative preparation.

Multiple factors affect the results of surgery for unstable angina. Myocardial preservation is a therapeutic approach for high-risk patients. The use of cold potassium cardioplegia improves the early result of aortocoronary bypass for unstable angina.

REFERENCES

1. Adams, P.X., Cunningham, J.N., Brazier, J. et al. Technique and experience using potassium cardioplegia during myocardial revascularization for preinfarction angina. *Surgery* 83:12, 1978.

2. Gerhardt, W., Ljringdahl, L., Borjesson, J. et al. Creatinine kinase B-subunit activity in human serum. I & II. *Clin Chem Acta.* 78:29, 1977.

3. Unstable Angina Pectoris. National Cooperative Study Group to compare medical and surgical therapy. *Am J Cardiol.* 42:201, 1978.

4. Weisel, R.D., Goldman, B.S., Lipton, I.H. et al. Optimal myocardial protection. *Surgery* 84:812, 1978.

5. Koster, J.K., Cohn, L.H., Collins, J.J. et al. Continuous hypothermic arrest versus intermittent ischemia for myocardial protection during coronary revascularization. *Ann Thorac Surg.* 24:330, 1977.

6. Craver, J.M., Sams, A.B., and Hatcher, C.R. Potassium induced cardioplegia. *J Thorac Cardiovasc Surg.* 76:24, 1978.

14 Intraaortic Balloon Pump Counterpulsation: Physiologic Principles and Applications in Unstable Angina

Bernard S. Goldman, MD

The intraaortic balloon pump (IABP) has had a significant impact on the management of unstable angina during the past six years. Although its initial role was to support the failing circulation in cardiogenic shock, the observation that IABP effectively aborted ischemic pain and reversed ischemic ECG changes resulted in widespread (and perhaps overzealous) usage in a wide variety of patients with unstable angina.[1,2] Recently, however, indications for IABP in the management of unstable angina have been better defined.[3,4]

Diastolic augmentation was shown to increase coronary blood flow by Kantrowitz in 1953[5] and counterpulsation was shown to decrease the tension-time index and myocardial oxygen consumption by Clauss in 1961.[6] Moulopoulos combined these concepts in 1962 with the introduction of a balloon catheter into the descending thoracic aorta to effect counterpulsation with diastolic augmentation and left ventricular systolic unloading, by alternate inflation and deflation of the balloon.[7] IABP was first applied clinically by Kantrowitz in 1967 to patients with left ventricular power failure.[8] Gold demonstrated in 1973 that IABP abolished episodes of recurrent ischemic pain and normalized ischemic ST-T wave changes in patients with medically refractory unstable angina, allowing hemodynamic stabilization, safe catheterization, and subsequent coronary artery bypass grafting with markedly reduced risk.[1]

PHYSIOLOGIC PRINCIPLES OF INTRAAORTIC BALLOON PUMP ASSIST

The beneficial effects of the IABP result from improved left ventricular function due to both diastolic augmentation and the reduction of left ventricular work. A salutary effect on acute myocardial ischemia accrues from positive changes in total coronary blood flow, myocardial oxygen consumption, and coronary collateral blood flow.[9]

The balloon catheter is inserted in retrograde manner into the descending thoracic aorta by direct exposure of a common femoral artery. Recently a percutaneous technique has been described.[10] There may be significant complications in patients with peripheral vascular occlusive disease (vide infra). The Avco balloon is helium-filled and tri-segmented, allowing displacement of blood in either direction during balloon inflation: the Datascope balloon is filled with CO_2 and is basically unidirectional due to a distal occlusive balloon. Our own experience at the Toronto General Hospital has been with the Avco unit, which is triggered by the sensed R-wave signal, permitting balloon deflation during systolic contraction. This effectively is "afterload" reduction decreasing peak left ventricular (LV) systolic pressure, mean ejection impedance, and thereby reducing left ventricular pressure work. The ejection fraction is improved with a decrease in left ventricular end-systolic volume; similar reductions of left ventricular end-diastolic volume and end-diastolic pressure aid to decrease peak left ventricular wall tension.[11] The effects of IABP on LV contractility at angiography in a patient with severe acute coronary insufficiency are demonstrated in Figure 14-1. Balloon inflation towards the onset of the T-wave provides diastolic pressure/time augmentation with increased aortic root pressure during the period of maximal nutrient coronary blood flow. The physical requirements for effective counterpulsation have been elaborated by Weber and Janicki.[12] Huckell and Adelman provided clinical information on the hemodynamic changes of balloon pump assist during cardiac catheterization and angiography.[13]

Recent studies in our laboratory have demonstrated slight decreases in subepicardial and subendocardial pressures during balloon counterpulsation in dogs (Painvin A., Hill, T.J., and Weisel, R.D., unpublished data). MacGregor has recently confirmed earlier work of Powell,[14] Weber,[12] and Gill.[15] Using radioactive microspheres in an animal made hypotensive by preload reduction, he demonstrated an improvement in subendocardial and collateral blood flow to a myocardial zone rendered ischemic by critical coronary artery stenosis.[13-15] (MacGregor, D.C., unpublished data.) Coronary blood flow studies in the human have had variable results due to fluctuations in aortic root pressure, left ventricular wall thickness, and the severity and extent of the coronary stenoses. Surgeons are familiar with the observed increase in coronary graft flow measured at operation with an electromagnetic flowmeter and an ISBP functioning in situ — indirect evidence for an increase in coronary blood flow. Gunstensen has suggested that IABP ensures maximal coronary vasodilatation and collateral blood flow by observations made during vein graft occlusion on IABP. Reactive hyperemia produces an increase in vein graft flow after temporary graft occlusion due to hypoxic dilatation of the distal arterial bed; with an IABP functioning there has been little or no reactive hyperemia noted, indirectly supporting the thesis that the perfusion bed is maximally dilated from counterpulsation (Gunstensen, J., and Goldman, B.S., unpublished data). Furthermore, IABP has been shown to reverse anaerobic myocardial metabolism and to reduce the extent and magnitude of myocardial ischemic injury either by an increase of coronary collateral flow to the ischemic zone or a local decrease in myocardial oxygen consumption.[9,16-20]

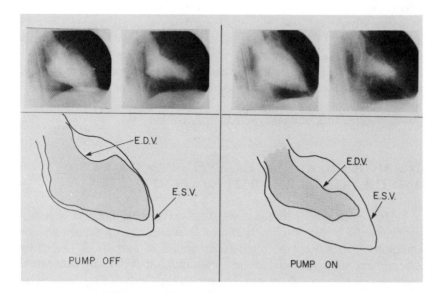

Figure 14-1   Representative cineangiogram frames in diastole and systole showing akinetic anterior wall off intraaortic balloon pump assistance (IABPA) and marked improvement in segmental wall motion on IABPA, in a patient with severe refractory ischemia.

PATHOPHYSIOLOGY OF ACUTE MYOCARDIAL ISCHEMIA

The mechanism of unstable angina is uncertain. Although vasospasm may play a critical role, most feel that a mechanical basis is important. Multiple plaque hemorrhages of recent onset have been demonstrated by Caulfield in arteries that supply myocardium corresponding to the site of ST-segment changes.[21] Compromise of major collaterals to a totally blocked vessel is a common angiographic finding. Unexplained changes in wall tension, systolic blood pressure, or heart rate may increase myocardial oxygen demand beyond the compromised supply. The imbalance between myocardial oxygen demand and oxygen delivery results in ischemia, manifested as worsening anginal pain, often prolonged and at rest, and usually accompanied by reversible ST-T wave changes in the affected myocardial perfusion zone. There are well-documented metabolic, functional, and morphologic consequences of significant reduction in total or regional coronary blood flow.[22] If the deprivation of nutrient blood flow, oxygen supply, and substrate provision persists, with accumulation of metabolic wastes, decreased myocardial oxygen consumption, and depletion of cellular glycogen, then cell injury will occur. When a significant number of myocardial cells become irreversibly injured, myocardial infarction results.[23] Ischemic myocardium loses its contractile ability and local alterations of pH or concentrations of potassium and calcium ions may alter conduction. The clinical correlates of prolonged, severe ischemia may be systemic hypoperfusion and ventricular dysrhythmias accompanying the anginal pain and ECG changes.[24] Ischemic impairment of myocardial contractility results in an increase in LV end-diastolic volume, LV wall tension and end-diastolic pressure, and further increases in myocardial oxygen demand. This vicious cycle leads to progressive impairment of left ventricular function and, if uninterrupted, may lead to infarction, left ventricular power failure, and, ultimately, circulatory collapse.[23]

THE MYOCARDIAL OXYGEN SUPPLY:DEMAND RATIO
AND THE INTRAAORTIC BALLOON PUMP

The relationship between myocardial oxygen requirement and coronary arterial blood flow has been simply expressed as a supply:demand equation[25,26] based on the physiologic studies of Sarnoff.[27] The major determinant of myocardial oxygen consumption is LV pressure work, which may be directly related to the tension time index (TTI) during ventricular systole. The principal determinant of coronary blood flow and oxygen supply is the area under the diastolic pressure trace minus the end-diastolic pressure: the diastolic pressure time index (DPTI). Thus, DPTI/TTI reflects myocardial oxygen supply:demand. The equation has been called the endocardial viability ratio (EVR) since the subendocardium is the myocardial zone at greatest jeopardy. This is especially so in patients with hypertension, left ventricular hypertrophy, tachycardia, or poor left ventricular function with a raised end-diastolic pressure. Experimental evidence exists for subendocardial necrosis when the EVR is less than 0.7 in animals with normal coronary arteries.[25] Although hematocrit and oxygen tension may alter the equation, the presence of coronary stenoses with significant gradients across the perfusion bed suggests that the EVR is an underestimation. Mechanical circulatory assistance with an intraaortic balloon pump uniformly improves the EVR by diastolic augmentation and reduction of LV afterload. The EVR has been suggested as a clinical monitor of the need for, and the success of, intraaortic balloon pumping.[28-30] The effects of intraaortic balloon pump assistance (IABPA) on the EVR are graphically displayed in Figure 14-2.

EFFECTS OF IABP ON MYOCARDIAL OXYGEN SUPPLY (DPTI) AND DEMAND (TTI)

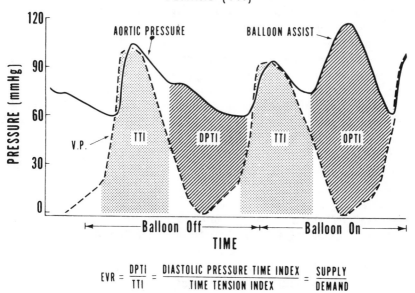

$$EVR = \frac{DPTI}{TTI} = \frac{DIASTOLIC\ PRESSURE\ TIME\ INDEX}{TIME\ TENSION\ INDEX} = \frac{SUPPLY}{DEMAND}$$

Figure 14-2 A representation of the method of calculating endocardial viability ratio (EVR). The left ventricular (VP) and the aortic pressures are shown. The area beneath the systolic portion of the curve or time-tension index is representative of myocardial oxygen consumption. The area beneath the diastolic pressure, DPTI (diastolic pressure time index), directly correlates with oxygen availability to the myocardium (supply). EVR is calculated in this manner or in a simple fashion from the arterial blood pressure and the left atrial pressure. (From: Bolooki, H. Clinical application of intra-aortic balloon pump. Mt. Kisco, N.Y.: Futura Publishing, 1977, p 18. Reproduced with permission.)

Adelman performed hemodynamic studies in 14 patients undergoing heart catheterization while on the intraaortic balloon pump.[13] The balloon was inserted prior to catheterization primarily because the patients had suffered complicated myocardial infarctions or severe intractable angina. All patients were being evaluated for possible cardiac surgery. The aortic, left and right heart pressures, cardiac output, left ventricular ejection fraction as calculated from angiograms, and the endocardial viability ratio were measured while the patient was on counterpulsation and after the balloon had been temporarily stopped for five minutes.

There was no significant change in the right heart, pulmonary artery, pulmonary capillary wedge, left ventricular systolic and end-diastolic or the aortic systolic, diastolic and mean pressures on or off counterpulsation. The cardiac output did not increase appreciably in the three patients in whom this was measured. There was also no significant change in left ventricular volumes or ejection fractions in six patients who had ventricular angiograms on and off counterpulsation, although one patient showed a dramatic improvement in ejection fraction on the balloon (see Figure 14-1). This patient had severe intractable angina that was controlled by balloon support; the improved left ventricular contraction was felt to be due to a reversal of ischemic left ventricular dysfunction in addition to some unloading of the left ventricle.

The only significant overall hemodynamic change on IABP was in the endocardial viability ratio. This ratio improved from 1.29 ± 0.51 to 1.90 ± 0.82 ($P < 0.001$), an average increase of 0.62 ± 1.52 on the balloon. With the exception of one patient in cardiogenic shock the increase in the endocardial viability ratio was greater than 30% (mean 48%). This change was primarily due to an increase in the diastolic pressure time index rather than a decrease in the tension time index. These findings indicated the major effect of balloon pumping may be to increase subendocardial perfusion.

THE TORONTO GENERAL HOSPITAL EXPERIENCE WITH THE INTRAAORTIC BALLOON PUMP IN UNSTABLE ANGINA

Our earliest experience with coronary artery bypass grafting at TGH was satisfying in patients with stable angina pectoris.[31] However, the morbidity and mortality in patients termed "preinfarction" angina was disturbingly high. Williams et al, in a retrospective study, were able to distinguish those patients who had no mortality with crescendo-type unstable angina, from those with acute coronary insufficiency who suffered a significantly higher mortality.[32] The latter patients had three distinguishing features: the acute coronary insufficiency was recurrent and unremitting, requiring prolonged hospitalization, often in numerous intensive care units; the pathologic examinations of autopsied hearts revealed "chronic" subendocardial infarction with myocytolysis, focal necrosis, and even fibrosis; and the endocardial viability ratio in these patients was consistently less than 0.6. The pathologic findings correlated with those of Page et al[24]: histologic examinations in their patients dying of left ventricular power failure demonstrated scattered areas of myocardial necrosis of varying histologic ages throughout the left ventricle, ie, the left ventricular power failure from infarction evolved over time with progression from initially ischemic viable myocardium to necrosis. Thus, we began to use the intra-aortic balloon pump for patients with "preinfarction" syndrome. Our first report demonstrated an improved survival in this group, but with an excess perioperative infarction rate. Of 19 patients with acute coronary insufficiency on IABP undergoing coronary bypass, there was only one death, but five perioperative infarcts (26.3%).[33] This was remarkably similar to the report of Weintraub and associates who operated on twelve patients with no deaths, but three perioperative infarcts (25.0%).[2] Since our patient referral pattern had not changed, (patients with recurrent and unremitting acute coronary insufficiency often had prolonged hospitalizations elsewhere with inadequate medical therapy) it is likely and indeed probable that they had already sustained microinfarcts before IABP, catheterization, and surgery. The unsuspected presence of established myocardial infarction in patients with acute coronary insufficiency has been documented and recently confirmed by radionuclide imaging.[34]

The logistic and physical deterrents that existed at TGH to early referral, urgent catheterization, and early coronary bypass prompted vigorous use of the balloon pump, primarily for temporal support. IABP allowed the privilege of time without the penalty of ongoing ischemic damage. The balloon pump was primarily used before anesthetic induction because of the demonstration of creatine phosphokinase release in patients under anesthesia, but before sternotomy.[35] The indications that had evolved at TGH by 1974 were based on: the patient's clinical status; the angiographic finding; and logistic requirements, at a time when the medical and anesthetic management were admittedly not ideal for patients with refractory ischemia.[36] Such indications as prolonged resting pain beyond 20 to 30 minutes with ECG changes, presence of significant left main coronary stenosis, significant impairment of left ventricular function, or the possibility of incomplete myocardial revascularization were similar to those indications reported by Bolooki[37] and Cooper.[38]

Of 42 patients with acute coronary insufficiency, supported by IABP at TGH in that period, the balloon pump was inserted before angiography in 11, with two deaths, (one in an operable patient and one of the six inoperable patients); 31 preanesthetic balloon pumps were inserted before coronary artery bypass surgery with two deaths. Thus, of 36 operated patients, there were three deaths (8.5% mortality) and three perioperative infarcts (8.5% morbidity) in the survivors. This patient population included seven patients with significant left main coronary stenosis, 14 with a poor ejection fraction (less than 40%), six with a low endocardial viability ratio (less than 0.7), and three with already elevated serum glutamic oxaloacetic transaminase value.[36]

Douglas et al reported on the subsequent experience at the TGH for surgery in 92 patients with resistant acute coronary insufficiency.[39] IABP was utilized predominantly in patients with refractory ischemic pain and left main coronary stenosis, severe three-vessel coronary disease, poor left ventricular function, or when the potential for incomplete revascularization existed. The operative mortality was slightly less for the 56 patients on IABP (5.4%) than the 36 patients without IABP (8.3%), and the perioperative infarction rate was equivalent (5.4% vs 5.5%) despite the fact that the IABP patients were generally considered a higher risk group.

Langou et al[40] reported similar results in a retrospective study of 194 patients seen between 1975 and 1977. The medical responders (64 patients) had no operative mortality while the medical nonresponders (130 patients) fared less well; those with balloon pump support had an operative mortality of 5.3% and those without balloon pump assist had an operative mortality of 14.5%. The overall perioperative infarction rate was 13%, 6% in responders, 6.6% in nonresponders on IABP, and 29% in nonresponders without IABP.

The past two years have allowed a crystallization of indications and a resultant marked decrease in IABP usage. This is due to the almost simultaneous application of better medical therapy in the hospital with vigorous use of long- and short-acting nitrates, nitroglycerin paste, intravenous nitroglycerin, and high-dose propranolol; earlier referrals; stabilization of patients in our CCU rather than in peripheral hospitals; invasive monitoring when accplicable; and marked improvements in techniques of anesthetic induction and intraoperative myocardial protection. Weisel has reviewed 420 patients with unstable angina operated upon in the past four years and noted a mortality for patients with either crescendo angina or acute coronary insufficiency equal to those patients with stable angina (4%).[41] Higher mortality and perioperative infarction rates were noted in those patients with unsuspected subendocardial, or indeed unrecognized, transmural myocardial infarction. This series is discussed earlier in this monograph. The use of the balloon pump in that series is illustrated in Figure 14-2. Currently, preoperative IABP is utilized in medical nonresponders who suffer truly refractory pain despite maximal and optimal therapy in our own CCU, who demonstrate concomitant ECG changes during pain, who may have laboratory, scan or ECG evidence for subendocardial insult, or if there is hemodynamic or electrical instability accompanying pain.

The recurrence of angina pectoris early after an established and recognized transmural acute myocardial infarction is evidence for threatened viable myocardium and significant coronary artery stenosis in the perfusion area adjacent to or remote from the infarct. When the pain occurs at rest, within the first one to two weeks following infarction, threatened extension may result in more muscle necrosis and left ventricular power failure with consequent high mortality. Threatened extension may be accompanied by ECG changes of ST-segment depression or elevation in the area of infarction or in a new area with or without slight enzyme rises. Medical treatment is often ineffective, and emergency coronary bypass may be complicated by a reperfusion injury. Catheterization and angiography may be hazardous due to the inherent instability of the patient. Gold, Bardet, and Haalebos and their colleagues[1,42,43] have documented the salutary effects of IABPA in this setting. The ischemic pain is aborted; the hemodynamics are stabilized, providing afterload reduction without compromise of coronary perfusion pressure; and safe diagnostic catheterization follows with subsequent revascularization of ischemic zones, whether adjacent or contralateral to the infarcted region. These patients do as well as those with unstable angina (acute coronary insufficiency) without an increase in the incidence of postoperative left ventricular power failure.

Thus, the intraaortic balloon pump in unstable angina is now clearly utilized in 1) impending infarction (severe, resistant acute coronary insufficiency); 2) subendocardial infarction with persisting rest pain; 3) certain patients with acute coronary insufficiency and poor anatomy, eg, significant left main coronary stenosis (+ or − right coronary artery occlusion) and poor left ventricular function (ejection fraction less than 30%); and 4) the syndrome of impending extension of acute myocardial infarction. The four stricter requirements offset any morbidity attendant upon balloon pump insertion. The complications of IABP are elucidated in the next section.

REFERENCES

1. Gold, H.K., Lemback, R.C., Sanders, C.A. et al. Intra-aortic balloon pumping for control of recurrent myocardial ischemia. *Circulation* 47:1197, 1973.

2. Weintraub, R.M., Voukydis, P.C., Arolsty, D.M. et al. Treatment of pre-infarction angina with intra-aortic balloon counterpulsation and surgery. *Am J Cardiol.* 34:809, 1974.

3. Weisel, R.D., Goldman, B.S., Teasdale, S. et al. Changing patterns of intra-aortic balloon pump assistance. *Can J Surg.* 21:125, 1978.

4. Miczoch, J., Pahcinger, D., Probst, P. et al. IABP in patients with unstable angina presented at 2nd European IABP Congress, Vienna, June 6–7, 1979.

5. Kantrowitz, A., and Kantrowitz, A. Experimental augmentation of coronary flow by retardation of the arterial pressure pulse. *Surgery* 34:678, 1953.

214

6. Clauss, R.H., Bertwell, W.G., Albertal, G. et al. Assisted Circulation. I. The arterial counterpulsator. *J Thorac Cardiovasc Surg.* 41:447, 1961.

7. Moulopoulos, S.D., Topaz, S., and Kolff, W.J. Diastolic balloon pumping (with carbon dioxide) in the aorta: A mechanical assistance to the failing circulation. *Am Heart J.* 63:669, 1962.

8. Kantrowitz, A., Tjonneland, S., Freed, P.S. et al. Initial clinical experience with intra-aortic balloon pumping in cardiogenic shock. *JAMA.* 203:113, 1968.

9. Cohn, K.H. *The Treatment of Acute Myocardial Ischemia. An Integrated/Surgical Approach.* Mt. Kisco, N.Y.: Futura Publishing Co., 1979, p. 152.

10. Subramanian, V.A., McCabe, J.C., Hoover, E. et al. Preliminary clinical experience with percutaneous intra-aortic counterpulsation: a new technique. Presented at 2nd European IABP Congress, Vienna, June 6–7, 1979.

11. Lembach, R.C., Buckley, M.J., Austen, W.G. et al. Effects of intra-aortic balloon pumping on coronary flow and metabolism in man. *Circulation* 43(suppl 1):77, 1971.

12. Weber, K.T., Janicki, J.S., and Walker, A.A. Intra-aortic balloon pumping: an analysis of several variables affecting balloon performance. *Trans Am Soc Artif Intern Organs.* 18:486, 1972.

13. Huckell, V.F., Adelman, A.G., Feig, K.E. et al. Hemodynamic studies during intra-aortic balloon counterpulsation. *Clin Res.* 23:605A, 1975.

14. Powell, W.J., Daggett, W.M., Maro, A.E. et al. Effects of intra-aortic balloon counterpulsation on cardiac performance, oxygen consumption and coronary blood flow in dogs. *Circ Res.* 26:753, 1970.

15. Gill, C.C., Wechsler, A.S., Newman, G.E. et al. Augmentation and redistribution of myocardial blood flow during acute ischemia by intra-aortic balloon pumping. *Ann Thorac Surg.* 16:445, 1973.

16. Summers, D.N., Kaplett, M., Norris, J. et al. Intra-aortic balloon pumping: Hemodynamic and metabolic effects during cardiogenic shock in patients with triple coronary obstructive disease. *Arch Surg.* 99:733, 1969.

17. Mueller, H., Ayres, S.M., Gianelli, S., Jr. et al. Effect of isoproterenol, 1-norepenephrine, and intra-arotic counterpulsation on hemodynamics and myocardial metabolism in shock following acute myocardial infarction. *Circulation* 45:335, 1972.

18. Sugg, W.L., Webb, W.R., and Ecker, R.R. Reduction of extent of myocardial infarction by counterpulsation. *Ann Thorac Surg.* 7:310, 1969.

19. Goldfarb, D., Fuesinger, G.C., Conti, C.R. et al. Preservation of myocardial viability by diastolic augmentation after ligation of the coronary artery in dogs. *Surgery* 65:32, 1968.

20. Maroko, P.R., Bernstein, E.F., Dibby, P. et al. Effects of intra-aortic balloon counterpulsation on the severity of myocardial ischemia injury following acute coronary occlusion. *Circulation* 45:1150, 1972.

21. Caulfield, J.B., Gold, H.K., and Leinbach, R.C. Coronary artery lesions associated with unstable angina (abstract). *Am J Cardiol.* 35:126, 1975.

22. Cerra, F.B., Lajos, T.L., Moutes, M. et al. Structural-functional correlates of reversible myocardial anoxia. *J Surg Res.* 16:140, 1974.

23. Mundth, E.D. Mechanical and surgical interventions for the reduction of myocardial ischemia. *Circulation* 53(suppl 1):176, 1976.

24. Page, D.L., Caulfield, J.J., Kastor, J.A. et al. Myocardial changes associated with cardiogenic shock. *N Engl J Med.* 285:133, 1971.

25. Buckberg, G.D., Fixler, D.E., Archie, J.P. et al. Experimental subendocardial ischemia in dogs with normal coronary arteries. *Circ Res.* 30:67, 1972.

26. Archie, J.P. Mechanical determinants of myocardial blood flow and its distribution. *Ann Thorac Surg.* 20:39, 1975.

27. Sarnoff, S.J., Braunwald, E., Welch, G.H. et al. Hemodynamic determinants of oxygen consumption of the heart with special reference to the tension-time index. *Am J Physiol*. 192:148, 1958.

28. Bregman, D., Parodi, E.N., Edie, R.N. et al. Intraoperative unidirectional intra-aortic balloon pumping in the management of left ventricular power failure. *J Thorac Cardiovasc Surg*. 70:1010, 1975.

29. Gunstensen, J., Scully, H.E., Kelly, T. et al. The prognostic significance of the endocardial probability ratio (DPTI/TTI) in aorto-coronary bypass surgery. *Can J Surg*. 19:93, 1976.

30. Phillips, P.A., Marty, A.T., Miyamoto, A.M. A clinical method for detecting subendocardial ischemia after cardiopulmonary bypass. *J Thorac Cardiovasc Surg*. 69:30, 1975.

31. Morch, J., Morton, B., McLaughlin, P. et al. Late results of aortocoronary bypass grafts in 100 patients with stable angina pectoris. *Can Med Assoc J*. 3:529, 1974.

32. Williams, W.G., Aldridge, H.E., Silver, M.D. et al. Pre-infarction angina—what is it? Edited by J.C. Norman. In *Coronary Artery Medicine and Surgery*. New York: Appleton-Century-Crofts, 1975.

33. Goldman, B.S., Gunstensen, J., Gilbert, B.W. et al. Increasing operability and survival with intra-aortic balloon pump assist. *Can J Surg*. 19:69, 1976.

34. Weintraub, R.M., Aroesty, J.M., Paulin, S. et al. Medically refractory unstable angina pectoris I. Long term follow-up of patients undergoing intra-aortic balloon counterpulsation and operation. *Am J Cardiol*. 43:877, 1979.

35. Isom, O.W., Spencer, F.C., Fergenbaum, H. et al. Pre-bypass myocardial damage in patients undergoing coronary revascularization: an unrecognized vulnerable period. *Circulation* 52(suppl 2):119, 1975.

36. Gunstensen, J., Goldman, B.S., Scully, H.E. et al. Evolving indications for preoperative intra-aortic balloon pump assistance. *Ann Thorac Surg*. 22:535, 1976.

37. Bolooki, H., Williams, W., Thurer, R.J. et al. Clinical and hemodynamic criteria for use of the intra-aortic balloon pump in patients requiring cardiac surgery. *J Thorac Cardiovasc Surg*. 72:756, 1976.

38. Cooper, G.N., Jr., Singh, A.K., Vargas, L.L. et al. Preoperative intra-aortic balloon assist in high risk revascularization patients. *Am J Surg*. 133:463, 1977.

39. Douglas, B.C., Adelman, A.G., Huckell, V.F. et al. Unstable angina: a clinical, angiographic and surgical profile. *Cardiovasc Med*. 3:167, 1978.

40. Langou, R.A., Geba, A.S., Hammond, G.L. et al. Surgical approach for patients with unstable angina pectoris: role of the response to initial medical therapy and intra-aortic balloon pumping in perioperative complications after aorto-coronary bypass grafting. *Am J Cardiol*. 42:629, 1978.

41. Weisel, R.D., Goldman, B.S., Baigrie, R.S. et al. Surgery for unstable angina. Presented at Royal College of Physicians and Surgeons, Montreal, Canada, February 1969.

42. Bardet, J., Regaud, M., Kahn, J.C. et al. Treatment of post myocardial infarction angina by intra-aortic balloon pumping and emergency revascularization. *J Thorac Cardiovasc Surg*. 74:299, 1977.

43. Haalebos, M.M.P., Braud, M.V.D., Michels, H.R. et al. Intra-aortic balloon pumping (IABP) and coronary artery bypass grafting (CABG) for impending extension of acute myocardial infarction (IEMI). Presented at 2nd European IABP Congress, Vienna, June 6–7, 1979.

15 Complications of the Intraaortic Balloon Pump

Jean Bardet, MD,
Jean Christian Farcot, MD,
Michel Rigaud, MD, and
Jean Pierre Bourdarias, MD

Since the first clinical results published by Kantrowitz and Kantrowitz in 1953,[1] circulatory assist by intraaortic balloon pumping (IABP) has been broadly used in various applications (eg, cardiogenic shock,[2-7] refractory preinfarction and postinfarction angina,[8-13] and cardiac failure after cardiopulmonary bypass[14-19]). Unfortunately this technique has complications that can negate its potential advantages. In severely ill patients with a lethal prognosis, IABP must be used despite these potential complications because there is no other alternative. However, in other indications, where the use of IABP is open to discussion, the risk of complications must be weighed against its potential advantages. The aim of this review is to analyze these complications.

Difficulty with inserting the balloon in the thoracic aorta via the femoral artery is not specifically a complication but is the first problem encountered, and the main cause of further vascular complications. Usually, most surgeons thread the catheter up the femoral artery through a 10-mm woven Dacron graft, which is subsequently anastomosed to the common femoral artery in end-to-side fashion.[20-23] Often this technique is lengthy and the time of intervention favors local wound infection. Thus it was abandoned in 1974, and since then the catheter has been passed through a femoral arterial purse-string suture only.[24]

Inability to insert the balloon is appreciated differently in each clinical report. Hochberg[25] found, in more than 400 cases surveyed, only three failures to insert the balloon (0.75% incidence). But it must be noted that in his inquiry, he received only a 65% response. One can suppose that the failure rate is considerably higher in the group of nonresponders.

In other publications, the rate of failure to insert the balloon is higher. In the report of McCabe et al,[23] the balloon could not pass into the aorta in 21 patients out of 100 despite a bilateral approach in 13. Lefemine et al[22] reported unsuccessful attempts at passage through the femoral artery in 7 out of 65 surgical patients (11%) and in 5 out of 29 medical patients (17%). In the Ambroise-Paré Hospital experience (Table 15-1), out of 158 medical patients considered to be candidates for counterpulsation, failure to insert the balloon through one groin occurred in 17 cases. In these patients, the balloon was ultimately passed via the contralateral femoral artery in eight cases. The overall inability rate (failure rate) was 5.7%.

Table 15-1
Experience with Insertion of an Intraaortic Balloon
at the Ambroise Paré Hospital (June 1979)

Indications for IABP	Totals No.	%	Failure to Insert the Balloon No.	%	Long-term Survival No.	%
Total patients	158	100	9	5.7	91	61
Cardiogenic shock	74	46.8	6	8.1	21	30
Left ventricular aneurysm	12	7.5	–	–	8	67
Postinfarction angina	35	22.2	1	2.8	30	88
Preinfarction angina	28	17.7	2	7.1	24	92
High-risk coronary	9	5.7	–	–	8	89

The reasons for failure to place a balloon catheter by the femoral route are varied. The main cause is atherosclerotic narrowing or complete stenosis of the femoral or iliac artery. Even in the absence of significant stenoses, the balloon may not be inserted because of excessive tortuosity of the arteries whereby the catheter tip may actually wedge or engage in the contralateral iliac artery. Also, as in any surgical procedure, one must take into account the experience of the surgeon. In our last 50 patients, where the balloon was inserted 35 times by the same surgeon, we had only one failure. On the other hand, of the 15 cases where the balloon was inserted as an emergency procedure by one of seven different surgeons on duty, we had four failures. When the catheter cannot be passed despite considerable manipulation and a bifemoral approach, a smaller balloon (20 cc) should be used.[22,23]

Other suggestions to facilitate insertion have been proposed. Bregman et al described the use of a flexible tip intraaortic balloon catheter that can negotiate aortoiliac occlusive disease by bending the tip and rotating the balloon until it passes easily. With this technique it was possible to insert the balloon in eight patients where passage was previously impossible.[26] Wolfson et al[27] reported their clinical experience with an Avco intraaortic balloon that was modified to allow pressure monitoring, injection of contrast medium, and passage of a guide wire. This modified intraaortic balloon was successfully placed in 15 of the 16 patients in the series, including four of five in whom prior attempts to place a standard Avco balloon catheter had failed. Lain[28] proposed dilation of narrowed arteries by simply passing a venous size 8 to 10 Fogarty catheter. Aortography[28] and/or examination by Doppler technique, before attempting balloon insertion, would allow one to diagnose arterial stenosis or obstruction, thus designating the better side to place the catheter. Otherwise, mainly in surgical patients, the balloon can be inserted through other routes: the iliac artery system by a retroperitoneal approach,[29] the axillary artery,[7,24,28] subclavian artery,[22] innominate artery,[28] aortic arch, or asending aorta.[20,23,28-32]

In our experience of 158 patients, the complications of IABP can be divided into three groups: 1) vascular, 2) infective, and 3) neurologic (Table 15-2). The overall incidence of complications has been reported to be between 4% and 36%, with most in the 10% to 16% range.[20] These data are generally calculated on the basis of total successful insertions, which would seem to understate the problems as 1) many patients with unsuccessful insertion attempts develop further complications, and 2) some patients who die soon after counterpulsation was established have little opportunity to develop complications. Scheidt et al[7] in a cooperative study of 87 patients reported 13 ischemic limb problems, an incidence of 15%. Actually, this rate is 37% if calculated on the basis of the 35 patients who lived long enough to have the balloon removed.

The main complications of IABP are vascular. Some vascular complications of IABP are related to the insertion of the balloon. Indeed McCabe et al[23] reported one-third of vascular complications in a group where the balloon catheter could not adequately be positioned. Dissection of the femoral, iliac artery or aorta is the most frequent complication due to the insertion of the balloon. Arterial dissection does not necessarily prevent adequate counterpulsation.

McCabe et al[23] reported that out of seven dissections five were unsuspected since counterpulsation was performed, despite the fact the balloon catheter had passed through, or lay in, a false lumen. More often,

Table 15-2
Complications of IABP Experience
at the Ambroise Paré Hospital (June 1979)

Vascular			
During IABP (158 patients)		*After IABP* (91 survivors)	
Not severe	36	Claudication	3
Dissection	2	Limb loss	1
Thrombosis	2		
Total	40	Total	4

Infective			
Local wound problems (113 weaned patients)		*Septicemia* (158 patients)	
Delay of wound healing	25	Death	7
Purulent sepsis of the groin	1	Survivor	1
Total	26	Total	8

Neurologic (158 patients)			
Hemiplegia		*Meningeal hemorrhage*	
Death	1	Death	1
Survivor	1		
Total	2	**Total**	1

arterial dissection is responsible for vascular insufficiency and requires balloon removal. Tyras and Williams[33] reported one case of paraplegia following IABP due to embarrassment of the spinal cord blood supply by the dissection. In 158 attempts to insert the balloon we have had two cases of arterial dissection. In both cases, there was acute limb ischemia and the balloon had to be removed. Other studies reported a 1.1% to 8.8% dissection rate.[7,13,20,22,23,31,32,34,35]

Perforation of the arterial wall from insertion of the catheter is seldom seen. It has never been observed in our experience or in that of Lefemine et al.[22] McCabe and his co-workers[23] reported a free perforation of the left common iliac artery that resulted in massive retroperitoneal hemorrhage and contributed to the death of the patient despite emergency repair.

Alpert and colleagues[20] reported three instances of local trauma at the insertion site. Two of these required endarterectomy and patch graft angioplasty, and in one case, a segmental resection and interposition of vein graft was necessary.

Both Rainer and Paton observed one case of intimal injury (reported in Alpert et al[20]). In the latter report, the patient died of catastrophic intraperitoneal hemorrhage. Arterial dissection and intimal injury are directly proportional to the time and force used to place the catheter. Of course, the risk of arterial complications depends on the experience of the surgeon. In cardiogenic shock it might be justified to push the catheter forward more forcibly, accepting a higher risk of complications than in other indications.

Arterial insufficiency is a frequent complication when the balloon is already in place. This may be due to arterial dissection and mechanical trauma of any portion of the arterial wall. It may also be caused by thrombotic or arterial occlusion by the catheter itself if the arterial lumen is small or narrowed by arteriosclerotic disease. This complication is enhanced by low cardiac output and hypotension. It was encountered in up to 50% of patients with cardiogenic shock.[22] Usually, arterial insufficiency is not severe; we reported[24] a 22% improvement rate of ischemic legs after a rise of aortic blood pressure or after the use of peripheral vasodilating drugs. Some authors found a longer duration of IABP in patients with limb ischemia than in patients without vascular complications.[9,34] This difference was not found in our experience, nor in that of McCabe et al.[23]

Unfortunately, arterial insufficiency may be very severe. In 149 patients where IABP was efficient, we nonetheless had to remove the balloon in four cases due to alarming arterial ischemia. There were two cases of arterial dissection and two cases of extensive thrombosis. In one of the latter, emergency Fogarty embolectomy catheters were successfully passed in both directions and the balloon could then be inserted into the contralateral groin. The systematic use of heparin decreases the risk of extensive thrombosis. Furthermore, we have not encountered this complication since the balloon has been passed directly into the common femoral artery without the woven Dacron graft. To avoid balloon removal and discontinuance of counterpulsation if leg complications do appear, Barsamian[36] recently proposed a femorofemoral crossover graft. Alpert et al[20] have also reported this technique.

Limb loss during or after IABP is the worst peripheral vascular complication of IABP. Hochberg[25] found mention of two amputations in 386 case reports; Bolooki et al[37] have found amputation necessary in two of 158 patients and we have had one amputation in 158 patients. Beckman et al[9] reported three amputations in 273 patients. In addition, one patient in the Beckman study died before amputation was performed. In seven reports,[4,9,20,22-25] the incidence of this complication was 0.75%. Intermittent claudication of later onset was noted in 3 out of 91 surviving patients in our experience, only one requiring arterial repair. Among the 40 survivors of Pace et al[34] six developed claudication and only one required reconstructive surgery. Two patients in the cooperative study of Scheidt and his colleagues[7] underwent iliofemoral bypass after the removal of the balloon. In several studies, in order to diminish the incidence of secondary claudication a Fogarty embolectomy catheter was passed in both directions at the time of the balloon extraction as a routine procedure[9,20,23,24] originally suggested by Saini and Berger.[38] Alpert[20] recommended frequent observation of limbs containing a balloon catheter with a Doppler ultrasound probe.[22]

Other complications of IABP have been studied less often than have the vascular complications. Wound problems are frequent when the balloon is passed through the groin. Delay in wound healing was observed in 25 patients previously reported in our institution.[24] It is due to persistent lymphedema and lymphocele and is responsible for local infection. This infection is generally torpid, superficial, and not severe. Even when bacteria are locally sampled general antibiotic therapy is usually not required, but only local wound care. A purulent infection of the groin is rare, but can be catastrophic. We observed one case occurring a few days after removal of the balloon, with abrupt external bleeding from arterial disruption since the Dacron suture line was involved in acute infection. Fortunately, emergency surgery was able to control hemorrhage and the patient survived, but he experienced claudication. A few cases of local infection have been reported in the literature[23,25,27]; they are usually not serious. McCabe et al[23] described five cases of wound infection and three problems related to the lymphatics. Beckman and his co-workers,[9] reported eight cases of localized wound sepsis. The use of a woven Dacron graft favors local infection and we have noted fewer infections now that we insert the balloon directly in the femoral artery without a Dacron graft. Furthermore, it is prudent to ligate or cauterize any potential source of lymphatic leakage. In addition, some authors recommend irrigating the wound with antibiotic solution before closure.[9,32] The incidence of generalized sepsis with positive blood cultures depends on the indication and duration of IABP. In our institution, we have had eight cases of septicemia. In all cases, the patients were in cardiogenic shock and had assisted ventilation. Furthermore, they were invasively monitored in multiple ways, including urinary output, central venous pressure, and radial artery pressure. The duration of IABP was always more than eight days. Seven of eight patients in this group died, but hemodynamic status unreponsive to IABP was responsible for death rather than septicemia. Nevertheless, we no longer maintain circulatory assist for more than eight days because of the risk of septicemia. McCabe et al[23] reported two cases of generalized infection and Beckman et al[9] two other instances. However, despite prolonged IABP of more than a week in 13 patients, Hagemeijer[39] noted only one case of severe infection responsible for death.

Neurologic complications of IABP are rare. We have observed two instances of hemiplegia and one meningeal hemorrhage.[24] In these three cases, the role of anticoagulant therapy must be considered. All patients in our experience received appropriate heparin therapy to avoid thrombotic complications, but this can promote bleeding. As reported, we now use low-molecular-dextran-weight infusion, and platelet counts in any patient are never below 30,000.[24] In the three patients with neurologic complications, platelet counts were between 50,000 and 100,000. Thrombocytopenia is not a problem in patients undergoing IABP and reverses soon after removal. McCabe et al[23] observed no bleeding disorders directly attributable to an absolute drop in platelet count alone. Hemiplegia can result from cerebral embolism as well. However, in our patients who died and underwent autopsy, we did not observe emboli in other organs, particularly not in the kidneys as reported elsewhere.[7] The use of nonthrombogenic material for the balloon and catheter, anticoagulant therapy, and permanent motion of the balloon without arrest for many hours seems to avoid this risk of systemic embolism. Finally, some authors have reported rupture of the catheter[40] or balloon, which is responsible for gas embolism.[41]

In conclusion, these complications are invariably the result of arterial disease, low cardiac output, and human or technical limitations. The incidence of inability to insert the balloon and the incidence of complications diminish with the experience of the surgeon, the use of low-molecular-weight dextran and heparin with appropriate control of anticoagulation levels. Doppler monitoring of the circulation should provide more critical observation and increased limb safety. The potential advantage of the balloon device must always be weighed against its potential risks in a given patient.

REFERENCES

1. Kantrowitz, A., Kantrowitz, A. Experimental augmentation of coronary flow by retardation of the arterial pressure pulse. *Surgery* 34:678, 1953.

2. Bardet, J., Bourdarias, J.P., Kahn, J.C. et al. Assistance circulatoire par contrepulsion intra-aortique. Resultats a long terme dans une serie de 108 cas. *Coeur Med Interne.* 16:391, 1977.

3. Bardet, J., Masquet, C., Kahn, J.C. et al. Clinical and hemodynamic results of intra-aortic counterpulsation and surgery for cardiogenic shock. *Am Heart J.* 93:280, 1977.

4. Bregman, D., and Goetz, R.H. Clinical experience with a new cardiac assist device: the dual chambered intra-aortic balloon assist. *J Thorac Cardiovasc Surg.* 62:577, 1971.

5. Heimbecker, R.O. Surgery for massive myocardial infarction. *Prog Cardiovasc Dis.* 11:338, 1969.

6. Leinbach, R.C., Gold, H.K., Dinsmore, R.E. et al. The role in cardiogenic shock. *Circulation* 48(suppl 3):95, 1973.

7. Scheidt, S., Wilner, G., and Mueller, H. Intra-aortic balloon counter pulsation in cardiogenic shock. Report of a co-operative clinical trial. *N Engl J Med.* 288:979, 1973.

8. Bardet, J., Rigaud, M., Kahn, J.C. et al. Treatment of post-myocardial infarction angina by intra-aortic balloon pumping and emergency revascularization. *J Thorac Cardiovasc Surg.* 74:299, 1977.

9. Beckman, C.B., Geha, A.S., Hammond, G.L. et al. Results and complications of intra-aortic balloon counterpulsation. *Ann Thorac Surg.* 24:550, 1977.

10. Gold, H.K., Leinbach, R.C., Sanders, C.A. et al. Intra-aortic balloon pumping for control of recurrent myocardial ischemia. *Circulation* 47:1197, 1973.

11. Huret, J.F., Agier, B., Rosier, S.P. et al. Delayed semi-elective coronary bypass surgery for unstable angina pectoris. *J Thorac Cardiovasc Surg.* 75:476, 1978.

224

12. Levine, F.H., Gold, H.K., Leinbach, R.C. et al. Management of acute myocardial ischemia with intra-aortic balloon pumping and coronary bypass surgery. *Circulation* 58(suppl 1):69, 1978.

13. O'Rourke, M.F., and Shepherd, K.M. Protection of the aortic arch and subclavian artery during intra-aortic balloon pumping. *J Thorac Cardiovasc Surg.* 65:543, 1973.

14. Berger, R.L., Saini, V.K., Ryan, T.J. et al. Intra-aortic balloon assist postcardiotomy cardiogenic shock. *J Thorac Cardiovasc Surg.* 66:906, 1973.

15. Buckberg, S.D., Olinger, G.N., Mulder, D.G. et al. Depressed post-operative cardiac performance. Prevention by adequate myocardial protection during cardiopulmonary bypass. *J Thorac Cardiovasc Surg.* 70:974, 1975.

16. Buckley, M.J., Craver, J.M., Gold, H.K. et al. Intra-aortic balloon pump assist for cardiogenic shock after cardiopulmonary bypass. *Circulation* 47 & 48(suppl 3):90, 1973.

17. Cleveland, J.C., Lefemine, A.A., Madoff, I. et al. The role of intra-aortic balloon counterpulsation in patients undergoing cardiac operations. *Ann Thorac Surg.* 20:652, 1975.

18. Gandjbakhch, I., Bardet, J., Belghiti, J. et al. Interet de la contre-pulsion intra-aortique comme support circulatoire en chirurgie cardiaque. (A propos de 60 observations.) *Arch Mal Coeur.* 70:565, 1977.

19. Lambert, J.J., Cohn, L.W., Lesch, M. et al. Intra-aortic balloon counter-pulsation. Indications and long term results in postoperative left ventricular power failure. *Arch Surg.* 109:766, 1974.

20. Alpert, J., Bhaktan, E.K., Gielchinsky, I. et al. Vascular complications of intra-aortic balloon pumping. *Arch Surg.* 3:1190, 1976.

21. Biddle, T.L., Stewart, S., and Stuart, I.D. Dissection of the aorta complicating intra-aortic balloon counterpulsation. *Am Heart J.* 92:781, 1976.

22. Lefemine, A.A., Kosowsky, B., Madoff, I. et al. Results and complications of intra-aortic balloon pumping in surgical and medical patients. *Am J Cardiol.* 40:416, 1977.

23. McCabe, J.C., Abel, R.M., Subramanian, V.A. et al. Complications of intra-aortic balloon insertion and counterpulsation. *Circulation* 57:769, 1978.

24. Bardet, J., Rigaud, M., and Bourdarias, J.P. Assistance circulatoire par contre-pulsion intra-aortique. Difficultes et complications. *Ann Cardiol Angeiol.* 26:219, 1977.

25. Hochberg, H. Transactions of the second meeting of users of the AVCO intra-aortic balloon pump. Roche Medical Electronics, 1975.

26. Bregman, D., Bolooki, H., and Malm, J.P. A simple method to facilitate difficult intra-aortic balloon insertions. *Ann Thorac Surg.* 15:636, 1973.

27. Wolfson, S., Karsh, D.L., Langou, R.A. et al. Modification of intra-aortic balloon catheter to permit introduction by cardiac catheterization techniques. *Am J Cardiol.* 41:733, 1978.

28. Lain, K. Transactions of the second meeting of users of the AVCO intra-aortic balloon pump. Roche Medical Electronics, 1975.

29. Lamberti, J.J., Cohn, L.H., and Collins, J.J., Jr. Iliac artery cannulation for intra-aortic balloon counterpulsation. *J Thorac Cardiovasc Surg.* 67:976, 1974.

30. Krause, A.M., Bigelow, J.C., and Scottpage, V. Transthoracic intra-aortic balloon cannulation to avoid repeat sternotomy for removal. *Ann Thorac Surg.* 21:562, 1976.

31. Piwnica, A., Bercot, M., Menasche, P.H. et al. Insuffisence cardiaque aigue au decours de la circulation extracorporelle. Methodes et indications actuelles de l'assistance circulatoire. *Ann Cardiol Angeiol.* 26:195, 1977.

32. Roe, B.B., and Chatterjee, K. Transaortic cannulation for balloon pumping: report of a patient undergoing closed-chest decannulation. *Ann Thorac Surg.* 21:568, 1976.

33. Tyras, O.H., and Williams, V.L. Paraplegia following intra-aortic balloon assistance. *Ann Thorac Surg.* 25:164, 1978.

34. Pace, P., Tilney, N., Couch, N. et al. Peripheral arterial complications of intra-aortic balloon counterpulsation. *Circulation* 54(suppl 2):13, 1976.

35. Dunkman, W.B., Leinbach, R.C., Buckley, M.J. et al. Clinical and hemodynamic results of intra-aortic balloon pumping and surgery for cardiogenic shock. *Circulation* 46:465, 1972.

36. Barsamian, E.M., Goldman, M., Crane, C. et al. Femoro femoral bypass graft in intra-aortic balloon counterpulsation. *Arch Surg.* 3:1070, 1976.

37. Bolooki, H., Williams, W., Thurer, R.J. et al. Clinical and hemodynamic criteria for use of the intra-aortic balloon pump in patients requiring cardiac surgery. *J Thorac Cardiovasc Surg.* 72:756, 1976.

38. Saini, V.K., and Berger, R.L. Technic of aortic balloon catheter deployment with the use of a Fogarty catheter sed-chest decannulation. *Ann Thorac Surg.* 14:440, 1972.

39. Hagemeijer, F. Prolonged intraaortic balloon pumping for low output after myocardial infarction. Presented at the first European Intraaortic Balloon Pump Congress, Rotterdam, The Netherlands, May, 1978.

40. Karayannacos, P.E., Shapiro, I.L., Kakos, G.S. et al. Counterpulsation catheter fracture: an unexpected hazard. *Ann Thorac Surg.* 23:276, 1977.

41. Weber, K.T., and Janicki, J.S. Intra-aortic balloon counterpulsation. *Ann Thorac Surg.* 17:602, 1974.

16 Urgent Surgical Therapy for Unstable Angina

Wilbert J. Keon, MD

The tenet that the less known about the disease, the more names given to it has certainly applied in recent years to the clinical entity commonly termed "unstable angina." Wearn, in an article published in 1923, is given credit for the first recorded description of unstable angina: "... the onset (of infarction) may occur after a number of angina attacks, which together with dyspnea may constitute the only previous warnings of involvement with coronary arteries."[1] As medical knowledge expanded and this syndrome became more familiar, a confusing number of descriptive terms were coined. Some of the more common terms developed were preinfarction angina, intermediate syndrome, impending myocardial infarction, crescendo angina, coronary insufficiency, and status anginosus.

This syndrome has received increased attention with the advent of direct coronary revascularization. Many of the terms employed presupposed that infarction was an inevitable outcome and that the syndrome was intermediate in severity on the continuum of stable angina progressing to myocardial infarction. Although these manifestations broadly described a continuum, it is possible to identify fairly discreet subsets of patients.

Wood[2] identifies 10% of patients with atherosclerotic disease as presenting with preinfarction or unstable angina. Cairns[3] reports that anywhere from 22% to 80% of patients with unstable angina progress to infarction and Klieger et al[4] state that 12% of infarction patients develop cardiogenic shock. Given the ability to revascularize ischemic segments of the myocardium, the problem then becomes one of determining the position of a given patient in the evolution of his disease process at a given time. Thus, if surgical therapy is to be undertaken, it can be done at the most optimal time.

The confusing terminology and multiplicity of criteria used in different centers makes it difficult but not impossible to compare the high-risk subgroups in patients in whom the prognosis is poor. Several centers have similar if not identical criteria for categorizing unstable angina patients. The criteria used at the University of Ottawa Cardiac Unit are:

1. Stable angina with recent spontaneous increase in severity.
2. Angina of recent onset with progressive increase in severity leading to either recurrent pain at rest lasting at least 15 minutes and not relieved by nitrates, or ischemic ST-T wave changes during chest pain with no evidence of recent infarction.

We use the term unstable angina for descriptive purposes only, recognizing its limitations and ambiguity.

Reports on Unstable Angina

Early reports advocating emergency surgical treatment of unstable angina were favorable.[2-9] Surgical experience illustrated an acceptably low operative mortality rate with good symptomatic relief. Subsequent reports demonstrated excellent surgical results with low operative mortality (1.6% to 8.0%), acceptable perioperative infarction rate, and excellent amelioration of symptoms as outlined in Table 16-1.

However, there have been some conflicting results reported on the surgical management of these patients with respect to timing of surgical therapy,[17] and with respect to long-term mortality. Bert,[18] Matloff,[19] and Bender[20] report significant increase in long-term survival of surgically treated patients whereas others report little or no difference.[14,21-24]

A number of observations can be made about angiography and aortocoronary bypass surgery in unstable angina.[16] The risk of coronary angiography varies from center to center but it is clearly higher during the acute stage of the illness than is the risk in stable angina.[25] The operative mortality rates again vary, ranging from 2.5% to 22.0%, but, in every center reporting, the rate is distinctly higher in unstable angina during the

Table 16-1
Results of Surgical Treatment for Unstable Angina

Author	No. of Patients	Operative Mortality (%)	Perioperative Infarction (%)	Follow-up (Mean time in mos)	Asymptomatic (%)	Improved (%)	Graft Patency (%)
Cheanvechai et al[5]	63	6.4	9.5	—	—	92	—
Geha et al[8]	48	2	4	12	81	—	—
Bertolasi et al[10]	62	8	13	31	70	86	—
Golding et al[11]	100	4	21	42	78	—	86
Hultgren et al[12]	52	1.9	15	24	60	95	—
Huret et al[13]	63	1.6	11	22	71	77	84
Miller et al[14]	67	10	10	—	—	89	—
NIH Randomized Trial[15]	141	5	18	36	—	85	—
Cohn[16]	23	0	4.6	10	82	13.5	—
Keon[7]	144	5.6	7	12	64	97.5	85

acute stage than in stable angina operated upon electively in the same institution.[25] The incidence of perioperative infarction is significant (up to 25%) and is the major cause of death.[14] The early follow-up of postoperative patients is highly favorable with complete relief of symptoms in 50% to 87%, improvement in 75% to 93%, and a low incidence of late death.[26] There is clearly less graft patency than in elective surgical procedures and it ranges from 56.0% to 92.3% of grafts studied.[25]

Researchers agree that emergency angiography and surgery can be performed with relatively low risk for unstable angina. Although the possibility of perioperative myocardial infarction is higher than in a medically treated group, the symptomatic improvement is substantially better for the surgically treated group.

It appears that a pattern of management for unstable angina is beginning to emerge whereby most physicians attempt to stabilize the patient with medical therapy. There is a tendency to treat those patients who fail to respond by undertaking early angiography and bypass surgery but only a prospective randomized trial conducted over an extended time period will elucidate the risk:benefit ratio.

Experience at the University of Ottawa Cardiac Unit

Between December 1970 and December 31, 1978, surgeons at the University of Ottawa Cardiac Unit performed 2682 surgical procedures for direct myocardial revascularization. Two hundred fifty procedures (9.3%) were classed as emergencies. The patients were divided into four groups: unstable angina (144), acute myocardial infarction (65), cardiogenic shock (28) and angiographic emergency (13) according to our criteria published in 1976.[4]

The conventional operative techniques with cold cardioplegia have been used for patients with unstable angina. However, if an acute infarct is present with compromised pump function, surgery is performed on the still-beating heart with emphasis on myocardial resuscitation during the surgical procedure.

The bulk of our emergency surgery (58%) has been performed on patients presenting with unstable angina. This group consisted of 21 (14.5%) females and 123 (85.5%) males with a mean age of 49.1 years. Twenty (14%) presented with single-vessel disease, 41 (28%) with double-vessel disease, and 83 (58%) with triple-vessel disease. One hundred thirty-one (91%) patients received total revascularization with either bypass grafts or internal mammary artery implants, or both. The mean number of grafts per patient was 2.9 and the mean increase in intraoperative blood flow measured by an electromagnetic flowmeter in 66 patients was 204 ml/min. Only 10 of the patients did not receive total revascularization, six of these early in our experience with emergency surgery. Fifty-one patients had additional procedures; 14 had left mammary implants, 32 endarterectomies, two resections, and two plications of left ventricular aneurysms and two aortic valve replacements.

The left ventricular function of all our patients is classified and designated as normal or given a class of dysfunction ranging from I to IV, Class IV having the most serious impairment. This is a joint decision between respective surgeons, cardiologists, and radiologists involved in the case. The evaluation is based on left ventriculography done in the right anterior oblique projection and on hemodynamic data (Figure 16-1).

The left ventricle is arbitrarily divided into four segments; one hypokinetic segment constitutes a Class I ventricle, two hypokinetic segments corresponding to Class II, and so forth. Among the many hemodynamic values accumulated for each case, the ejection fraction results are weighed most heavily in assessing the left ventricular contractility. The majority of Class IV ventricles exhibit an ejection fraction of less than 0.2 and all patients with Class III or IV are less than 0.4.

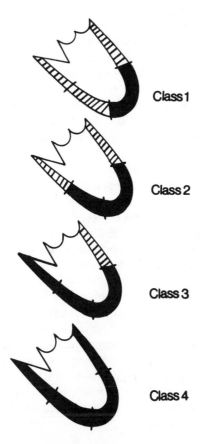

Figure 16-1 Angiographic classification of ventricular contractility.

The distribution of patients by ventricular function is illustrated in Table 16-2. Of 144 patients with unstable angina, six did not have ventriculography performed due to the severity of their physical condition at angiography. Twenty-four (17.4%) were classified as normal, 48 (34.8%) as Class I, 48 (34.8%) as Class II, 10 (7.2%) as Class III, and 8 (5.8%) as Class IV. A total of 87% of the patients had normal or mild to moderate impairment of ventricular function. This contrasts with patients who had emergency surgery for acute myocardial infarction where normal to moderate impairment of ventricular function was found in 62.9% of the patients. Ten patients were unclassified and a ventriculogram was not done due to emergency.

There were eight (5.6%) hospital deaths. Five were classified as operative deaths (within 48 hours of surgery) and the cause attributed to low cardiac output syndrome in two cases, perioperative myocardial infarction in one case, subendocardial hemorrhagic necrosis in one case, and rupture of thoracic aneurysm in one case. The remaining three early deaths, within 30 days of surgery, were caused by low cardiac output in one case, myocardial infarction in another, and in the third by cardiorespiratory failure. Three more deaths occurred, one at four months caused by rupture of a mycotic aneurysm, one at ten months by a myocardial infarction, and one at 18 months from an unknown cause. The early mortality of 5.6% is slightly higher than that of 3.5% for nonemergency cases. However, the late mortality is similar at 7.6% and 9.0% respectively. Thirteen patients had a combination of severe three-vessel disease (one with left main) and poor left ventricular function. The mortality of this group was considerably higher at 30.8% (4 of 13).

Seven patients (4.8%) required circulatory assistance with the intraaortic balloon pump. The IABP was used preoperatively in an attempt to stabilize the patient during catheterization. It was used postoperatively when the patients exhibited signs of acute pump failure. Six of these patients were hospital deaths, five had severely compromised ventricular function and the sixth had moderately impaired ventricular function and mitral valve disease. Three of the deaths were attributed to low cardiac output (one with infarction) and one each to rupture of a thoracic aortic aneurysm, perioperative myocardial infarction and subendocardial hemorrhagic necrosis. The total perioperative infarction rate using ECG and enzyme criteria was ten (7%), two of which were fatal (20%). In unstable angina, if the coronary lesions are amenable to surgery, corrective surgery should be done as an emergency procedure. We advocate the use of the balloon pump postoperatively in patients with signs of pump failure or intraoperative infarction. However, we do not believe that routine use of IABP is warranted in most of these patients because of the associated morbidity from the balloon itself.

Table 16-2
Emergency Myocardial Revascularization – Classification of Ventricles

	Total No. of Patients	Normal		Class I		Class II		Class III		Class IV	
Unstable angina	138	24	(17.4)*	48	(34.8)	48	(34.8)	10	(7.2)	8	(5.8)
Acute myocardial infarction	62	3	(4.8)	9	14.5	27	(43.6)	14	22.6	9	(14.5)
Cardiogenic shock	27	1	(3.6)	–	–	2	(7.4)	2	(7.4)	24	(89.0)
Angiographic emergency	13	5	(38.5)	3	(23)	4	(31)	1	(7.5)	–	–

*Numbers in parentheses denote percentages.

The physical layout of the University of Ottawa Cardiac Unit (Figure 16-2) lends itself to emergency surgery. With the coronary care unit and catheterization laboratories adjacent to the operating rooms, there is a minimum of delay and logistic problems in processing of patients from one stage of investigation and treatment to the next.

It is interesting to note that 11 (7.6%) of the unstable angina emergency cases required further elective coronary artery bypass grafting performed between two months and six years after the first emergency operation. Two patients, neither of whom had incomplete revascularization at first operation, required reoperation because of the progression of disease. This reoperation was performed at a mean of 18 months. Five patients had second surgery due to compromised or occluded grafts. This was performed at a mean of 13 months. Four patients required reoperation for a combination of progression of disease and compromised or occluded grafts and the duration between operations for this group of patients was 52 months. The reoperation rate for all other patients undergoing coronary artery bypass grafting was only 3.6%.

Follow-up (three months to four years postoperatively) on 112 of the 113 survivors, demonstrated symptomatic improvement using the New

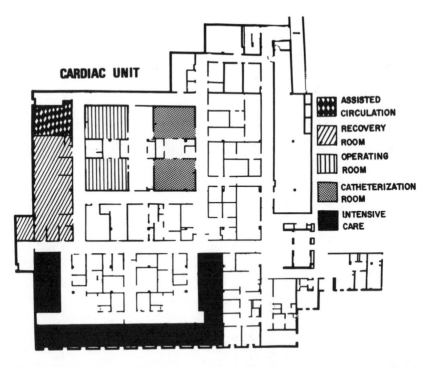

Figure 16-2 Schematic drawing of the intensive care area of the University of Ottawa Cardiac Unit.

York Heart Association classification as illustrated in Figure 16-3. Seventy-two patients (64.3%) improved by three classes, 32 patients (28.5%) improved by two classes and five patients (4.5%) improved by only one class. The remaining three patients (3.7%) demonstrated no symptomatic improvement.

The work status of 92 patients at one year follow-up is illustrated in Table 16-3. Sixty-five patients (70.7%) were working full-time, with ten patients (10.9%) working part-time. Of the 17 not working, seven (7.6%) were retired, their mean age being 57 years, seven (7.6%) were unable to work because of angina, and three (3.3%) were physically able to work but could not find employment.

Discussion

Improvement in surgical techniques and a better understanding of the indications for and potential hazards of coronary artery surgery have resulted in improved operative results and lower morbidity and mortality. More complications are expected with surgery performed on an emergency basis whether it is for unstable angina or for its possible sequelae, acute

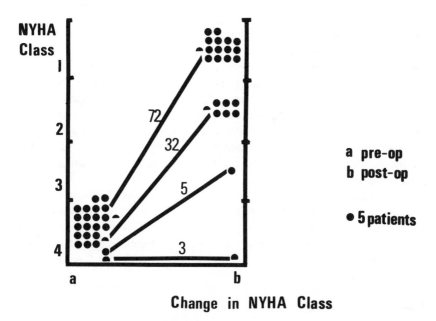

Figure 16-3 Change in New York Heart Association class in myocardial revascularization for unstable angina.

Table 16-3
Emergency Myocardial Revascularization for Unstable Angina
Work status at one year (92 patients)

Working	
Full time	65 (70.7%)
Part time	10 (10.9%)
Not working	
Able	3 (3.3%)
Not able	7 (7.6%)
Retired*	7 (7.6%)

*Mean age 57 yr, range 38 to 70 yr.

myocardial infarction, with or without cardiogenic shock. When examining the results of urgent surgery for unstable angina, one must first consider the objectives of surgical therapy in patients presenting with this syndrome: prevention of death; prevention of myocardial infarction and preservation of salvageable ischemic myocardium; relief of pain; and promotion of a useful life.

Cheanvechai et al[5] report that there is little risk in performing angiography in the acute phase. Surgery performed in the presence of acute myocardial infarction or shock, or both, is more complicated and life-threatening. Indeed, in our experience, with early surgical intervention we have found decreased operative mortality in patients refractory to medical management and before myocardial injury occurs.

Cairns et al[3] in a summary of nine authors reports that the early (one to three months) infarction rate for medically treated unstable angina patients ranged from 7% to 80%, resulting in a mortality of 0.8% to 60.0% and a late mortality from 6 to 14 months of 15% to 73%. The perioperative infarction rate of 7% compares favorably with these figures, as does the mortality rate of 20% for perioperative infarction. In addition to acceptable survival and longevity figures, symptomatic improvement in surgically treated patients has been shown to be significantly better than in those treated medically.

With an 84% follow-up on all survivors, we have demonstrated improvement in 97.5% of the patients, with 64% remaining asymptomatic. Chatterjee et al[27,28] have demonstrated that symptomatic improvement in surgical survivors who have not experienced perioperative infarction has been associated with significantly improved left ventricular function after successful surgery.

Conclusions

To advocate surgery for all unstable angina or acute myocardial infarction patients is foolhardy and would ignore many problems associated with timing, logistics and resources. Currently, only patients with unstable angina refractory to intensive medical management are treated surgically.

Coronary heart disease requires lifelong management. It is no longer rational to consider medical and surgical modes of therapy as antagonists. Neither method professes to offer a cure. Modern treatment requires the intelligent use of both. Aggressive management with angiography and emergency surgery is both feasible and indicated in selected cases, offering significant therapeutic advantages to patients who are unresponsive to medical management. We agree with Cheanvechai, however, that it should be done at an institution equipped to accomplish this without delay.

REFERENCES

1. Wearn, W.T. Thrombosis of the coronary arteries with infarction of the heart. *Am J Med Sci.* 165:250, 1923.

2. Wood, P. Acute and subacute coronary insufficiency (abstract). *Br Med J.* 1:1179–1786, 1961.

3. Cairns, J.A. Current management of unstable angina. *Can Med Assoc J.* 119:447–479, 1978.

4. Klieger, R.E., Martin, T.F., Miller, J.D. et al. Mortality of myocardial infarction treated in CCU. *Heart Lung* 4:215–226, 1975.

5. Cheanvechai, D., Effler, D.B., Loop, F.L. et al. Emergency myocardial revascularization (abstract). *Am J Cardiol.* 31:125, 1973.

6. Hill, J.D., Kerth, W.H., Kelly, J.J. et al. Emergency aortocoronry bypass for impending or extending myocardial infarction. *Circulation* 43(suppl 1):1–105, 1971.

7. Keon, W.J., Bédard, P., Akyurekli, Y. et al. Emergency coronary surgery, evolving indications. *J Cardiovasc Surg.* 17:140–146, 1976.

8. Geha, A.S., Bauer, A.E., Krone, R.J. et al. Surgical treatment of unstable angina by saphenous vein and internal mammary artery bypass grafting. *J Thorac Cardiovasc Surg.* 71:348–354, 1976.

9. Favaloro, R.G., Effler, D.B., Cheanvechai, C. et al. Acute coronary insufficiency, surgical treatment by saphenous vein graft technique. *Am J Cardiol.* 28:598–607, 1971.

10. Bertolasi, C.A., Tronge, J.E., Riccitelli, M.A. et al. Natural history of unstable angina with medical or surgical therapy. *Chest* 40:596–605, 1976.

11. Golding, L.A., Loop, F.D., Sheldon, W.C. et al. Emergency revascularization for unstable angina. *Circulation* 58:1163–1166, 1978.

12. Hultgren, H.N., Pfeiffer, J.F., Angell, W.W. et al. Unstable angina: comparison of medical and surgical management. *Am J Cardiol.* 39:734–740, 1977.

13. Huret, J.F., Agier, B., and Rosier, S.P. Delayed semi-elective coronary bypass surgery for unstable angina pectoris. *J Thorac Cardiovasc Surg.* 75(3):476–482, 1978.

14. Miller, D.C., Canom, D.S., Fogarty, G.J. et al. Saphenous vein coronary artery bypass in patients with pre-infarction angina. *Circulation* 47:234–241, 1973.

15. Hutter, A.M., Jr., Russell, R.O., Jr., Resnekov, L. et al. Unstable angina pectoris: national randomized study of surgical versus medical therapy: results in one, two and three-vessel disease (abstract). *Circulation* 56(suppl):60, 1977.

16. Cohn, L. The surgical treatment of acute myocardial ischemia. Mount Kisco, N.Y.: Futura Publishing Co., 1973.

238

17. Conti, R., Brawley, R., Pitt, B. et al. Unstable angina: morbidity and mortality in 57 consecutive patients evaluated angiographically (abstract). *Am J Cardiol.* 31:127.

18. Bert, G., Caplitt, M., Padmanabhan, N. et al. Management of preinfarction angina. *J Thorac Cardiovasc Surg.* 71:110–117, 1976.

19. Matloff, J.M., Sustaita, H., Chatterjee, K. et al. The rationale for surgery in preinfarction angina. *J Thorac Cardiovasc Surg.* 69:73–81, 1975.

20. Bender, H.W., Fisher, R.D., Faulkner, S.L. et al. Unstable coronary artery disease. *Ann Thorac Surg.* 19:521–528, 1975.

21. Bonchek, L.I., Rahimtoola, S.H., Anderson, R.D. et al. Late results following emergency saphenous vein bypass grafting for unstable angina. *Circulation* 50:972–977, 1974.

22. Seybold-Epting, W., Oglietti, J., Wukasch, D.C. et al. Early and late results after surgical treatment of pre-infarction angina. *J Am Thorac Surg.* 21:97–101, 1976.

23. Hultgren, H.N. Medical versus surgical treatment of unstable angina. *Am J Cardiol.* 38:479–485, 1976.

24. Emergency surgery needless in unstable angina patients. *Medical Post,* March 27, 1977, p 1.

25. Conti, R., Brawley, R.K., Griffiths, L.S.C. et al. Unstable angina pectoris: morbidity and mortality in 57 consecutive patients evaluated angiographically. *Am J Cardiol.* 32:745–750, 1973.

26. Bertolasi, C.A., Tronge, J.A., Carreno, C.A. et al. Unstable angina — prospective and randomized study of its evolution with and without surgery. Preliminary report. *Am J Cardiol.* 33:201–208, 1974.

27. Chatterjee, K., Swan, H.J.C., Parmley, W.W. et al. Depression of left ventricular function due to acute myocardial ischemia and its reversal after coronary saphenous vein bypass. *N Engl J Med.* 286:1117–1122, 1972.

28. Chatterjee, K., Swan, H.J.C., Parmley, W.W. et al. The influence of direct myocardial revascularization on left ventricular asynergy and function in patients with coronary heart disease — with or without previous myocardial infarction. *Circulation* 47:276–286, 1973.

17 Surgical Therapy for Unstable Angina

Lawrence H. Cohn, MD,
John J. Collins, Jr., MD,
J. Kenneth Koster, Jr., MD
Gilbert H. Mudge, MD,
Stanley Lee-Son, MD, and
Stephen Van Devanter, MD

An important subset of patients with arteriosclerotic heart disease are those with unstable angina. This syndrome has had a number of synonyms over the years[1,2] but the term unstable angina is now generally used to identify those patients intermediate between chronic stable angina and a myocardial infarction.[3] The incidence of this syndrome is as high as 40% in some series of coronary revascularization patients.[4] As a number of improvements in medical therapy for acute and chronic arteriosclerotic heart disease have taken place over the past decade there has been increasingly successful application of coronary bypass surgery for unstable angina.[5-10] Successful surgical treatment of unstable angina was first reported in 1970 by Hill and his co-workers.[11] Similar publications indicating the efficacy of emergency coronary bypass surgery in patients with this syndrome soon followed from the Cleveland Clinic and from Stanford University.[12,13] These early reports indicated that coronary bypass surgery done expeditiously, in centers where coronary bypass surgery was established, was effective in relieving myocardial ischemia. It was also associated with only a slightly higher operative mortality than elective coronary bypass surgery. Application of this aggressive surgical approach, however, did not yield uniformly good results.[14-18] These reports along with the increasing awareness of the efficacy of propranolol for unstable angina[3] stimulated a more comprehensive and rational approach to the patient with unstable angina encompassing combined medical and surgical therapy. This chapter will review our integrated medical/surgical approach for patients with unstable angina, will present a retrospective analysis of patients operated on for unstable angina at the Peter Bent Brigham Hospital from 1970 to 1978, and outline details of our anesthetic and operative management of patients with unstable angina.

MATERIAL AND METHODS

The definition of unstable angina in our clinic is 1) prolonged anginal pain, either at rest or of an increased intensity incompletely relieved by nitrates; 2) ECG and ST- and T-wave abnormalities either permanent or transient with episodes of pain but without new Q-wave formation; 3) normal serum glutamic oxaloacetic transaminase (SGOT), creatine phosphokinase, and negative creatine phosphokinase isoenzymes; and 4) angiographic documentation of one or more obstructions of the coronary arteries greater than 80% lumen diameter. Using these criteria we identified 221 patients (operated on for unstable angina from July 1970 to July 1978) of 1348 (16%) total coronary bypass graft operations. (This excludes those with concomitant valve replacement or cardiogenic shock.) There were 177 men and 44 women ranging in age from 27 to 78, with a mean age of 54 years. Intensive medical therapy was administered to all patients. This consisted of admission to the coronary care unit, adequate pain control by morphine sulfate, sedation with diazepam or nitrous oxide inhalation anesthetic, oxygen therapy, intravenous, sublingual, and/or dermal nitrates, oral vasodilators, and high-dose beta-adrenergic blockade with propranolol hydrochloride. Efforts were made with this regimen to achieve a heart rate of less than 60 beats/min and systolic arterial pressure less than 95 mm Hg. Based on the response to this medical regimen, patients could be retrospectively divided into one of two groups: those who underwent semi-elective coronary bypass surgery after being stabilized and "cooled down" to a pain-free situation (114), and those who did not stabilize with maximal medical therapy and who had to undergo urgent or emergent surgical revascularization (107). Surgery in the latter group was usually performed for one of the following indications: continuing pain despite maximal medical therapy, hemodynamic abnormalities, and/or arrhythmic instability. These patients would undergo urgent cardiac catheterization immediately followed by coronary bypass surgery.

All patients with unstable angina underwent both selective coronary angiography and left ventriculography. Single-vessel disease was found in 26 patients, double-vessel disease in 55 patients, and triple-vessel disease in 140 patients. Left main coronary stenosis was documented in 81 of the 221 patients (35%). The left ventricular ejection fraction was calculated in 150 of 221 (68%) patients and ranged from 0.11 to 0.85 with a mean of 0.59; 12 patients had ejection fractions of less than 0.40. Table 17-1 shows the distribution of the arteriographic lesions in the medically controlled and medically uncontrolled patient groups. There is no significant difference in the frequency of one-, two-, or three-vessel disease between the medically controlled and medically uncontrolled groups. There was, however, a higher percentage of patients with left main coronary stenosis in the group that could not be medically stabilized (49% vs 29%).

Table 17-1
Distribution of Arteriographic Lesions in the Medically Controlled and Uncontrolled Groups

	No. of Patients	1-Vessel Disease	2-Vessel Disease	3-Vessel Disease	Left Main Coronary Stenosis	
Medically controlled	114	13	32	69	33	(29%)
Medically uncontrolled	107	13	23	71	48	(49%)
	221	26	55	140	81	(37%)

Figure 17-1 shows the ECG response of a typical patient stabilized with intensive medical therapy with high-dose propranolol; the patient was operated upon semielectively. In Figure 17-2 are ECG and angiographic findings of a patient who underwent emergency surgery immediately after coronary angiography because of continued rest pain and ECG changes despite maximal medical therapy.

Postoperative evaluation was carried out as of April 1, 1979, providing a minimum follow-up of nine months, a maximum of 98 months, and a mean follow-up of 36 months. In addition to physical condition, postoperative assessment included incidence of late myocardial infarction, presence or absence of angina pectoris, and work status of each patient.

OPERATIVE TECHNIQUE

All patients were operated on using cardiopulmonary bypass involving single cannulation of the right atrium for venous drainage and cannulation of the ascending aorta for arterial perfusion. Hemodilution was carried out in the oxygenator with a Ringer lactate-albumin prime to a hematocrit of approximately 20% to 25%; blood was added only if patients were anemic prior to surgery. Flow rates on cardiopulmonary bypass varied from 1.25 to 1.75 l/min/m² with moderate systemic hypothermia.

During the eight years of this series there was an evolution in myocardial protection techniques; the most common techniques utilized were 1) ventricular fibrillation with segmental coronary isolation, 2) intermittent ischemic arrest with periods of reperfusion, 3) continuous ischemic arrest with local cardiac hypothermia, and 4) continuous ischemic arrest with local cardiac hypothermia plus intraaortic hyperkalemic cardioplegia. Hypothermic ischemic arrest with topical hypothermia and hyperkalemic cardioplegic solution (300 ml every 30 min of ischemic time) is now most commonly used. The hyperkalemic solution consists of 30 mEq potassium/liter of Ringer's lactate and bicarbonate to insure a slightly basic pH, and is slightly hyperosmotic compared to blood. The myocardial protection technique is shown in Figure 17-3. During the single period of aortic cross-clamp all distal venocoronary anastomoses are done using a single running suture of 6-0 monofilament Prolene beginning at the heel of the

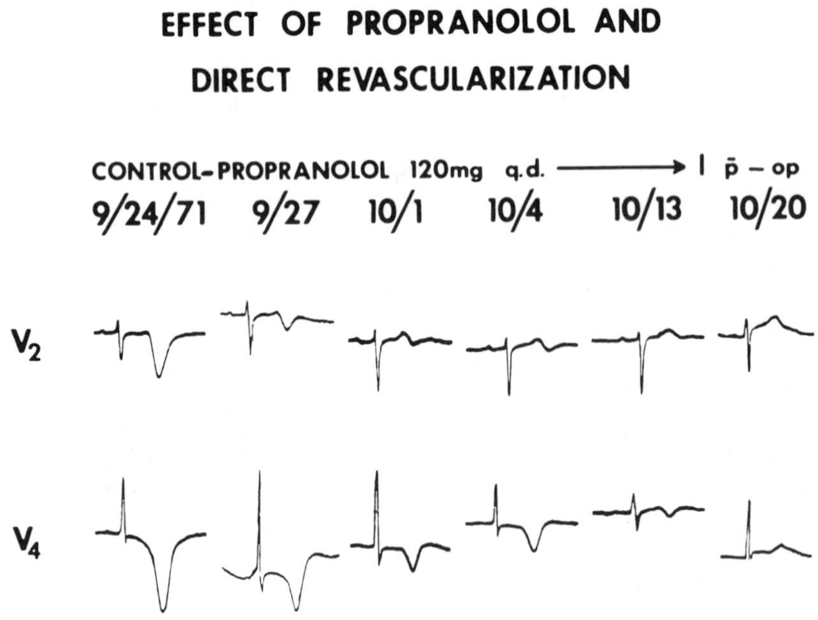

EFFECT OF PROPRANOLOL AND
DIRECT REVASCULARIZATION

Figure 17-1 Effect of propranolol on direct revascularization in a patient with unstable angina. Stabilization of ECG by propranolol is noted over a two-day period. (Copyright 1978, American Medical Association. *Arch Surg.* 113:1312, 1978. Reproduced with permission.)

anastomosis running around the toe and completing the anastomosis on the other side of the vein heel to minimize operating time and ischemia. After all distal anastomoses are complete, the heart is perfused and defibrillated and a partially occluding aortic clamp is placed so that proximal aorta to venous anastomoses can be performed while the heart is being resuscitated and reperfused. Cardiopulmonary bypass is then discontinued. A left ventricular vent was not routinely used unless there was an exceptionally large bronchial arterial collateral flow or significant aortic regurgitation.

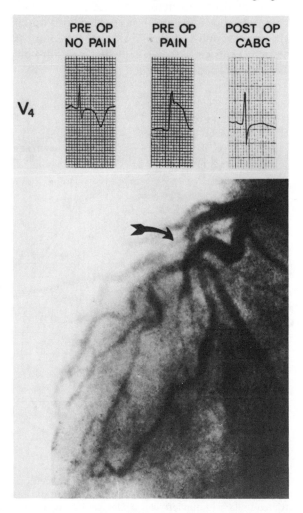

Figure 17-2 Electrocardiographic and angiographic findings in a patient with unstable angina refractory to medical therapy requiring emergency coronary bypass after coronary revascularization. Arrow points to critical lesion of left anterior descending. (Copyright 1978, American Medical Association. *Arch Surg.* 113:1312, 1978. Reproduced with permission.)

The anesthetic regimen consists of intravenous morphine sulfate (3 mg/kg) with nitrous oxide and thiopental for induction. Because of the metabolism of morphine, overnight ventilation is required with extubation usually on the morning of the first postoperative day; this is usually done when ventilatory mechanics and the arterial blood gas picture is satisfactory. A left atrial pressure monitoring line is used occasionally, particularly in those patients who cannot be stabilized prior to surgery. A right atrial line is also placed at operation through the right atrial appendage. Digoxin is administered prophylactically in maintenance doses postoperatively, and all patients received preincision intravenous cephalosporin antibiotics for two days intravenously and two days orally. A temporary pacing wire is placed on the right ventricle. Mediastinal chest tubes are placed with the integrity of both pleural spaces being maintained.

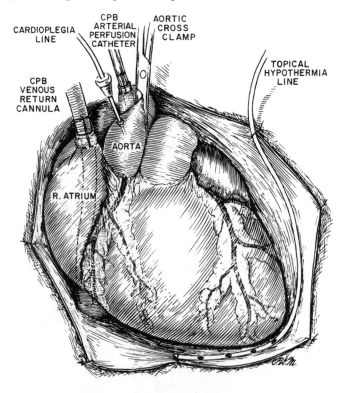

Figure 17-3 Cardiopulmonary bypass technique and current method of myocardial protection during coronary bypass surgery. A single right atrial cannula and distal ascending aortic cannula without left ventricular vent is used for most patients. Topical hypothermia is accomplished by perfusing 4°C lactated Ringer's solution through the pericardium, through the nasogastric tube, and cardioplegia intermittently perfuses cold hyperkalemic cardioplegic solution into the aortic root. (Cohn, L. [Ed.]. *The Treatment of Acute Myocardial Ischemia.* New York: Futura Publicaions, 1979. Reproduced with permission.)

Intraaortic balloon counterpulsation was utilized in 20 patients. In 12 it was placed preoperatively prior to catheterization and surgery, while in eight patients it was placed during operation because of perioperative ischemia. The device was inserted through the femoral artery with a Dacron tube conduit and connected to an Avco balloon pump console.

Table 17-2 shows the number of graft operations in each of the two groups and the mean grafts per patient. Thirty-six patients had a single bypass graft, 79 had a double graft, 84 had triple grafts, 19 a quadruple graft, two had a quintuple graft, and one patient had six bypass grafts.

Table 17-2
Bypass Graft Operations in Medically Controlled and Uncontrolled Patients with Unstable Angina

	No. of Patients	Coronary Bypass Grafts						Mean Grafts per Patient
		1	2	3	4	5	6	
Medically controlled	114	20	38	39	14	2	1	2.5
Medically uncontrolled	107	16	41	45	5	0	0	2.4
Totals	221	36	79	84	19	2	1	

RESULTS

The operative deaths and late deaths in both the medically controlled and medically uncontrolled groups are summarized in Table 17-3. Perioperative myocardial infarction was defined as the appearance of a new Q wave or loss of R-wave voltage in the postoperative ECG, usually combined with elevations in SGOT greater than 100 mg%, or positive creatine phosphokinase myocardial isoenzymes, or both. The follow-up period was nine to 98 months, with a mean of 36 months. In the medically stabilized group the operative mortality was one of 114 patients (0.9%). There were seven perioperative myocardial infarctions (6.1%) and two late deaths (1.8%). In the medically uncontrolled group 107 patients (urgent or emergent surgery) there were seven operative deaths (6.5%), eight perioperative myocardial infarctions (7.5%), and five late deaths (5.5%). The overall statistics of the 221 patients with unstable angina showed eight operative deaths (3.2%), 15 perioperative myocardial infarctions including fatal infarctions (6.9%), and eight late deaths (3.6%). Table 17-4 summarizes operative mortality vs extent of coronary artery disease; triple-vessel mortality (5 out of 140) (3.5%); there were two operative deaths out of 55 patients with double-vessel disease and one of 26 in single-vessel disease patients.

Table 17-3
Operative and Late Deaths in Patients with Unstable Angina

	No. of Patients	Operative Deaths	Late Deaths
Medically controlled	114	1 (0.9%)	3
Medically uncontrolled	107	7 (6.5%)	5
Totals	221	8 (3.6%)	8 (3.6%)

Table 17-4
Operative Mortality vs Extent of Coronary Artery Disease in Patients with Unstable Angina

	No. of Patients	Operative Deaths	Late Deaths
1-Vessel Disease	26	1	1
2-Vessel Disease	55	2	3
3-Vessel Disease	140	5	4
Totals	221	8	8

Table 17-5 summarizes data on the 81 of 221 patients (35%) who had significant obstruction of the left main coronary artery. The stable left main group consisted of 33 patients with one operative death (3%), while the medically unstable left main group had 48 patients with five operative deaths (10.4%) for an overall operative mortality of 6 of 81 patients (7.4%). Of the eight operative deaths in the entire series six patients had left main coronary stenosis. Actuarial life-table analyses of survival data are illustrated in Figures 17-4, 17-5, 17-6. In Figure 17-4 survival curves for the medically controlled, medically uncontrolled, and entire group are shown; the overall survival at 98 months was 87%, 89% for the stable group, and 83% for the emergent group (p < 0.06). There was no statistical significance between survival of patients with one-, two-, or three-vessel involvement, nor for the survival of non-left-main vs left main coronary occlusion (p < 0.07). Of the 20 patients who had intraaortic balloon counterpulsation (IABCP) four died (20%); all four had the balloon placed intraoperatively for acute myocardial ischemia. All 12 patients who had IABCP preoperatively, including five with left main stenosis, are long-term survivors.

Postoperative angina, late nonfatal myocardial infarction, and work capacity was determined from the 200 surviving patients, excluding the operative deaths (8), the late deaths (8), and those patients lost to follow-up (4). The incidence of recurrent angina is summarized in Table 17-6; 141 of 200 patients (70%) had no angina whatsoever, 48 (24%) patients had mild, but markedly improved angina, and 11 (6%) had the same or worse degree of angina. Table 17-7 summarizes the work status of the 200 patients available for follow-up; 75 (37.5%) patients are currently working at some form of gainful occupation, 38 patients could work but choose not to, 50 patients have retired, and 37 patients are on disability.

DISCUSSION

The overall therapeutic plan for patients with unstable angina has undergone important changes since the first successful surgical report in 1971.[11] At the outset, unstable angina or, as it was most often termed in

Table 17-5
Mortality in Patients with Unstable Angina
Having Left Main Coronary Stenosis

	No. of Patients	Operative Deaths	Late Deaths
Medically controlled	33	1 (3%)	0
Medically uncontrolled	48	5 (10.4%)	3
Totals	81	6 (7.4%)	3 (3.7%)

Table 17-6
Incidence of Recurrent Angina

Degree of Recurrent Angina	No. of Patients
None	141
Mild	48
Unchanged	11
	200

Table 17-7
Postoperative Work Status of Patients with Unstable Angina

	No. of Patients
Working	75
Could work	38
Retired	50
Disabled	37
	200

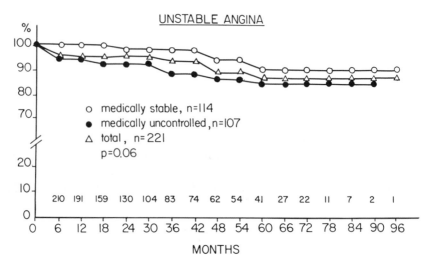

Figure 17-4 Actuarial survival for patients with unstable angina divided into the medically controlled and medically uncontrolled group compared to the total.

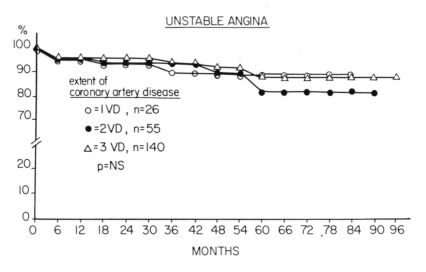

Figure 17-5 Actuarial delineation of survival of patients with unstable angina divided into one-, two-, and three-vessel disease.

1971, "preinfarction angina," was thought to be a surgical emergency requiring acute revascularization because of acute myocardial ischemia. Theoretically this approach would appear to be ideal but because of imperfect operating techniques, inadequate myocardial preservation and less efficient anesthetic management of myocardial ischemia lead to high mortality in some centers. It was suggested by Fischl and co-workers[3] that propranolol should be effective in patients with unstable angina in whom there was a serious imbalance between myocardial oxygen supply and demand. This concept was cautiously tested during the early years of this series and led to the present increasing use of this regimen in all such patients. This view, however, was not initially shared by others; some institutions believed that the use of propranolol in patients who were about to undergo coronary bypass surgery was contraindicated. For example, Viljoen, et al[19] advised that propranolol be discontinued three weeks prior to coronary bypass surgery. Our policy has been to continue propranolol up to the operation, having found discontinuation of propranolol to be extremely detrimental in some patients.[20,21] Our clinical data and that of others[22,23] have demonstrated that many patients with unstable angina, including those with left main coronary stenosis, can be brought under in-hospital control with intensive medical treatment. The number of patients with unstable angina who are currently operated upon as emergencies is relatively small compared to the earlier years of this series. We employ maximal medical therapy in an attempt to stabilize these patients to a pain-free, stable ECG

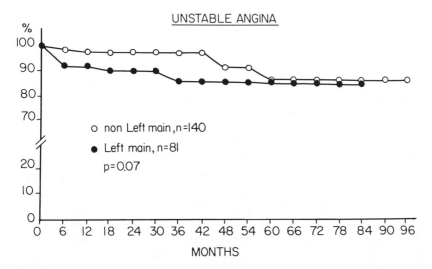

Figure 17-6 Patients with unstable angina divided into actuarial survival curves depending upon the presence or absence of left main coronary stenosis.

state. In addition to bedrest in the coronary care unit, high-dose propranolol; nitrous oxide inhalation; sedation; and dermal, oral, and intravenous nitrates are administered. Once the pain-instability cycle can be
broken, patients may undergo coronary angiography and surgery with risk
comparable to that of elective coronary revascularization. On the other
hand, angiography and urgent coronary bypass surgery is done on an
urgent and emergency basis for patients who do not respond to this regimen
and are suspected of having a left main coronary stenosis. Some surgeons
have been concerned about postoperative myocardial depression that may
result from propranolol administered at high doses up until the time of
surgery. This has not been our experience. If bradycardia or depressed
myocardial function is noted after cardiopulmonary bypass, these abnormalities can be easily reversed with dopamine. The number of patients with
depressed ventricular function after propranolol is rare and probably
reflects the less-than-adequate myocardial protection administered to these
critical patients in earlier years.[22,23]

Controversy concerning the ideal form of management of patients
with unstable angina was the subject of a large multicenter prospective randomized medical/surgical study.[24] These results have been recently
reported and have provoked considerable comment.[25] Despite the large
number of potential patients for entry into the study from the nine
cooperating centers, only 288 patients in a 48-month period were entered.
All had transient ST- and T-wave changes, 90% had pain at rest in the
hospital, and 76% had multivessel coronary disease. These data are discussed in detail by Conti and Curry (see Chapter 21) but it was found that
both the medical and surgical mortality in the hospital was low and that the
infarction rate was the same in both groups. The long-term survival of both
the medical and surgical patients was similar and not statistically different.
A great deal of emphasis was placed on the effect of the different modalities
on longevity. However, the real purpose of the study was to determine if
medical therapy could stabilize a significant percentage of patients who
otherwise would have undergone urgent or emergency surgery. The study
clearly demonstrated that the majority of patients treated medically could
be stabilized and undergo semielective surgery. It is important to note that
in the subsequent months after the patients were divided into medicine or
surgery groups, 36% of the medically designated patients crossed over to
have surgery within a very short time after entrance into the study. These
data clearly do not allow any valid conclusions to be made about the
longevity statistics of medical vs surgical therapy for this condition. The
data suggest the ultimate need for operation in the large majority of patients with unstable angina, whether or not they can be stabilized with
medical therapy after admission. Other randomized medical/surgical
studies in single centers have been carried out and similarly do not show
statistically significant differences in longevity over relatively short-term

periods with few exceptions.[26-29] In all of these studies there is documentation of the safety of medical stabilization for the acute patients but a high crossover rate from medical to surgical therapy during the early months. These papers also are consistent with the early clinical observations by Krauss et al[30] and Gazes et al,[31] which showed a very high one-year infarction and mortality rate in patients with unstable angina in an era prior to coronary angiography and propranolol.

The role of preoperative intensive pharmacologic beta blockade cannot be stressed too much. We believe that in most cases propranolol will satisfactorily control myocardial oxygen demands to a level consistent with that of available oxygen supply. With more aggressive use of multidrug therapy and the marked improvement in all forms of medical treatment, the number of patients truly medically refractory becomes smaller each year. These refractory patients are usually those with left main coronary stenosis or very proximal tight stenosis of the left anterior descending artery. In some instances, despite maximal pharmacologic intervention, the safety of the patient may be enhanced by the use of the intraaortic balloon counterpulsation device.[32] Some have recommended that this device be used in most patients with unstable angina prior to surgery.[33-37] We do not concur with routine use and have used IABCP preoperatively only selectively for those who remain unstable despite maximal pharmacologic manipulation. In our unstable angina group there were 12 of 221 (5%) patients in whom the balloon was used preoperatively. Of these 12, five had left main coronary stenosis. Implantation of the balloon pump commits the patient to an urgent operation and the major arterial complication rate of balloon counterpulsation is significant.[38] In our own hospital 20% of patients had peripheral vascular complications associated with the use of IABCP. Therefore, we continue to employ IABCP selectively as do others.[6,7]

The left main coronary patient group has been found to be a heterogeneous clinical group because of the wide variety of clinical presentation. Patients with left main coronary stenosis may have no angina, stable chronic angina, or totally refractory unstable angina, a reflection of the absence or presence of coronary collaterals.[39] In our earlier clinical experience the appearance of a left main lesion was felt to be an indication for urgent surgery. As with most syndromes in coronary heart disease both cardiologists and cardiac surgeons have acquired a better "feel" for the nuances of the various anatomic and clinical syndromes. The timing of operation is not quite so rigid, and is much more judicious and appropriate to the environment and the individual patient situation.

Finally, the marked improvement in surgical results throughout the world is an outcome of improved anesthesia and improved myocardial protection for patients undergoing coronary bypass surgery.[40-44] As we have indicated, propranolol is continued up to the time of surgery without problems; occasional bradycardia noted on induction should be treated with atropine. Anesthetic safety is enhanced by careful hemodynamic monitoring and the maintenance of the rate × pressure product less than 12000[42] and in some instances the monitoring of a special precordial "V" lead has been helpful in predicting the onset of ischemia before any hemodynamic change occurs.[40] The time from which the unstable angina patient leaves his hospital bed to the time he is on cardiopulmonary bypass is the most critical period for patients with unstable angina; better knowledge of the determinants of ischemia during this period and more sensitive intraoperative monitoring devices have made this period considerably safer. Myocardial protection has also improved significantly in the last five years since the introduction of hyperkalemic cardioplegia by Gay and Ebert,[45] which cools the endocardium as well as epicardium in a very short time. After cardioplegic arrest there is complete cessation of any mechanical work and a small amount of substrate continues to be metabolized during anoxia. Though our series has a perioperative infarction rate of 6% for the entire series, this reflects our entire experience extending back to 1970, when myocardial protection was less effective. Our perioperative infarction rate is now about 3% in cases of coronary artery bypass grafting for unstable and stable angina while the numbers of grafts per patients have increased.

In conclusion, all patients with unstable angina should be subjected to an intensive maximal medical effort to "cool down" the ischemic myocardium and deranged hemodynamics. As this and many other series now show, stabilization of unstable angina is quite possible in the majority of patients. Emergency surgery need not be performed except in situations where maximal medical therapy has been carried out without cessation of pain and where there is continuing hemodynamic or arrhythmic instability. Ultimately, surgical therapy is the treatment of choice for unstable angina, whether done urgently in the few cases that require it, or whether it be done in the semielective state as most instances allow. Coronary artery bypass grafting for unstable angina has a low perioperative infarction rate, a low operative mortality, and excellent long-term survival. In those situations where there is suspected left main coronary stenosis and marked instability of the patient's clinical, electrical, and hemodynamic course, selective use of preoperative balloon counterpulsation should be employed.

REFERENCES

1. Fowler, N.O. "Preinfarctional" angina: a need for an objective definition and for a controlled clinical trial of its management. *Circulation* 44:755–757, 1971.

2. Cohn, P.F., and Cohn, L.H. Medical/surgical treatment of unstable angina. Edited by L.H. Cohn. In *The Treatment of Acute Myocardial Ischemia: An Integrated Medical/Surgical Approach*. Mt. Kisco, N.Y.: Futura Publishing Co., 1979.

3. Fischl, S.J., Herman, M.V., and Gorlin, R. The intermediate coronary syndrome: clinical, angiographic, and therapeutic aspects. *N Engl J Med.* 288:1193–1198, 1973.

4. Hatcher, C.R., Jr., King, S.B., III, and Kaplan, J.A. Surgical management of unstable angina. *World J Surg.* 2:689–700, 1978.

5. Cohn, L.H., Alpert, J., Koster, J.K.K., Jr. et al. Changing indications for the surgical treatment of unstable angina. *Arch Surg.* 113:1312–1316, 1978.

6. Olinger, G.N., Bonchek, L.I., Keelan, M.H., Jr. et al. Unstable angina: the case for operation. *Am J Cardiol.* 42:634–640, 1978.

7. Golding, L.A.R., Loop, F.D., Sheldon, W.C. et al. Emergency revascularization for unstable angina. *Am J Cardiol.* 41:356, 1978.

8. Geha, A.S., Baue, A.F., Krone, R.J. et al. Surgical treatment of unstable angina by saphenous vein and internal mammary artery bypass grafting. *J Thorac Cardiovasc Surg.* 71:348, 1976.

9. Schroeder, J.S., Lamb, I., Hu, M. et al. Coronary bypass surgery for unstable angina pectoris: long-term survival and function. *JAMA.* 237:2609, 1977.

10. Matloff, J.M., Suistaita, H., Chatterjee, K. et al. The rationale for surgery in pre-infarction angina. *J Thorac Cardiovasc Surg.* 69:73, 1975.

11. Hill, J.D., Kerth, W.H., Kelly, J.J. et al. Emergency aorto-coronary bypass for impending or extending myocardial infarction. *Circulation* 43:105–110, 1971.

12. Favaloro, R.G., Effler, D.B., Cheanvechai, C. et al. Acute coronary insufficiency (impending myocardial infarction and myocardial infarction). *Am J Cardiol.* 28:598–607, 1971.

13. Cohn, L.H., Fogarty, T.J., Daily, P.O. et al. Emergency coronary artery bypass surgery. *Surgery* 70:821–829, 1971.

14. Hultgren, H.N., Pfeifer, J.F., Angell, W.W. et al. Unstable angina: comparison of medical and surgical management. *Ann Thorac Surg.* 19:521–528, 1975.

15. Bertolasi, C.A., Tronge, J.E., Riccitelli, M.A. et al. Natural history of unstable angina with medical or surgical therapy. *Chest* 70:596–605, 1976.

16. Seybold-Epting, W., Oglietti, J., Wukasch, D.C. et al. Early and late results after surgical treatment of preinfarction angina. *Ann Thorac Surg.* 21:97–102, 1976.

17. Berndt, T.B., Miller, D.C., Silverman, J.F. et al. Coronary bypass surgery for unstable angina pectoris. *Am J Med.* 58:171–176, 1975.

18. Conti, R.C., Brawley, R.K., Griffith, L.S.C. et al. Unstable angina pectoris: morbidity and mortality in 57 consecutive patients evaluated angiographically. *Am J Cardiol.* 32:745–750, 1973.

19. Viljoen, J.F., Estafanous, G., and Kellner, G.A. Propranolol and cardiac surgery. *J Thorac Cardiovasc Surg.* 64:826–830, 1972.

20. Alderman, E.L., Coltart, J., Wettach, G.E. et al. Coronary artery syndromes after sudden propranolol withdrawal. *Ann Intern Med.* 81:625–627, 1974.

21. Diaz, R.G., Somberg, J., Freeman, E. et al. Myocardial infarction after propranolol withdrawal. *Am Heart J.* 88:257–258, 1974.

22. Caralps, J.M., Mulet, J., Wienke, H.R. et al. Results of coronary artery surgery in patients receiving propranolol. *J Thorac Cardiovasc Surg.* 67:526–529, 1974.

23. Jones, E.L., Kaplan, J.A., Korney, E.R. et al. Propranolol therapy in patients undergoing myocardial revascularization. *Am J Cardiol.* 38:696–700, 1976.

24. Russell, R.O., Moraski, R.E., Kouchoukos, N. et al. Unstable angina pectoris: national cooperative study group to compare medical and surgical therapy. I. Report of protocol and patient population. *Am J Cardiol.* 37:896–902, 1976.

25. Hutter, A.M., Jr., Russell, R.O., Jr., Resnekov, L. et al. Unstable angina pectoris — National Randomized Study of surgical versus medical therapy: Results in 1, 2 and 3 vessel disease. *Circulation* 55(suppl 3):60, 1977.

26. Selden, R., Neill, W.A., Ritzmann, L.W. et al. Medical versus surgical therapy for acute coronary insufficiency: a randomized study. *N Engl J Med.* 293:1329–1333, 1975.

27. Hultgren, H.N., Pfeifer, J.F., Angell, W.W. et al. Unstable angina: comparison of medical and surgical management. *Am J Cardiol.* 39:734–740, 1977.

28. Bender, H.W., Jr., Fisher, R.D., Faulkner, S.L. et al. Unstable coronary artery disease: comparison of medical and surgical treatment. *Ann Thorac Surg.* 19:521–528, 1975.

29. Bertolasi, C.A., Tronge, J.E., Carreno, C.A. et al. Unstable angina: prospective and randomized study of its evolution, with and without surgery. *Am J Cardiol.* 33:201–208, 1974.

30. Krauss, K.R., Hutter, A.M., Jr., and DeSanctis, R.W. Acute coronary insufficiency: course and followup. *Circulation* 45 & 46:66–71, 1972.

31. Gazes, P.C., Mobley, E.M., Jr., Faris, H.M., Jr. et al. Preinfarctional (unstable) angina: a prospective study — ten-year followup. *Circulation* 48:331–337, 1973.

32. Lamberti, J.J., Cohn, L.H., Lesch, M. et al. Intraaortic balloon counterpulsation for postoperative left ventricular power failure: indications and long-term results. *Arch Surg.* 109:766, 1974.

33. Cooper, G.N., Jr., Singh, A.K., Vargas, L.L. et al. Preoperative intraaortic balloon assist in high risk revascularization patients. *Am J Surg.* 133:463–468, 1977.

34. Gold, H.K., Leinbach, R.C., Buckley, M.J. et al. Refractory angina pectoris: followup after intra-aortic balloon pumping and surgery. *Circulation* 54:41–46, 1976.

35. Scully, H.E., Gunstensen, J., Williams, W.G. et al. Surgical management of complicated acute coronary insufficiency. *Surgery* 80:437–442, 1976.

36. Weintraub, R.M., Voukydis, P.C., Aroesty, J.M. et al. Treatment of preinfarction angina with intra-aortic balloon counterpulsation and surgery. *Am J Cardiol.* 34:809–814, 1974.

37. Langou, R.A., Geha, A.S., Hammond, G.L. et al. Surgical approach for patients with unstable angina pectoris: role of the response to initial medical therapy and intra-aortic balloon pumping in perioperative complications after aortocoronary bypass grafting. *Am J Cardiol.* 42:629–633, 1978.

38. Pace, P.D., Tilney, N.L., Lesch, M. et al. Peripheral arterial complications of intra-aortic balloon counterpulsation. *Surgery* 82:685, 1977.

39. Cohn, L.H., Koster, J.K.K., Mee, R.B. et al. Surgical management of stenosis of the left main coronary artery. *World J Surg.* 2:701–708, 1978.

40. Kaplan, J.A., and King, S.B. The precordial electrocardiographic lead (V_5) in patients who have coronary artery disease. *Anesthesiology* 45:570, 1976.

41. Dunbar, R.W., Kaplan, J.A., and King, S.B. Vasodilator treatment of heart failure after cardiopulmonary bypass. *Anesth Analg (Cleve).* 54:842, 1975.

42. Kaplan, J.A., Dunbar, R.W., and Jones, E.L. Nitroglycerin infusion during coronary artery surgery. *Anesthesiology* 45:14, 1976.

Kaplan, J.A., Dunbar, R.W., Bland, J.W., Jr. et al. Propranolol and cardiac surgery: a problem for the anesthesiologist? *Anesth Analg (Cleve).* 54:571, 1975.

44. Moore, C.H., Lombardo, T.R., Allums, J.A. et al. Left main coronary artery stenosis: hemodynamic monitoring to reduce mortality. *Ann Thorac Surg.* 26:445–451, 1978.

45. Gay, W.A., Jr., and Ebert, P.A. Functional, metabolic and morphologic effects of potassium induced cardioplegia. *Surgery* 74:284, 1973.

18 Factors Influencing Morbidity and Mortality During Surgery For Unstable Angina

Richard D. Weisel, MD
Robert J. Cusimano,
Ronald S. Baigrie, MD,
Bernard S. Goldman, MD
George Christakis,
Robert Zeldin, MD, and
Ronald J. Baird, MD

DEFINITION OF THE PROBLEM

Unstable angina has been defined as "an increase in the frequency and severity of symptoms during the month prior to presentation."[1] Included in this broad definition are patients with new onset angina, crescendo angina, and patients with rest angina. By this definition, there is an increasing number of patients with unstable angina being referred for aortocoronary bypass (ACB) surgery. At the University of Toronto hospitals, the incidence of unstable angina has risen from 20% among 726 patients undergoing ACB in 1970-1971, to 55% among 2210 patients undergoing ACB in 1978-1979. This broad category includes both patients requiring urgent revascularization because of uncontrolled symptoms and patients undergoing elective surgery for new onset angina. Therefore it is not surprising that the risks of ACB remain higher for patients with unstable than for patients with stable angina. Between 1975 and 1979 at the Toronto General Hospital, there was a 3% mortality for the 1286 patients with stable angina and a 6% mortality for the 772 patients with unstable angina. Because the number of patients with unstable angina is increasing, a careful review of the factors producing their higher risk of surgery is mandatory.

HIGH-RISK SUBGROUPS

The most important factor influencing the results of surgery for unstable angina is the patient's presentation to the coronary care unit. An extensive review of 876 patients undergoing surgery for unstable angina at the Toronto General Hospital between July 1, 1974 and June 30, 1979, was conducted to identify prognostic factors. Gazes[2] was the first to report an increased hospital mortality for patients who continued to complain of rest pain despite medical attention. Bertolasi[3] reported an increased mortality (35%) for patients with the intermediate syndrome as compared to a low (5%) mortality for those treated for progressive angina. The National Cooperative Study Group[4] reported a significant increase in the hospital mortality rate among patients with triple-vessel as compared to single-vessel disease (6% vs 0%). In addition, there was an increased incidence of in-hospital acute myocardial infarction among those with triple-vessel disease (12% vs 6%). A recent report by Wiles et al[5] indicated that hospital mortality following ACB for unstable angina was increased in patients who failed a trial of maximal medical therapy as well as those with hypertension and triple-vessel disease. Armstrong[6] has investigated the prognostic value of recent ischemic ECG changes and increases in CK-MB values when they are measured serially in the coronary care unit. If both ECG and CK-MB were normal, there was a 14% incidence of subsequent ischemic episodes, but there was no infarction or mortality. If both ECG and CK-MB were abnormal, there was an 8% infarction rate and a 15% mortality within one year.

These studies demonstrate the significance of identifying high-risk subgroups for medical or surgical therapy for unstable angina. The results of surgical intervention cannot be considered independent of a careful evaluation of the risk factors in the patient population under investigation.

The importance to the surgeon of identifying high-risk subgroups must be emphasized. Patients who have an incomplete response to medical therapy are frequently presented for surgical consideration. Most have extensive coronary artery disease and, provided the lesions are amenable to surgical correction, ACB is considered as a semielective procedure. The surgeon must define the risks in order to decide the appropriate timing and his alternatives for the carrying out of his procedure. Patients with unstable angina who have no electrocardiographic or enzyme abnormalities may undergo elective bypass surgery with risks comparable to patients with stable angina. However, patients who have evidence of extensive preoperative ischemic injury present a greater challenge. These patients may benefit from a planned delay in revascularization. An appropriate delay may be four to six weeks following their acute ischemic episode. Patients who continue to have ischemic events despite optimal medical therapy cannot await a "cooling off" period. For these patients, the surgeon must critically evaluate the conduct of his procedure to minimize the operative risks. The use of preoperative intraaortic balloon pump assistance or preoperative hemodynamic monitoring for anesthesia induction may be helpful. Only a careful analysis of the anticipated risks of surgery will permit appropriate timing and adequate preoperative preparation.

Definition of High-Risk Subgroups

Retrospective review identified three factors that appeared to differentiate patients with unstable angina with a higher surgical risk. First, the pattern and duration of pain that induced the patient's presentation differentiated high- from low-risk groups. All patients had an increasing frequency and severity of their ischemic symptoms. Those with short (< 20 min) episodes of pain usually had provoked, rather than resting, symptoms. An occasional patient with short pain episodes developed symptoms with minimal provocation and had evidence (by ECG or enzyme changes) of severe myocardial ischemia. These patients are an exception to our categorization attempts. Patients with prolonged pain episodes developed their symptoms spontaneously. An occasional individual had provoked episodes of prolonged rest pain and these patients were difficult to categorize.

A careful examination of the electrocardiograms also permitted differentiation. New ischemic changes included ST depression (or, in eight patients, elevation) greater than 2 mm and, occasionally, T-wave changes. Electrocardiograms were obtained with pain in the majority of patients. However, most patients who developed ischemic ECG changes with their initial pain episodes had persistence of these abnormalities after the pain was finally controlled by medical management.

Serum enzyme elevation was an influential factor. Measurements were made daily for three days after admission to the coronary care unit or until the symptoms were controlled. Enzyme elevations were within the normal range, slightly elevated (less than 1.5 times normal) or substantially elevated (greater than 3 times normal). Occasionally, patients showed distinct elevations of cardiac enzymes within the normal range. These patients may have had subclinical myocardial necrosis. However, more extensive arborization of the categories was not attempted.

Analysis of these three factors permitted differentiation of unstable angina patients into five subgroups. Patients with crescendo angina (CA) had an increasing frequency and severity of symptoms; however, their episodes were short and usually provoked. They did not have changes in ECG or enzymes while being treated for their acute ischemic episode. These patients underwent semielective or elective revascularization. The second group was "classical" acute coronary insufficiency (ACI). These patients had prolonged episodes of rest pain despite medical attention. The majority had reversible new ischemic electrocardiographic changes associated with their pain episodes. A careful review of the results of their surgery did not uncover a substantial difference between those with reversible ischemic ECG changes and those without. Therefore, the ACI group includes patients with prolonged episodes of rest pain with or without reversible ECG changes. Many patients had prolonged episodes of rest pain and new ischemic ECG changes that persisted despite treatment for their acute ischemic episode. Patients who had electrocardiographic, but not enzymatic, criteria for a subendocardial myocardial infarction were categorized as "probable" infarction (PI). Patients with both persistent electrocardiographic abnormalities and minimal enzyme elevations associated with episodes of rest pain had a subendocardial infarction (SEI). Patients with an unstable anginal pattern whose initial electrocardiogram and enzyme results suggested a transmural myocardial infarction were classified as either an evolving or "extending" transmural infarction or as postinfarction unstable angina. The few patients operated on under these circumstances had medically resistant symptomatology and a higher risk for their urgent surgery.

This classification of high-risk groups with unstable angina varies considerably from most recent reports. Patients with new onset angina or a crescendo pattern to chronic stable angina are seldom admitted to our coronary care unit. Instead, the majority of patients are admitted because of a strong suspicion of an acute myocardial infarction. Patients with new onset or crescendo angina are rarely referred for urgent surgery.

Patients admitted to the coronary care unit with prolonged episodes of rest pain are a diverse group. Those with reversible ischemic electrocardiographic changes and no serum enzyme elevations have been included in the National Cooperative Study.[4] Results of surgical treatment in this group of patients were not different than those with prolonged episodes of rest pain without ECG changes with pain. Serial CK-MB analysis in the CCU has demonstrated evidence of limited myocardial necrosis in 20% of both groups with acute coronary insufficiency (those with and those without reversible ischemic ECG changes with their pain). We have therefore found it appropriate to combine the two groups into the category of ACI.

Patients with prolonged episodes of rest pain who have new ischemic electrocardiographic changes that do not resolve as the pain is controlled appear to have a higher perioperative morbidity and mortality than patients with ACI. Although these patients do not have enzyme elevations, it is likely that they have had a limited subendocardial infarction. They are therefore classified as probable infarction. These patients would have been excluded from the National Cooperative Study of unstable angina but were apparently included in the studies of Bertolasi[3] and Armstrong.[6] Some have considered these patients to have persistent unstable angina following a myocardial infarction. This designation seems unreasonable since their extent of preoperative ischemic injury is distinctly less than those with a definite subendocardial infarction or, indeed, those with definite transmural infarction.

Patients with a documented subendocardial infarction (SEI) have a high risk of continued medical therapy. There have been, however, few reports on the results of surgical therapy (within one month) of this event. Patients with unstable angina and prolonged episodes of rest pain therefore have a spectrum of preoperative ischemic injury that extends from patients without ECG changes to those with fixed ST- and T-wave abnormalities and slightly elevated enzymes. We have therefore developed three groups that represent this spectrum (ACI, PI, and SEI). Although not strictly comparable to other recent studies of unstable angina, these three high-risk subgroups provide the greatest challenge to the surgeon and evaluation of their high-risk status is therefore essential.

Additional Risk Factors

In addition to the type of unstable angina, other factors contributing to the surgical risk were also investigated (Table 18-1). First, the extent of coronary artery disease was assessed by a preoperative coronary artery score. A value was provided to each of the three major coronary distributions based on the most severe lesion in the major artery in that distribution. A score of 1 was applied when the stenosis was 25% to 50%, 2 when the stenosis was 51% to 74%, 3 when the stenosis was 75% to 89%, 4 when the stenosis was 90% to 99%, and 5 when the stenosis was 100%. In addition, the occurrence of left main stenosis or left main equivalent was recorded. The left ventriculogram was graded on a scale of 1 to 4. The New York Heart Association classification was employed to grade the functional status (1 to 4). The timing of surgery was also found to be an important determinant of the results. A score of 1 to 4 was developed for surgical timing: 1 = elective, 2 = semielective (same hospitalization as the acute ischemic episode), 3 = urgent (12 to 48 hr following an event), 4 =

emergent (0 to 12 hr following an event). The indication for the preoperative intraaortic balloon pump assistance was recorded. Intraoperative factors that were evaluated include the number of coronary arteries bypassed, the postoperative coronary artery score (where a bypass to a previously diseased vessel reduced the score for that vessel to 0), the aortic cross-clamp time, the pump time, and the type of myocardial protection employed.

Table 18-1
Factors Considered in Reviewing Results of Aortocoronary Bypass Surgery for Patients with Unstable Angina

---

Type of unstable angina (extent of injury)
Left main coronary artery stenosis
Urgency of surgery
Class according to New York Heart Association
Grade of left ventricular contractility
Extent of coronary artery disease
Number of bypass grafts
Intraoperative anoxic time
Pump time
Use of balloon pump preoperatively

POSTOPERATIVE MORBIDITY AND MORTALITY

The hospital morbidity and mortality following aortocoronary bypass for unstable angina were determined following a careful clinical review, an evaluation of postoperative hemodynamic data, an independent review of postoperative electrocardiograms, and serum enzymes. Five categories of complications were developed. The first was a perioperative myocardial infarction. This complication occurred when a new Q wave developed or when R wave progression was lost in patients whose clinical status and postoperative enzymes were consistent with the diagnosis of a perioperative myocardial infarction. Second, definite ischemia was diagnosed when ischemic ECG changes persisted in the postoperative period and enzyme elevations were greater than routinely encountered. Third, suspected ischemia occurred when electrocardiographic and enzyme changes were present but were not diagnostic of perioperative ischemic episode. Fourth, low output syndrome was diagnosed postoperatively when inadequate perfusion did not respond to volume loading and intraaortic balloon pump assistance and/or inotropic drugs were required to maintain the circulation. Fifth, no cardiac complications occurred when none of the above were encountered.

RESULTS

Morbidity and Mortality

There was a 4% hospital mortality, a 9% incidence of perioperative myocardial infarction, and a 10% incidence of low output syndrome in 876 patients undergoing aortocoronary bypass for unstable angina from 1974–1979. Figure 18-1 demonstrates the relation between the unstable angina categories and the postoperative result of surgery. The morbidity and mortality of aortocoronary bypass for acute coronary insufficiency was not statistically different than for crescendo angina. However, postoperative morbidity and mortality increased substantially for patients with persistent ischemic electrocardiographic changes. These patients had the highest perioperative morbidity and mortality.

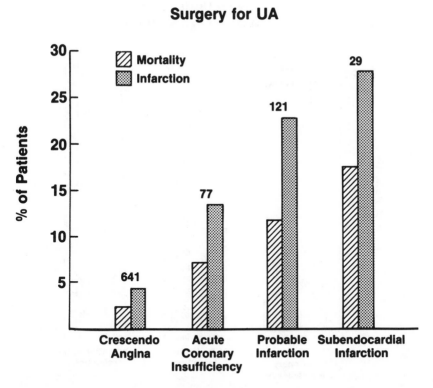

Figure 18-1 The hospital mortality and incidence of perioperative myocardial infarction (new Q waves) is illustrated for the 867 patients undergoing aortocoronary bypass surgery for unstable angina from 1974–1979. An increase in perioperative morbidity and mortality is demonstrated to correspond with increasing evidence of preoperative ischemic injury.

Left Main Stenosis

There was a 15% incidence of left main coronary artery stenosis or left main equivalent. Left main stenosis did not influence the risks of coronary artery surgery for crescendo angina. However, among the 227 patients who had either acute coronary insufficiency, probable infarction, or subendocardial infarction, there was a 27% incidence of left main stenosis or left main equivalent. The mortality for that group was 9% and the perioperative infarction rate was 13%. In contrast, those patients who did not have left main stenosis had a mortality of 7% and a perioperative infarction rate of 9%. The difference was not statistically significant. A dramatic trend is seen in Figure 18-2, which demonstrates a trend towards increasing mortality and morbidity for patients with left main stenosis who have more extensive preoperative ischemia.

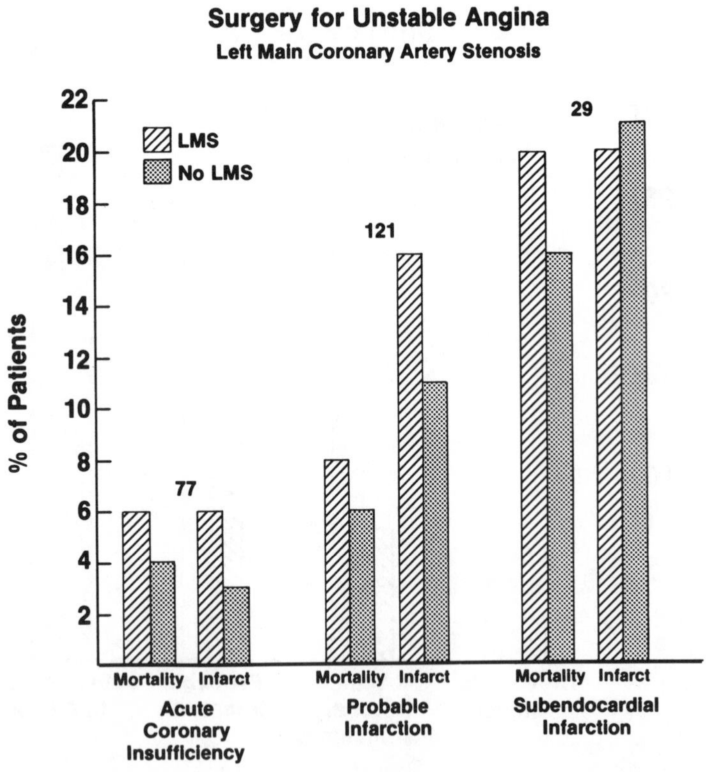

Surgery for Unstable Angina

Left Main Coronary Artery Stenosis

Figure 18-2 The hospital mortality and incidence of perioperative myocardial infarction is illustrated for the 227 patients with left main coronary artery stenosis (or equivalent) who had prolonged episodes of rest pain (ACI, PI, or SEI). Twenty-seven percent of patients in these groups had left main stenosis. The mortality and perioperative morbidity was found to be related to the extent of preoperative ischemic injury.

Decreased Left Ventricular Function

Thirty-eight percent of patients with acute coronary insufficiency, probable infarction, or subendocardial infarction had a left ventricle grade of 3 or 4. The mortality and morbidity for this group of patients was not substantially different from those with a left ventricular grade of 1 or 2. The type of unstable angina was found to be a more significant predictor than the grade of left ventricular function.

Timing of Surgery

The urgency of surgical intervention in any given case of unstable angina was a function of the symptoms, extent of preoperative ischemia, availability of the operating room, and the personalities of referring cardiologists and operating surgeons. The effects of "urgency" are therefore difficult to interpret in a retrospective review. The timing of surgical intervention in patients with unstable angina shifted dramatically after March 1977. Prior to that date, 44% of patients undergoing aortocoronary bypass for ACI, PI, or SEI underwent an urgent operation. After that date, 27% underwent urgent surgery. The shift resulted from a conscious effort to provide more intensive and more prolonged medical management of patients with unstable angina. Instead of the primary treatment modality, surgery became the treatment of last resort. Figure 18-3 illustrates the effects this change in policy had on the mortality of ACB for unstable angina. Since 1977, there has been a marked rise in the perioperative mortality for patients with PI or SEI. Patients with ACI who require urgent operation continue to enjoy a result comparable to those undergoing semielective surgery.

Ischemia Following Aortocoronary Bypass

Surviving patients who do not have the classic criteria for a perioperative myocardial infarction were occasionally found to have substantial evidence of ischemic injury. Figure 18-4 illustrates the incidence of definite and suspected ischemia in each of the subgroups.

Since there is a substantial overlap between infarction and ischemia, Figure 18-5 provides a more comprehensive picture of the results of aortocoronary bypass for unstable angina. This illustration depicts the lack of either ECG or enzyme changes in the immediate postoperative period. There is a definite relationship between the category of unstable angina and postoperative ischemic injury.

Intraaortic Balloon Pump Assistance (IABPA)

Intraaortic balloon pump assistance was used extensively between 1974 and 1977 to protect patients undergoing urgent surgery for unstable angina. Improved medical management since 1977 has substantially reduced the need for preoperative balloon pump assistance. In addition, there has been a shift in the selection criteria for balloon usage. Patients with extensive preoperative ischemia, left main stenosis, poor left ventricular function, or intractable symptomatology are now felt to be candidates for

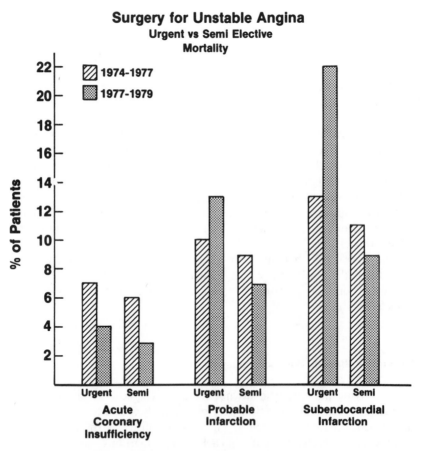

Figure 18-3 The hospital mortality is illustrated for patients undergoing urgent (less than 48 hours) and semielective (same hospitalization) ACB for unstable angina and prolonged episodes of rest pain. In March 1977, the Toronto General Hospital changed from a policy of urgent revascularization to a policy of delayed surgery for patients with medically resistant unstable angina. The result has been an increased mortality of urgent cases.

balloon usage. IABPA is generally reserved for patients with probable or subendocardial infarction who require urgent surgery and have other complicating conditions. Table 18-2 demonstrates a relatively stable perioperative mortality and morbidity in patients who require preoperative IABPA despite the increasing selectivity in its usage.

Low Output Syndrome

The postoperative incidence of low output syndrome was found to correlate directly with the extent of preoperative ischemic injury as represented by the categories of unstable angina. Figure 18-6 illustrates the incidence of low output syndrome in various categories of unstable angina. The use of preoperative IABPA was found to substantially reduce the postoperative incidence of low output syndrome in patients with probable or subendocardial infarction.

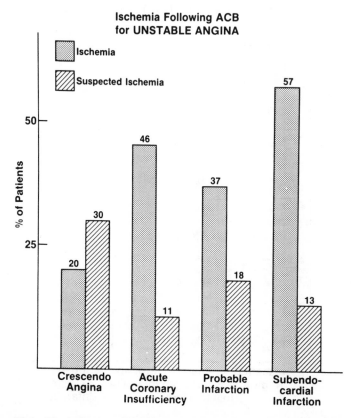

Figure 18-4   The incidence of definite (by electrocardiographic and enzyme criteria) and suspected ischemia is illustrated for each of the subgroups of unstable angina.

A careful history of the presentation and evaluation of the initial cardiograms and cardiac enzymes permit identification of high-risk subgroups with unstable angina. The incremental influence of left main coronary artery stenosis, poor left ventricular function, the response to therapy, and the type of procedure performed is difficult to evaluate by a single variant analysis. However, the influence of each of these factors has been suggested. A multivariant analysis is required to provide an adequate description of the incremental influence of each of these factors.

MULTIVARIANT ANALYSIS

A multivariant analysis requires a mathematical model that will describe the events under investigation. The mathematical model employed should permit an adequate interaction of the variables and a description of

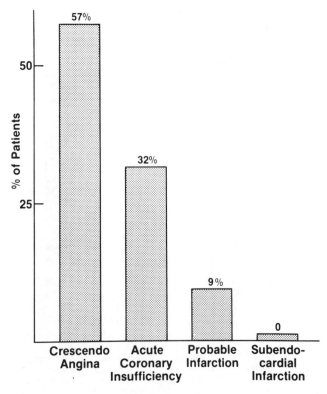

Figure 18-5 The incidence of patients without evidence of perioperative ischemia is illustrated for each of the subgroups of unstable angina.

Table 18-2
The Influence of Preoperative Intraaortic Balloon Pump Assistance Employed in Patients with Probable or Subendocardial Infarction on Hospital Mortality, Perioperative Myocardial Infarction, and Postoperative Low Output Syndrome

| | With Preoperative IABPA | | | | | Without Preoperative IABPA | | | | |
	No. of Patients	%	Mortality %	Perioperative Myocardial Infarction %	Low Output Syndrome %	No. of Patients	%	Mortality %	Perioperative Myocardial Infarction %	Low Output Syndrome %
1974–76	15	39	7	33	13	23	61	13	30	43
1977–78	15	25	13	20	20	44	75	7	18	27
1979	2	25	0	0	0	28	93	7	14	14

the results independent of these interactions. We have employed a linear logistics model to evaluate the incidence of perioperative myocardial infarction (MI) after aortocoronary bypass for unstable angina. MI is a binary variable since there are only two possible responses. The occurrence of a postoperative infarction was given a score of 1 if present and 0 if absent. The linear logistics model assumes that there is a sigmoid relation between the binary variable (MI) and the factors that influence it. Either continuous or discrete variables may be employed. The equation of the sigmoid curve that describes the relationship is illustrated in Figure 18-7. The relative relationship of each variable to the probability of infarction is given by the coefficients of the linear logistic equation.

Forty preoperative and intraoperative factors were accumulated for each patient on an IBM 370 computer at the University of Toronto computer center. The linear logistics technique attempted to find the fewest number of variables that provided the best prediction of perioperative infarction. Each variable was tested independently and then combined with all other variables to find the fewest number, which when combined, provided the best prediction. Five factors were found to be significant by this

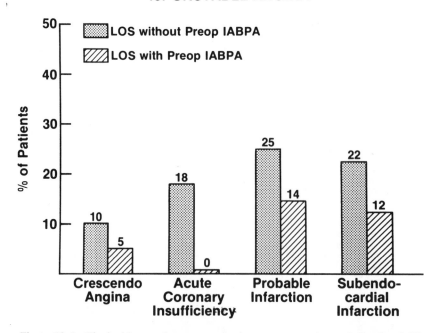

Figure 18-6 The incidence of postoperative low output syndrome following ACB for unstable angina is illustrated. The use of preoperative intraaortic balloon pump assistance reduced the incidence of postoperative low output syndrome in each high risk subgroup of unstable angina.

multivariant analysis: 1) the category of unstable angina, 2) New York Heart Association class, 3) preoperative coronary artery disease score, 4) left ventricular grade by angiography, and 5) pump time. The equation for this relationship is given below. This equation relates the probability of perioperative infarction to each of the five variables. The specific probability equation for predicting the likelihood of a perioperative myocardial infarction in a patient undergoing aortocoronary bypass for unstable angina is illustrated. The acute coronary insufficiency (ACI) subgroup, the extent of coronary artery disease (CAD) New York Heart Association (NYHA) class, and left ventricular grade (LVG) are found to directly influence the operative result. The length of the pump run is the only intraoperative variable found to have influenced the postoperative result in this group of patients.

$$\text{LOG}\left(\frac{p}{1\text{-}p}\right) = \text{ACI} + 0.23\,(\text{CAD}) - (\text{LVG}) + \text{NYHA} + 0.02\,(\text{Pump Time})$$

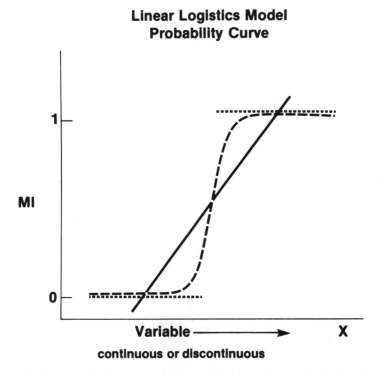

Linear Logistics Model Probability Curve

Figure 18-7 The sigmoid configuration of the probability curve for the biphasic variable myocardial infarction is illustrated. Logistic analysis provides a statistical means to determine factors influencing the results of aortocoronary bypass for unstable angina.

270

An example of the use of this probability equation will be helpful. Consider a patient with "classical" acute coronary insufficiency (2), and New York Heart class (4), with the LV grade (4), a coronary artery score of (9), and a pump time of 141 minutes. The equation predicts the probability that this patient will have a myocardial infarction as 76%.

SUMMARY

A comprehensive review of 876 patients undergoing aortocoronary bypass surgery for unstable angina has suggested certain factors that appear to affect significantly the hospital morbidity and mortality. The most important consideration is the extent of preoperative ischemic injury as diagnosed by three clinical parameters: the pattern and duration of pain, electrocardiographic changes, and cardiac enzyme elevations. These parameters permit differentiation of five categories of patients presenting for surgery with unstable angina. The risks of revascularization were found to be directly related to the extent of preoperative injury, as represented by these clinical classes. In addition, there is an incremental influence of the functional class, left ventricular grade, and the extent of coronary artery disease. Intraoperative factors appear to have less influence on the overall result.

From these studies certain recommendations can be made. Patients with unstable angina should have a careful evaluation within the first 24 hours to determine the extent of ischemic injury. An attempt should be made to control symptoms with intensive medical management. Patients who fail the most aggressive medical regimen require urgent revascularization. Preoperative preparation should include adequate beta blockade and every attempt should be made to control symptoms during the immediate preoperative period. Factors that increase myocardial oxygen requirements should be reduced as much as possible. Preoperative balloon pump assistance can provide a smoother anesthesia induction in patients with extensive ischemia who are at high risk for perioperative injury. The use of cold potassium cardioplegia may improve the results of urgent surgery in patients refractory to medical management.

Patients whose symptoms are improved but not eliminated by medical management are a difficult group for the cardiologist. Our study would suggest that semielective, rather than urgent, surgery will provide better results for patients with extensive preoperative ischemia. A judicious delay of two to six weeks may be appropriate in patients whose symptoms are improved but not eliminated with medical management. Patients who have a normal resting electrocardiogram and who do not show evidence of cardiac enzyme release with their acute ischemic episode have risks of urgent revascularization similar to that of semielective revascularization or stable angina. The decision for the surgical timing in this group is not critical.

A multivariant analysis confirms the importance of identifying high-risk subgroups who are prone to perioperative morbidity and mortality. Careful assessment will permit improved results in these high-risk patients.

REFERENCES

1. Canadian Task Force on Coronary Artery Disease. *Can Med Assoc J.* 117:451, 1977.

2. Gazes, P.C., Mobley, E.M., Faris, H.M. et al. Preinfarction (unstable) angina—a prospective study—10 year follow up. *Circulation* 48:131, 1973.

3. Bertolasi, C.A., Tronge, J.E., Carreno, C.A. et al. Unstable angina—prospective and randomized study of its evolution, with and without surgery. *Am J Cardiol.* 33:201, 1978.

4. Unstable Angina Pectoris: National Co-operative Study Group to compare medical and surgical therapy. *Am J Cardiol.* 42:839, 1978.

5. Wiles, J.C., Peduzzi, P.N., Hammond, G.L. et al. Preoperative predictors of operative mortality for coronary bypass grafting in patients with unstable angina pectoris. *Am J Caridol.* 39:939, 1977.

6. Armstrong, P.W., Chong, M.A., and Parker, J.A. The spectrum of unstable angina. *Ann Roy Coll Phys Surg Can.* 12:28, 1979.

19 Early Postmyocardial Infarction Angina (Impending Reinfarction): Surgical Treatment Combined with Intraaortic Balloon Pumping

Jean Bardet, MD, and
Jean Pierre Bourdarias, MD

Impending reinfarction implies further ischemia peripheral to the area of initial myocardial infarction or development of a new area of infarction. Left ventricular power failure correlates with the amount of loss of left ventricular mass.[1-3] Recurrent anginal pain with electrocardiographic changes of ischemia in new areas 2 to 15 days after the onset of infarction indicates a high risk of increasing irreversible myocardial insult, with further depression of cardiac function. From pathologic studies it would seem that when the amount of left ventricular myocardium inactivated by recent or old infarcts exceeds 40% to 50%, lethal cardiogenic shock invariably occurs.[4-6] Medical, mechanical, and surgical treatments are directed, therefore, to preserving myocardium by supporting the circulation, decreasing myocardial oxygen demand, and, in some cases, by directly increasing coronary blood flow.

Patients with acute myocardial infarction and continued ischemic attacks at rest, despite adequate medical therapy, are at high risk of reinfarction and death.[7] Medical therapy in this group of patients is somewhat limited because of the narrower therapeutic range for administration of beta-blocking drugs and vasodilating agents. Lack of success in the medical management of this clinical setting has led to the employment of emergency surgical therapy. Early and occasional reports support the contention that myocardial revascularization may be indicated under such circumstances. This was associated, however, with a relatively high operative mortality rate. During the acute phase of myocardial infarction surgical mortality apparently depends on the interval from the onset of infarction to surgical treatment.[8] Furthermore, there is emerging evidence that the high mortality and morbidity rates are partly secondary to operating on an actively ischemic myocardium.[9] Circulatory assist by intraaortic balloon pump (IABP) has been effective in controlling pain in patients with refractory myocardial ischemia.[10-13] The ability of IABP to reverse ischemia when medical therapy has failed is related to its unique effect of simultaneously increasing coronary perfusion pressure and reducing myocardial oxygen demand.[14-16] With the experimental and clinical basis for controlling myocardial ischemia by IABP firmly established, the next logical step should be cardiac catheterization. This would determine whether or not coronary and left ventricular anatomy precludes bypass surgery. Thus, IABP and rapid and precise diagnostic coronary angiography, followed by direct myocardial revascularization, would represent an effective approach to early postinfarction refractory angina.

It is the purpose of this chapter to review some of the clinical observations that lend support to this concept. A survey of the world surgical experience and the authors' experience will also be included.

DEFINITION AND DIAGNOSTIC CRITERIA

We may define postinfarction angina as a syndrome of acute myocardial ischemia occurring during the acute phase of a transmural myocardial infarction (ie, more than two and less than 15 days after the onset of symptoms). Ischemia may involve either the myocardium peripheral to the initial area of myocardial infarction or the opposite left ventricular wall. Admittedly, progression of a relatively large ischemic area to frank myocardial infarction in addition to the original one may lead to further serious complications in a great number of patients.

The criteria generally accepted for the diagnosis of postinfarction angina are: 1) Recurrence of anginal pain at rest lasting 20 to 30 minutes or more, usually resistant to sublingual nitroglycerin, and only relieved by opiates; 2) Transitory ST-segment elevation and T-wave changes at the time of pain either in the area of the recent infarct *and* in the adjacent area, or in a different area (opposite left ventricular wall); 3) No further elevation of cardiac enzymes (CPK, SGOT, LDH) to levels diagnostic of myocardial infarction.

Transient ST-segment depression has also been used by some investigators as an indicator of myocardial ischemia. Strictly isolated episodes of ST-segment depression were rare in our experience and have been noted in only 2 out of 34 patients. Occasionally, however, episodes of ST-segment depression, following episodes of ST-segment elevation, were recorded in the same leads. Transient ST-segment depression may be either the direct manifestation of subendocardial ischemia in the involved leads, or the reciprocal of ST-segment elevation (transmural ischemia) recorded in the opposite leads. It is our opinion that the criteria for diagnosis should not include ST-segment depression unless its reciprocal origin can be definitely excluded. Using the above definition postinfarctional angina has been observed in only 2% to 3% of patients with acute myocardial infarction. A clear distinction should be made, however, between postinfarction angina and a different and more frequent clinical condition termed "infarct extension."[17-19] Myocardial infarct extension occurring several days after the acute event is generally thought to be the result of a second wave of necrosis after the initial ischemic insult. It is characterized clinically by recurrent chest pain associated with further ECG changes confined to the original area of infarction and re-elevation of myocardial enzymes. The frequency with which infarct extension has been observed is variable. Using the precordial mapping technique Reid et al[18] and Madias[20] reported an extension rate of approximately 50%. On a clinical basis, Rosati (in Pitt, B.[21]) estimated a rate of 11% to 17% in 797 episodes of acute myocardial infarction. More recently, Rothkopf et al[19] using CK-MB radioimmunoassay detected infarct extension in 14% of 43 patients. Hutchins and Bulkley[17] identified histologically infarct extension in 17% of the 76 specimens studied. The quantity of myocardium involved, however, was generally insufficient to compromise cardiac function further since it was limited to the surviving myocardium overlying the acute infarct ("contraction band necrosis").

NATURAL HISTORY

There is a paucity of information concerning the course of the patient with the postinfarction anginal syndrome. Also, the use of nonuniform diagnostic criteria has been responsible for some confusion about the nature, morbidity, and mortality of patients presenting with the clinical condition. In most studies dealing with unstable angina this small subset of patients was not individualized. Other reports include data on infarct extension with or without cardiogenic shock, mechanical complications of myocardial infarction, and early revascularization of acute myocardial infarctions complicating coronary angiography.

Smullens et al[22] studied 26 patients with evolving myocardial infarction and reported a 42% mortality rate in the 12 patients treated medically. Evolving myocardial infarction was defined as recurrent chest pain occurring two hours to two weeks after a myocardial infarction.

McGowan[7] analyzed three groups of patients with acute myocardial infarction. Nine patients had postinfarction angina associated with ST-segment elevation (group 1). Only episodes of pain occurring 24 hours or more after initial infarction were considered to represent ischemic episodes distinct from the initial infarction. Seventeen patients had postinfarction angina with ST-segment depression or no ST-segment changes (group 2). **Thirty-one patients had no postinfarction angina (group 3). The patients in** group 1 had a statistically significant increased incidence of early reinfarction (7 out of 9) and death (3 out of 9), when compared to the other groups, singly or combined. In group 2 there were two reinfarctions and two additional patients died within one month of their initial infarction. No further infarctions or deaths occurred in this group over an average follow-up of 12 months. Of the 31 patients in group 3, two had reinfarction and two died within four weeks after the initial infarct. In the authors' experience, three out of eight patients who could not be operated on died within six months after onset of symptoms.

Thus, although precise information is still lacking about the natural history and prognosis of acute myocardial infarction complicated by recurrent ischemia, many investigators feel that it is not benign, particularly when ischemic attacks are unresponsive to medical therapy. In patients with unstable angina refractory to maximum medical therapy a mortality rate as high as 20% at three months has been reported.[23] Nevertheless, in none of these high-risk patients was the preinfarctional state superimposed on a recent acute infarction. One would expect a somewhat higher risk in patients recovering from an acute infarction.

MEDICAL TREATMENT

The majority of patients with unstable angina respond to intensive in-hospital medical therapy with nitroglycerin and beta-blocking drugs.[24-27] However, a sizeable portion of the patients with postinfarction angina appear to have recurrent ischemic attacks refractory to conventional therapy. Little is known regarding the incidence with which medical therapy fails to control severe myocardial ischemia in this postinfarction group. Of the 93 patients with refractory angina studied by Levine et al[28] 33 (35%) were recovering (less than 10 days) from a transmural myocardial infarction. In the series reported by Weintraub and Aroesty[29] 12 out of 42 patients (29%) had angina resistant to medical therapy within days of an acute myocardial infarction. In the authors' experience, 34 (63%) of the 54 patients with refractory unstable angina were in the early phase (less than 15 days) of a recent infarction.

The precise underlying pathophysiology of this clinical syndrome has not yet been fully defined. Failure of medical therapy to control recurrent ischemia may actually be due to the inability of currently available drugs to affect the cause of ischemia. The vasospastic hypothesis appears now to be substantiated by objective data.[30,31] Although vasospastic angina has been treated successfully by nitrates,[32-34] and more recently by calcium antagonists,[35] the myocardial infarction rate remained as high as 21% in a recent study.[30] It is likely that other measures for the containment of ischemic injury should be considered, especially with prolonged episodes of ischemia. In our experience, and that of others,[36-38] IABP proved very useful to prevent recurrence of ischemic attacks. This finding suggests that the balloon pump may have a direct action on the functional component of coronary artery obstruction, but this theory requires further evaluation.

Medical treatment is more limited in postinfarction angina because of the known hazards in the administration of various drugs. Anticoagulant therapy was ineffective,[10,37] and did not prevent infarction in our nonoperative patients. Although ischemic pain could be temporarily interrupted by nitroglycerin in several patients,[10,29,37] usually ischemic attacks could not be prevented by oral isosobide dinitrate given in doses up to 5 mg sublingually every 2 hours or 10 mg orally every 3 hours.[37]

Beta blockade is widely used in the treatment of unstable angina, but is not devoid of risk in patients with acute myocardial infarction. Moderate doses (120 mg/day) of propranolol may be administered. Although they were adequate to reduce heart rate to < 70 beats/min, they did not prevent recurrence of ischemic attacks.[10,28,29] The dosage of propranolol could not be increased because of the potential for cardiac depression, which can be especially hazardous when ischemia progresses to infarction. Furthermore, in some patients, beta-blocking drugs either were contraindicated or had to be withheld because of left ventricular failure, bradycardia, and hypotension.

More recently vigorous therapy with vasodilator agents has been reported to be effective in stabilizing patients with recurrent chest pain, ST-segment elevation, and ventricular arrhythmias following acute myocardial infarction.[39] In the nine patients studied, ischemic attacks were unresponsive to antianginal and antiarrhythmic therapy. Most patients improved markedly within 30 minutes of nitroprusside infusion. One patient, however, died suddenly within 48 hours.

So far, only a small number of patients have been treated in this manner and these encouraging results must be confirmed by subsequent studies. In addition, the effects of vasodilator agents on regional myocardial blood flow in patients with coronary artery disease have not been fully elucidated. Recently, Mann et al[40] reported that nitroprusside administered intravenously to patients with chronic stable angina decreased regional myocardial blood flow substantially in nearly all patients, whether or not a well-developed collateral circulation was present. Since the primary effect of nitroprusside on the coronary circulation is vasodilation of resistance vessels, such an effect could result in redistribution of blood flow away from an ischemic area.[41-43] This coronary steal could explain the increase in ischemic injury that has been demonstrated in some patients with chronic angina[40] or acute myocardial infarction.[44-46] In contrast, after nitroglycerin, intramyocardial blood flow may be redistributed so that ischemic areas may actually have increased flow.[40,42,46]

SURGICAL TREATMENT

The failure of medical therapy to control recurrent postinfarction angina has led to the employment of prompt coronary revascularization. Although not yet well-defined, the risk of surgery in patients with acute myocardial infarction depends on the interval from the onset of infarction to surgical treatment, and the fact that the surgical procedure is performed on an actively ischemic myocardium. The available data regarding the surgical risk in this subset of patients with myocardial infarction, however, are scanty and most reports include small and varied patient groups.

Dawson et al[8] reported that the incidence of bypass surgery performed soon after myocardial infarction was high and remained so during the first 30 days. During the first week after infarction the surgical mortality in 21 patients was 38%; three-fourths of these patients had early complications of infarction including postinfarction angina, ventricular arrhythmias, or cardiogenic shock. Mortality decreased to 16% in 69 patients operated on 8 to 30 days after infarction; less than 50% of these patients had complications. After one month the mortality was 5.8%, no more than the overall operative mortality rate in 1700 operated patients.

Cheanvechai et al[47] reported on 30 patients operated on after an acute myocardial infarction. Twenty-four underwent surgery promptly after an in-hospital acute infarction in an attempt to salvage myocardium and six underwent surgery 3 to 14 days after infarction because of the development of postinfarction angina. Only one patient was in cardiogenic shock prior to surgery and the surgical mortality was 5.4%. Reul et al[48] reported a 50% operative mortality rate in eight patients with acute myocardial infarction without hypotension but with chest pain and diaphoresis. Hill et al[49] have operated on four patients unsuccessfully with this condition, in whom left ventricular failure developed. Sustaita et al[50] reported patients successfully operated on for recurrent severe angina within four to eight hours after infarction. Cohn et al[51] reported two patients with severe postinfarction angina, successfully revascularized within three weeks of their original infarction. All three patients operated on by Keon et al,[52] 2 to 30 days after an acute infarction, survived. More recently, only 2 out of 15 patients reported by Wellons et al[53] died during the immediate postoperative period. None of these patients was supported by the balloon pump preoperatively or postoperatively.

Finally, a review of the previously reported surgically treated cases[22,48-55] indicates that operative mortality rate was 22.2% (12 out of 54 patients). With increasing experience and refinement in surgical techniques one may expect a lower surgical mortality rate. Nevertheless, patients with recent infarction and severe recurrent ischemia undoubtedly face an increased operative risk.

INTRAAORTIC BALLOON PUMPING COMBINED WITH SURGICAL TREATMENT

It is generally agreed that IABP dramatically controls the ischemic symptoms, stabilizes myocardial energetics, and facilitates emergency coronary angiography and subsequent myocardial revascularization. This experience has led several investigators to advocate angiographic studies followed by revascularization with IABP support for patients whose postinfarction angina does not subside rapidly with adequate medical therapy.[10,29,37]

The ability of IABP to reverse or reduce ischemia is related to its unique effect of simultaneously increasing coronary perfusion pressure and reducing myocardial oxygen demand.[14,16,56] Review of the current clinical data also indicates that IABP may hold promise for reducing operative risk for patients with impending infarction. Scully et al[57] found that preoperative IABP improved survival rate in patients with acute coronary insufficiency. Feola et al[58] reported 36 patients with impending or evolving myocardial infarction with persistent chest pain, who were treated with IABP followed by bypass surgery. The operative mortality rate was 5.5%. In contrast, the operative mortality of 61 similar patients operated on without IABP was 13.1%. During the preoperative period, IABP increased lactate extraction and decreased left ventricular filling pressure. Intraoperatively, IABP increased coronary graft flow and the myocardial tissue oxygen tension was higher. Thus, in patients with acute ischemia these beneficial effects enhance the safety of semiemergent revascularization as recently confirmed by Langou et al.[59]

Furthermore, there is increasing evidence that the high perioperative infarction rate reported in some series of unstable angina is secondary to operating on an actively ischemic myocardium.[9,60] In patients with severe ischemia, anesthesia and anoxic arrest during the grafting procedure may potentially accelerate the progression of an ischemic area to frank infarction. A decline in morbidity may be expected if a longer period of stabilization is allowed, provided that all the necessary steps are taken to avoid the risk of preoperative loss of myocardium. Relevant to this point, IABP provides safety to the myocardium and appears to play a role in lowering the infarction rate.[59]

SURVEY OF SURGICAL EXPERIENCE IN THE LITERATURE

Levine et al[28] reported the use of IABP in 35 patients: 26 patients (79%) had no recurrence of pain during pumping and the remaining nine had recurrent pain with decreased frequency. During test interruption of IABP, 40% of patients showed recurrence of pain. Resumption of IABP was effective in all cases. Coronary angiography and ventriculography were performed in all patients without complication. One patient underwent angiography without IABP and the study was complicated by recurrent ischemia, ventricular tachycardia and hypotension. Serial enzymes studies suggested reinfarction. All patients underwent coronary bypass surgery with IABP support during induction of anesthesia and in the perioperative and postoperative periods. There were three operative deaths (8.5%) and only one patient (2.2%) showed now Q waves in the postoperative ECG.

Weintraub and Aroesty[29] reported similar results in 12 patients. IABP controlled ischemic episodes in most patients. Within 24 hours of stabilization, coronary angiographic studies were performed following which the patients underwent revascularization with a single operative death.

Bardet et al[10] used IABP to control refractory postinfarction angina in 32 patients. Drug therapy was left unchanged during the whole period of circulatory assist and patients were given propranolol (except when contraindicated) up to the day before operation. All patients showed some recurrence of ischemic attacks during pumping. All these patients had cardiac catheterization and 24 underwent bypass surgery. There was one operative death (4.2%) and one patient demonstrated reinfarction in the postoperative ECG.

To this time, 71 patients[28,29] including 26 patients of our own have been treated with IABP combined with coronary artery bypass surgery, with an operative mortality rate of 7% (five deaths) and a postoperative reinfarction rate of 3.5% (2 of 57 patients). These results compare favorably with those obtained by various surgical groups without the aid of the balloon pump (22%). Further experience with preoperative IABP should help to solve the question of whether or not IABP truly decreases operative risk in these highly selected patients.

EXPERIENCE AT THE AMBROISE PARÉ HOSPITAL

Thirty-four patients with postmyocardial infarction angina have been treated in our institution by IABP and 26 underwent semiemergent revascularization. There were 32 men and 2 women with a mean age of 56 years (range, 40 to 67 years). All had recently suffered from a transmural infarction documented by Q waves on the ECG and characteristic elevation of cardiac enzymes (creatine phosphokinase, lactic dehydrogenase, glutamic oxaloacetic transaminase). All patients were treated with bedrest, heparin, and long-acting nitrates. Twelve patients had painful episodes lasting more than 20 minutes despite the administration of moderate doses of propranolol (60 to 80 mg/day), whereas the other 22 had prolonged pain of more than one hour that required opiates for relief. A twelve-lead ECG recorded during pain showed ST-segment elevation. In 17 cases, recurring ischemia involved both the original site and a new area and in 17 cases it was limited to a new area, usually the opposite left ventricular wall. In addition, six of these patients had had an infarction more than six months previously. The mean interval between the initial infarction and impending reinfarction was six days (range, 2 to 15 days). In three patients, the initial infarction was complicated by severe arrhythmias and 22 patients had clinical signs of heart failure (class II or III of the Myocardial Infarct Research Unit [MIRU] classification). In 16 patients the mean pulmonary wedge was monitored via a Swan–Ganz catheter. Circulatory assist was initiated within 24 hours (range, 4 to 96 hours) using either an Avco or a Datascope console. A 30- to 40-cc intraaortic balloon catheter was introduced into the femoral artery by the usual technique. After 32 hours of IABP, on average, all patients underwent left ventricular cineangiography in the right and left anterior oblique projections and coronary artery angiography without interrupting balloon assist. Ventriculograms were analyzed according to a modified Leighton's technique.[1] Ejection fraction was calculated from the right anterior oblique frames. IABP was maintained for an average of 4.2 days (range, 2 to 10 days).

Balloon pumping did not cause any local or systemic complications. On circulatory assist, systolic blood pressure dropped from 127 ± 23 to 102 ± 25 mm Hg, whereas mean blood pressure rose slightly from 88 ± 14 to 92 ± 17 mg Hg. The peak diastolic pressure during balloon pumping was 132 ± 26 mm Hg. Anginal pain did not recur in any patient on IABP. No attempt was made to discontinue balloon assist in any patient on IABP. In one patient, however, IABP was temporarily discontinued for technical reasons and within a few minutes an anginal attack occurred associated with ST-segment changes. In three patients prior attacks of ventricular tachycardia and/or fibrillation did not recur. The mean left ventricular end-diastolic pressure was 20 ± 10 mm Hg, exceeding 12 mm Hg in 24 patients. Left ventriculography demonstrated moderate mitral regurgitation in nine patients. Twenty-six patients had akinetic or severely hypokinetic segments involving more than 25% of the end-diastolic perimeter. Two patients had an apical aneurysm. One patient had an anterior ventricular septal defect associated with a moderate left-to-right shunt. Nineteen patients had triple-vessel disease, 10 had double-vessel disease, and five had single-vessel disease. Significant stenosis (70%) of the left anterior descending artery was observed in 30 patients, of the right coronary artery in 29, and of the left circumflex artery in 23.

Eight patients did not undergo operations (Table 19-1). Four patients had severe lesions in all three major coronary arteries, which were not suitable for surgery, and they all had reinfarction 1 day, 8 days, and 3 months after removal of the balloon. Three died in cardiogenic shock and the fourth had severe heart failure. Four patients had only single-vessel disease of the right coronary artery and were not considered for surgery as the operative risk appeared greater than the possible benefit of revascularization. After removal of the balloon, pain did not recur in two patients, one suffered from a myocardial infarction and is alive and pain-free. The other has moderate exertional angina.

Table 19-1
In the Ambroise Paré Hospital Experience Eight Patients
with Impending Myocardial Reinfarction Did Not Undergo Operation

	No. of Patients
Inoperable (severe triple-vessel disease)	4*
Single stenosis of the right coronary artery	4†

*Three of these patients died from recurrent myocardial infarction and cardiogenic shock within three months.
†One patient experienced reinfarction, and one angina pectoris.

Twenty-six patients underwent surgery (Table 19-2). Fourteen had double-bypass grafts, 10 had single-bypass graft, and two patients had an aneurysmectomy, combined with a double-bypass graft in one and closure of a ventricular septal defect in the other. The left anterior descending coronary artery was bypassed in 21 patients, the right coronary artery and the left circumflex artery in nine patients each, and a diagonal branch in one. None of the patients died during the immediate postoperative period owing to precarious hemodynamics. However, IABP was required for two to eight days postoperatively in 13 patients. One patient died on the eighth day from gastrointestinal bleeding. Necropsy revealed a patent graft without further infarction. The other 25 patients survived the operation.

Table 19-2
In the Ambroise Paré Hospital Experience 26 Patients
with Impending Myocardial Reinfarction Underwent Surgery

	No. of Patients
Immediate postoperative complications	
Death	0
New infarction	1
Secondary postoperative complications	
Death (gastrointestinal bleeding 8th day)	1
New infarction	0
Long-term survivors: 25 patients (35 ± 13 months)	
Mild left ventricular failure	5
Angina pectoris	3

LATE OPERATIVE RESULTS

Follow-up evaluation available from three institutions has shown encouraging results. In the 16 postinfarction patients followed by Gold et al[37] for an average of 22 months, only three showed recurrence of mild exertional angina. There were no late deaths and no late infarctions. Of 93 patients with intractable unstable angina, including 26 patients with postinfarction angina, 88 survived the operation and have been followed for up to six years (average, 38.4 months) in a more recent study from the same group.[28] There were only three late deaths secondary to myocardial infarction and only one additional late infarction. Three of the four late infarctions occurred within the first 14 months of operation. Of the 84 remaining patients, 74% were free of angina. Similarly, Weintraub and Aroesty[29] reported no late deaths in 42 patients with preinfarction angina unresponsive to medical therapy, including 12 postinfarction patients. Over 75% had remained asymptomatic with a follow-up of 40 months (mean, 23 months). For our 25 surviving patients after an average follow-up of 35 months, only four patients demonstrated recurrence of exertional angina. There were no late deaths or late infarctions.

SUMMARY AND CONCLUSIONS

Patients with early postinfarction angina may benefit by a combined approach of circulatory assist, definition of coronary obstruction by angiography, and direct surgical revascularization (if there is reasonable residual left ventricular function). Review of current data indicates that impending reinfarction may be effectively treated by IABP combined with semiemergent coronary artery bypass grafting in those circumstances where medical therapy cannot contain the ischemic process. This group of patients will probably undergo further and perhaps fatal compromise of already altered left ventricular function if allowed to progress to reinfarction. The results indicate that when these patients are treated surgically, reinfarction may be prevented in the majority of cases, operative mortality is low (7%), and long-term results satisfactory. The major areas yet to be resolved in the pathophysiology and treatment of postmyocardial infarction angina are: the role of coronary spasm in this clinical setting, and the ability of the new available drugs (calcium antagonists) to arrest the process of myocardial infarction. Further clinical experience with the early application of pharmacologic intervention is needed, and might prove helpful, particularly in hospitals that are distant from centers capable of performing "combined therapy" (ie, balloon assist and surgery).

REFERENCES

1. Rigaud, M., Rocha, P., Boschat, J. et al. Regional left ventricular function assessed by contrast angiography in acute myocardial infarction. *Circulation* (in press).

2. Swan, H.J.C., Danzig, R., Sukumalchantra, Y. et al. Current states of treatment of power failure of the heart in acute myocardial infarction with drugs and blood volume replacement. *Circulation* 44(suppl IV):IV-277, 1969.

3. Wolk, M.J., Scheidt, S., Killip, T. Heart failure complicating acute myocardial infarction. *Circulation* 45:1125, 1972.

4. Alonso, D.R., Scheidt, S., Post, M. et al. Pathophysiology of cardiogenic shock. Quantification of myocardial necrosis, clinical, pathologic and electrocardiographic correlations. *Circulation* 48:588, 1973.

5. Harnarayan, C., Bennett, M.A., Pentecost, B.L. et al. Quantitative study of infarcted myocardium in cardiogenic shock. *Br Heart J.* 32:728, 1970.

6. Page, D.L., Caufield, J.B., Kastor, J.A. et al. Myocardial changes associated with cardiogenic shock. *N Engl J Med.* 285:133, 1971.

7. McGowan, R.L. Transient ST-segment elevation with postmyocardial infarction angina: prognostic significance. *Am Heart J.* 89:449, 1975.

8. Dawson, J.T., Hall, R.J., Hallman, G.L. et al. Mortality in patients undergoing coronary artery bypass surgery after myocardial infarction. *Am J Cardiol.* 33:483, 1974.

9. Golding, L.A.R., Loop, E.D., Sheldon, W.C. et al. Emergency revascularization for unstable angina. *Circulation* 58:1163, 1978.

10. Bardet, J., Rigaud, M., Kahn, J.C. et al. Treatment of post-myocardial infarction angina by intra-aortic balloon pumping and emergency revascularization. *J Thorac Cardiovasc Surg.* 74:299, 1977.

11. Bardet, J., Bourdarias, J.P., Kahn, J.C. et al. Assistance circulatoire par contrepulsion intra-aortique. Resultats a long terme dans une serie de 108 cas. *Coeur Med Interne.* 16:391, 1977.

12. Gold, H.K., Leinbach, R.C., Sanders, C.A. et al. Intra aortic balloon pumping for control of recurrent myocardial ischemia. *Circulation* 47:1197, 1973.

13. Weintraub, R.M., Voukydis, P.C., Aroesty, J.M. et al. Treatment of preinfarction angina with intraaortic balloon counterpulsation and surgery. *Am J Cardiol.* 34:809, 1974.

14. Braunwald, E., Covell, J.W., Maroko, P.R. et al. Effects of drugs and of counterpulsation on myocardial oxygen consumption. *Circulation* 30 & 40(suppl IV):220, 1969.

15. Maroko, P.R., Bernstein, E.F., Libby, P. et al. Effects of intraaortic balloon counter pulsation in the severity of myocardial ischemic injury following acute coronary occlusion. *Circulation* 45:1150, 1972.

16. Powell, W.J., Jr., Daggett, W.M., Magro, A.E. et al. Effects of intraaortic balloon counterpulsation on cardiac performance oxygen consumption and coronary blood flow in dogs. *Circ Res.* 26:753, 1970.

17. Hutchins, G.M., and Bulkley, E.H. Infarct expansion versus extension: two different complications of acute myocardial infarction. *Am J Cardiol.* 41:1127, 1978.

18. Reid, P.R., Taylor, D.R., and Kelly, D.T. Myocardial infarct extension detected by precordial ST-segment mapping. *N Engl J Med.* 290:123, 1974.

19. **Rothkopf, M., Boerner, M.J., Smitherman, T.C. et al.** Detection of myocardial infarct extension by CK-B radioimmunoassay. *Circulation* 59:268, 1979.

20. Madias, J.E. Precordial mapping in acute anterior myocardial infarction. *Clin Res.* 23:21, 1975.

21. Pitt, B. Natural history of myocardial infarction and its prodromal syndromes. *Circulation* 53(suppl II):II-177, 1976.

22. Smullens, S.N., Wiener, I., Kasparian, H. et al. Evaluation and surgical management of acute evolving myocardial infarction. *J Thorac Cardiovasc Surg.* 64:495, 1972.

23. Gazes, P.C., Mobley, E.M., Faris, H.M. et al. Preinfarction (unstable) angina—A prospective study: ten-year follow-up. Prognostic significance of ECG changes. *Circulation* 48(suppl II):II-331, 1973.

24. Day, L.J., Thibault, G.E., and Sowton, E. Acute coronary insufficiency—review of 46 patients. *Br Heart J.* 39:363, 1977.

25. Fischl, S.J., Herman, M.V., and Gorun, R. The intermediate coronary syndrome: clinical, angiographic, and therapeutic aspects. *N Engl J Med.* 288:1193, 1973.

26. Hultgren, H.N. Medical versus surgical treatment of unstable angina. *Am J Cardiol.* 38:479, 1976.

27. Huret, J.F., Agier, B., Rosier, S.P. et al. Delayed semi-elective coronary bypass surgery for unstable angina pectoris. *J Thorac Cardiovasc Surg.* 75:476, 1978.

28. Levine, F.H., Gold, H.K., Leinbach, R.C. et al. Management of acute myocardial ischemia with intraaortic balloon pumping and coronary bypass surgery. *Circulation* 58(suppl I):I-69, 1978.

29. Weintraub, R.M., and Aroesty, J.M. The role of intraaortic balloon pumping and surgery in the treatment of preinfarction angina. *Chest* 69:707, 1976.

30. Maseri, A., Severi, S., Des Nes, M. et al. "Variant" angina: one aspect of a continuous spectrum of vasospastic myocardial ischemia. Pathogenic mechanisms, estimated incidence and clinical and arteriographic findings in 138 patients. *Am J Cardiol.* 42:1019, 1978.

31. Oliva, P.B., and Breckenridge, J.C. Arteriographic evidence of coronary arterial spasm in acute myocardial infarction. *Circulation* 56:366, 1977.

32. Affaki, G., Waters, D.D., Theroux, P. et al. Intravenous nitroglycerin in refractory unstable angina. (abstract) *Am J Cardiol* 43:416, 1979.

33. Distante, A., Maseri, A., Severi, S. et al. Management of vasospastic crescendo angina by continuous infusion of isosorbide dinitrate. (abstract) *Circulation* 58(suppl II):II–153, 1978.

34. Page, A., Huret, J.F., Roudant, R. et al. La trinitrine intra-veineuse dans le traitement du syndrome de menace. *Nouv Presse Med.* 8(suppl 4):266, 1979.

35. Bardet, J., Baudet, M., Rigaud, M. et al. Diltiazem, a new calcium antagonist versus propranolol in treatment of spontaneous angina pectoris. (abstract) *Am J Cardiol.* 43:416, 1979.

36. Cooper, G.N., Singh, A.H., Vargas, L.L. et al. Preoperative intraaortic balloon assist in high risk revascularization patients. *Am J Surg.* 133:463, 1977.

37. Gold, H.K., Leinbach, R.C., Buckley, M.J. et al. Refractory angina pectoris: follow-up after intra-aortic balloon pumping. *Circulation* 54(suppl III):III–41, 1976.

38. Pasternak, R.C., Hutter, A.M., Jr., De Sanctis, R.W. et al. Variant angina: management and follow-up. (abstract) *Circulation* 58(suppl II):II–133, 1978.

39. Parodi, O., Maseri, A., and Simonetti, I. Management of unstable angina at rest by verapamil. A double-blind cross-over study in coronary care unit. *Br Heart J.* 41:167, 1979.

40. Mann, T., Cohn, P.F., Holman, B.L. et al. Effect of introprusside on regional myocardial blood flow in coronary artery disease. Results in 25 patients and comparison with nitroglycerin. *Circulation* 57:732, 1978.

41. Chiarello, M., Gold, H.K., Leinbach, R.C. et al. Comparison between the effects of nitroprusside and nitroglycerin on ischemic injury during acute myocardial infarction. *Circulation* 54:766, 1976.

42. Fam, W.M., and McGregor, M. Effect of nitroglycerin and dipyridamole on regional coronary resistance. *Circu Res.* 15:355, 1964.

43. Winbury, M.M., Howe, B.B., and Hefner, M.A. Effect of nitrates and other coronary dilators on large and small coronary vessels: an hypothesis for the mechanism of action of nitrates. *J Pharmacol Exp Ther.* 168:70, 1969.

44. Armstrong, P.W., Boromand, K., and Parker, J.O. Nitroprusside in acute myocardial infarction: correlative effects on hemodynamics and precordial mapping. (abstract) *Circulation* 54(suppl II):II–76, 1976.

45. Brown, T.M., Matthews, O.P., and Walter, P.F. Assessment of the effect of vasodilator therapy upon hemodynamics and ischemic injury in acute anterior myocardial infarction. (abstract) *Am J Cardiol.* 37:123, 1976.

46. Cohn, P.F., Maddox, D.E., Holman, B.C. et al. Effect of sublingual nitroglycerin on regional myocardial blood flow in patients with coronary artery disease. *Am J Cardiol.* 39:672, 1977.

47. Cheanvechai, C., Effler, D.B., Loop, E.D. et al. Emergency myocardial revascularization. *Am J Cardiol.* 32:901, 1973.

48. Reul, G.J., Morris, G.C., Howell, J.F. et al. Emergency coronary artery bypass grafts in the treatment of myocardial infarction. *Circulation* 47 & 48(suppl III):177, 1973.

49. Hill, D., Kerth, W.J., Kelly, J.J. et al. Emergency aortocoronary bypass for impending or extending myocardial infarction. *Circulation* 48 & 49(suppl I):105, 1971.

50. Sustaita, H., Chatterjee, K., Matloff, J.M. et al. Emergency bypass surgery in impending and complicated acute myocardial infarction. *Arch Surg.* 105:30, 1972.

51. Cohn, L.H., Fogarty, T.J., Daily, P.O. et al. Emergency coronary artery bypass. *Surgery* 70:821, 1971.

52. Keon, W.J., Bedard, P., Shankar, K.R. et al. Experience with emergency aortocoronary bypass grafts in the presence of acute myocardial infarction. *Circulation* 7 & 8(suppl III):151, 1973.

53. Wellons, H.A., Grossman, J., and Crosby, I.K. Early operative intervention for complications of acute myocardial infarction. *J Thorac Cardiovasc Surg.* 73:763, 1977.

54. Miller, D.C., Cannon, D.S., Fogarty, T.J. et al. Saphenous vein coronary artery bypass in patients with preinfarction angina. *Circulation* 47:234, 1973.

55. Pifarre, R., Spinazzola, A., Nemickas, R. et al. Emergency aortocoronary bypass for acute myocardial infarction. *Arch Surg.* 103:525, 1971.

56. Roberts, A.J., Alonso, D.R., Combes, J.R. et al. Role of delayed intraaortic balloon pumping in treatment of experimental myocardial infarction. *Am J Cardiol.* 41:1202, 1978.

57. Scully, H.E., Gunstensen, J., Williams, W.G. et al. Surgical management of complicated acute coronary insufficiency. *Surgery* 80:437–442, 1976.

58. Feola, M., Wiener, L., Walkinsky, P. et al. Improved survival afforded by intra-aortic balloon counterpulsation in patients with acute myocardial ischemia undergoing emergency surgical revascularization. (abstract) *Circulation* 54(suppl II):II-38, 1976.

59. Langou, R.A., Geha, A.S., Hammond, G.L. et al. Surgical approach for patients with unstable angina pectoris: role of response to initial medical therapy and intraaortic balloon pumping in perioperative complications after aortocoronary bypass grafting. *Am J Cardiol.* 42:629, 1978.

60. Cohn, L.H., Alpert, J., Koster, K. et al. Changing indications for the surgical treatment of unstable angina. *Arch Surg.* 113:1312, 1978.

20 Long-Term Follow-up of Patients Undergoing Aortocoronary Bypass Surgery for Unstable Angina

Allan G. Adelman, MD, and
Brian M. Chesnie, MD

This follow-up study was carried out on 92 patients who underwent aortocoronary bypass surgery for unstable angina at the Toronto General Hospital between November, 1974 and May, 1976. During this period we were much more aggressive with emergency and urgent aortocoronary bypass surgery for this condition than we are at present. These 92 patients were diagnosed as having unstable angina by their attending and catheterizing cardiologist prior to angiography. They were having recurrent attacks of angina or an accelerating pattern to their pain despite in-hospital treatment with bedrest, propranolol, and nitrates. Many of these patients were referred from other medical centers for evaluation of revascularization because their pain was refractory to medical management in a coronary intensive care unit. All patients were considered potential surgical candidates before catheterization was carried out.

PATIENTS

Prior to coronary angiography, 120 patients were diagnosed as having unstable angina.[1] In 28 of these patients aortocoronary bypass surgery was not done because ten did not have significant disease, ten were inoperable, and eight died or infarcted before surgery could be carried out (Figure 20-1). Of the 120 patients, 89% were men and 11% were women. Most patients were in their late 40s or early 50s, with an average age of 51.7 years. The women tended to be older than the men (58.6 vs 50.4 yr). Fifty-five percent had symptoms of coronary artery disease for at least one year and 85% had had angina for over three months. The majority (77%) had had pain at rest despite treatment with propranolol and nitrates in an intensive care unit and 72% had documented ischemic electrocardiographic changes during their attacks of pain.

Sixty-two of the 92 patients who underwent surgery were operated on within one week of angiography. Seventeen had their surgery performed within three weeks of angiography and only 13 had surgery performed

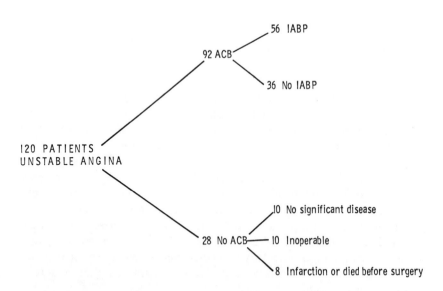

Figure 20-1 120 patients diagnosed as having unstable angina prior to coronary angiography. (From: Chesnie, B., Adelman, A.G., Douglas, B.C. et al. Results of aortocoronary bypass surgery in patients with unstable angina. *Can J Surg.* 22(2), 1979. Reproduced with permission.)

more than three weeks after coronary angiograms were done. Of the 92 patients undergoing aortocoronary bypass, 56 had prophylactic intraaortic balloon support at the time of surgery (see Figure 20-1). This was used at the discretion of the surgeon if the patients were felt to be at a higher risk because of their clinical condition, coronary artery anatomy, or because of poor left ventricular function. During this period, we tended to use the balloon much more frequently because our anesthetic techniques and methods of myocardial preservation were not so advanced as they are at the present time.[2]

RESULTS

Figure 20-2 shows the angiographic profile in the 92 surgical patients and in the balloon- and non-balloon-assisted subgroups. Only proximal stenosis equal to or greater than 75% in a major vessel are shown, as lesions less than this and distal disease were not assessed. Forty-one had triple-vessel, 31 double-vessel, and 20 single-vessel disease. A greater proportion of patients who were operated on with balloon support had triple- and double-vessel disease compared to those who did not have balloon support. Eighty-three of the 92 patients had a 75% or greater proximal stenosis of the left anterior descending artery. Fifteen had left main stenosis. The one patient with left main stenosis who was operated on without intraaortic balloon pump support died during surgery. Twelve of the 22 patients with grade III ventricles (ejection fractions less than 40%) and all six patients with grade IV ventricles (ejection fractions of less than 20%) had balloon support. In contrast, 15 of the 36 patients operated on without the balloon had normal ventricles. Thus, patients who were operated on with prophylactic intraaortic balloon support tended to be those with multiple-vessel disease, left main stenosis, and poor left ventricular function in addition to unstable angina.

The type of surgery performed on these patients is shown in Figure 20-3. Thirty patients had single-, 48 had double-, and 14 had triple-vessel aortocoronary bypass grafts. Fifteen patients had an associated endarterectomy. A much higher proportion (80%) of balloon patients had multiple bypasses whereas half of those operated on without balloon support had single bypasses. A left anterior descending aortocoronary bypass graft was carried out in 80 of the 83 patients who had a significant stenosis of this vessel.

There were five documented perioperative infarctions as evidenced by new Q waves on a postoperative electrocardiogram. There were three infarctions in the balloon group and two in the non-balloon group for an overall infarction rate of 5.4% (Table 20-1). There were six perioperative deaths, three in each group, for a surgical mortality of 6.5% The mortality rate was slightly but not significantly lower in the balloon group (5.4% vs 8.3%) despite the fact that these patients tended to have multiple-vessel disease, more severe left ventricular dysfunction, and multiple bypasses done. It also included all but one of the patients with main left stenosis.

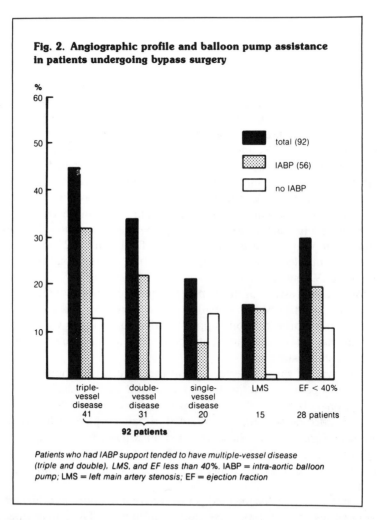

Figure 20-2 Angiographic profile and balloon pump assistance in patients undergoing bypass surgery. (From: Douglas, B.C., Adelman, A.G., Huckell, V.F. et al. Unstable angina: a clinical, angiographic, and surgical profile. *Cardiovasc Med.* 3(2):169, 175, 1978. Reproduced with permission.)

Table 20-1
Surgical Morbidity and Mortality in Patients
Undergoing Aortocoronary Bypass Surgery for Unstable Angina

No. of Patients	Total	IABP	No IABP
	92	56	36
Infarction	5 (5.4%)	3 (5.4%)	2 (5.5%)
Mortality	6 (6.5%)	3 (5.4%)	3 (8.3%)

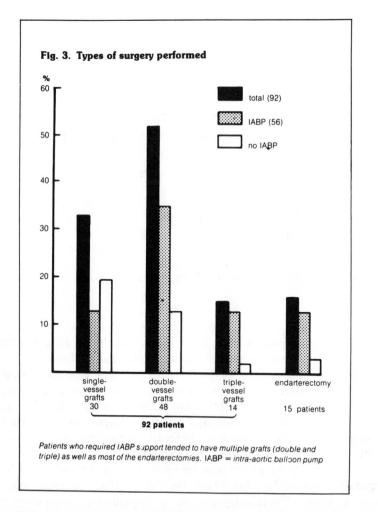

Figure 20-3 Types of surgery performed. (From: Douglas, B.C., Adelman, A.G., Huckell, V.F. et al. Unstable angina: a clinical, angiographic, and surgical profile. *Cardiovasc Med.* (3)2:169, 175, 1978. Reproduced with permission.)

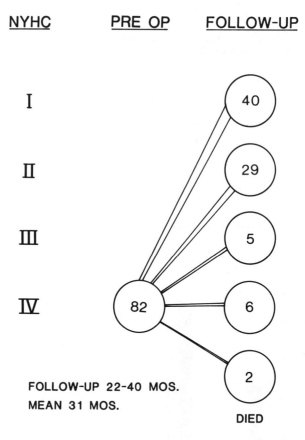

NYHC　　　PRE OP　　FOLLOW-UP

I

II

III

IV

82

40

29

5

6

2

FOLLOW-UP 22-40 MOS.
MEAN 31 MOS.

DIED

Figure 20-4 Follow-up of patients undergoing aortocoronary bypass surgery for unstable angina.

The average postoperative hospital stay was slightly longer in the patients operated on with balloon support compared to those operated on without the balloon (18 vs 14 days). There was some morbidity associated with balloon insertion. There were two cases of aortic dissection, two cases of femoral embolism, one transient ischemic attack, and one case of peroneal nerve palsy. Fortunately, the only long-term morbidity seen was one patient who had a moderate degree of intermittent claudication. This patient had suffered a femoral artery embolism.

The patients have now been followed either directly or through their primary physician for 22 to 40 months (Figure 20-4). The mean follow-up was 31 months. The primary method of follow-up was a simple questionnaire of symptomatology based on the New York Heart Classification (NYHC). Four of the surviving 86 postoperative patients have been lost to follow-up. Forty patients were completely asymptomatic and categorized as Class I, NYHC. Twenty-nine patients experienced some symptoms on more than normal activity, Class II, NYHC (Figure 20-4). This was defined as walking more than two city blocks or climbing two flights of stairs. Of these 29 patients, 15 had angina, 12 had angina and dyspnea, and two had dyspnea alone. One of the latter patients also had emphysema. Five patients experienced symptoms on less than two city blocks or climbing less than two flights of stairs (Class III, NYHC) (Figure 20-4). One of them had angina, one had dyspnea, and three had both. All six patients in Class IV, NYHC, had angina at rest (Figure 20-4).

There were only two late deaths. One patient who was bedridden postoperatively died six months after surgery with congestive heart failure. He had triple-vessel disease and required balloon support for severe left ventricular dysfunction. The other patient died in a motor vehicle accident. Overall, 82% of the patients who were operated on and followed for close to three years maintained their clinical improvement.

Of the 40 patients in Class I, 17 had single-, 20 had double-, and three had triple-vessel bypasses. Of the 17 patients with single-vessel bypasses, 14 had single-vessel disease and three had double-vessel disease. Of the 20 who had two vessels bypassed, 16 had double-vessel and four had triple-vessel disease. Of the 29 in Class II, eight had single-, 14 had double-, and seven had triple-vessel bypasses. Of 11 in Classes III and IV, two had single-, six had double-, and three had triple-vessel bypasses. The long-term results, therefore, did not seem to depend on the number of bypasses carried out, single, double, or triple, but there did appear to be better symptomatic improvement in the patients where the vessels bypassed matched the number of vessels that were critically diseased. There was also a similar proportion (in the range of 55) of patients in each class who had intraaortic balloon pump support.

DISCUSSION

Up to 20% of patients admitted to coronary care units[3] and undergoing angiography[4] have unstable angina. The 120 patients diagnosed as having unstable angina in this study represent about 10% of those undergoing angiography for coronary artery disease during this 18-month period in our institution. Ten were found to have no significant coronary artery disease, an incidence similar to that reported in other studies in which as many as 19% of patients undergoing angiography had no significant disease.[5] The prognosis in these patients is considered to be relatively benign despite the fact that they often present with pain and electrocardiographic changes similar to the patients with unstable angina. Two of the 10 patients with normal coronary arteries in this series had spontaneous spasm during coronary angiography suggesting that this may be the explanation for the unstable "angina" syndrome in some of these patients.

Of the 110 patients with significant coronary artery disease, 18 did not undergo aortocoronary bypass surgery because 10 were inoperable and 8 died or infarcted before surgery could be carried out. The 92 patients who underwent aortocoronary bypass surgery in this series therefore included all patients with unstable angina who were surgical candidates and who survived until surgery could be carried out during this 18-month period. The majority of these patients had multiple-vessel disease; the left anterior descending coronary artery was almost always affected (90% of cases). Scanlon et al[5] and Weintraub et al[6] noted a similar pattern in their studies, with 50 of 69 and 15 of 16 patients having left anterior descending involvement, respectively. Left main stenosis, which occurred in 17% of our patients and never as an isolated lesion, has been reported in 2.5% to 5.9% of patients undergoing angiography[7,8] and in about 15% of patients with unstable angina.[9,10] Recent studies have also emphasized that left main stenosis is usually associated with involvement of other vessels.[7,8,11,12]

In the mid-1970s most patients with unstable angina who underwent angiography at the Toronto General Hospital and who were considered surgical candidates were operated on within one week of investigation. In these patients, surgery was associated with a relatively low mortality (6.5%) and a low perioperative infarction rate (5.4%). This perioperative morbidity and mortality compared favorably with those of other surgical,[13-15] and most medical series[4,6,16] for this time period. Golding et al[17] recently reported a 4% mortality and a perioperative infarction rate of 17% at the Cleveland Clinic. Also, almost all surgical studies[13-15] indicate that surgery offers more immediate and effective relief of angina in these patients than does medical therapy.

Intraaortic balloon pumping has been used in unstable angina both as a method of pain relief and as an adjunct to revascularization surgery.[5,7,18] Although patients in this study were not randomized, the mortality in the group with the greater risk factors (ie, multiple-vessel disease, left main stenosis, and poor left ventricular function), was slightly but not significantly lower when the balloon was utilized (5.4% vs 8.3% in the non-balloon group). Patients with left main stenosis have been reported to have a relatively high mortality rate at surgery[19-22] but this mortality has improved with better awareness of the anesthetic induction hazard in these patients. In our study, 15 of the 16 patients with left main stenosis who were operated on with balloon pump assist survived surgery, and one patient without balloon pump assist died at surgery. It was concluded[23] that balloon pumping may be of value in patients with left main stenosis, poor left ventricular function, and multiple-vessel disease, but recent literature has suggested that further investigation is warranted.[24,25] Currently, prophylactic intraaortic balloon pumping is being used less frequently at the Toronto General Hospital, as is the case in most other centers, because of the development of better anesthetic and improved myocardial preservation techniques.

Of the 86 surviving postoperative patients, 82 were followed from 22 to 40 months, with a mean follow-up of 31 months. Prior to surgery, all patients were in Class IV, NYHC. At the time of follow-up, 40 patients were Class I, NYHC and 29 were Class II. Eighty-two percent of patients, therefore, experienced clinical improvement after surgery. In addition, there was an extremely low late mortality (2.4%) and one of the two patients who died postoperatively died of incidental causes. These findings are compatible with those of other centers.[26-28] Golding et al[17] had four late deaths (4.3%) and three late infarctions (3.1%) out of a total of 100 patients. Seventy-eight percent of their survivors were asymptomatic.

It is felt that the frequency with which patients obtain symptomatic relief and the duration of relief depends not only on the number of bypasses carried out and the patency of these grafts, but also on the degree of revascularization.[29] This refers to the number of vessels a surgical team is able to bypass that are critically diseased. For example, if two vessels are diseased and only one is able to be bypassed (the other being too diseased distally for grafting), then symptoms may not be completely relieved. The Cleveland Clinic reported that 86.6% of patients who had complete revascularization were Class I, NYHC or were asymptomatic postoperatively compared with only 55.7% of patients who had incomplete revascularization surgery.[30] Eighty-four percent (58 of 69) of our patients who were in Class I, NYHC postoperatively had complete revascularization.

This was a follow-up study of 92 patients with unstable angina who underwent emergency or urgent angiography and coronary bypass surgery during the mid-1970s. The diagnosis was based on an accelerating pattern of pain often unrelated to exertion and refractory to intensive medical management. This study indicates that these patients could be operated on with a relatively low operative mortality (6.5%) and infarction rate (5.4%) for this period in the evolution of aortocoronary bypass surgery for unstable angina. In addition, there was an extremely low late mortality (2.4%) with one of the two patients dying of incidental causes. Furthermore, the majority of patients (82%) were clinically improved and maintained this improvement over a follow-up period averaging close to three years.

The authors express appreciation to Ms. Donna Taylor for typing and editing the manuscript.

REFERENCES

1. Judkins, M.P.S. Selective coronary arteriograph. I. A percutaneous transfemoral technique. *Radiology* 89:815, 1967.
2. Goldman, B.S., Walker, P., Gunstensen, J. et al. Intra-aortic balloon pumps assist: adjunct to surgery for left ventricular dysfunction. *Can J Surg.* 19:128, 1975.

298

3. Kraus, K., Hitter, A.M., and DeSanctis, R.W. Acute coronary insufficiency. *Arch Intern Med.* 129:808, 1972.

4. Miller, D.C., Cannom, D.S., Fogarty, T.J. et al. Saphenous vein coronary artery bypass in patients with preinfarction angina. *Circulation* 47:234, 1973.

5. Scanlon, P.J., Nernickas, R., Moran, J.F. et al. Accelerated angina pectoris. *Circulation* 48:19, 1973.

6. Weintraub, R., Voukypis, P.C., Aroesty, J.M. et al. Treatment of preinfarction angina with intraaortic balloon counterpulsation. *Am J Cardiol.* 34:809, 1974.

7. Cohen, M.V., Cohen, P.E., Herman, M.V. et al. Diagnosis and prognosis of main left coronary artery obstruction. *Circulation* 45 & 46 (suppl 1):57, 1972.

8. Proudfit, W.L., Shirey, E.K., Sones, F. et al. Distribution of arterial lesions demonstrated by selective cinecoronary arteriography. *Circulation* 36:54, 1967.

9. Conti, R.C., Brawley, R.K., Griffiths, L.S., et al. Unstable angina pectoris: morbidity and mortality in 57 consecutive patients evaluated angiographically. *Am J Cardiol.* 32:745, 1973.

10. Plotnick, G., and Conti, R.C. Unstable angina: angiography, morbidity, and mortality of medically treated patients. *Circulation* 51 & 52(suppl 2):89, 1975.

11. Lavine, P., Kimbiris, D., Segal, B.L. et al. Left main coronary disease. *Am J Cardiol.* 30:791, 1972.

12. DeMotts, J.H., Bonchek, L.I., Rösch, J. et al. Left main coronary disease. *Am J Cardiol.* 36:136, 1975.

13. Bonchek, L.I., Rahmitoola, S.H., Anderson, R.P. et al. Late results following emergency saphenous vein bypass grafting for unstable angina. *Circulation* 50:972, 1974.

14. Cheanvechai, C., Effler, D.B., Loop, F.O. et al. Emergency myocardial revascularization. *Am J Cardiol.* 32:901, 1973.

15. Bolooki, H., Sommer, L., Kaiser, G.A. et al. Long-term follow-up in patients receiving emergency revascularization for intermediate coronary syndrome. *J Thorac Cardiovasc Surg.* 68:90, 1974.

16. Gazes, P.C., Mobley, E.M., Faris, H.M. Preinfarctional (unstable) angina—a prospective study: ten-year follow-up. *Circulation* 48:331, 1973.

17. Golding, L.A.R., Loop, F.D., Sheldon, W.C. et al. Emergency revascularization for unstable angina. (abstract) *Am J Cardiol.* 41:356, 1978.

18. Gold, H.K., Leinbach, R.C., Buckley, M.J. et al. Refractory angina pectoris: follow-ups after intra-aortic balloon pumping and surgery. *Circulation* 54(suppl 3):41, 1976.

19. Zeft, H.J., Manley, J.C., Huston, J.H. et al. Left main coronary artery stenosis: results of coronary bypass surgery. *Circulation* 49:68, 1974.

20. McCallister, B.D., Killer, D.A., Reed, W.R. et al. Results following coronary artery bypass in patients with left main coronary artery disease. *Am J Cardiol.* 35:153, 1975.

21. Talano, J.V., Scanlon, P.J., Khan, M. et al. Influence of surgery on survival in 145 patients with left main coronary disease. *Circulation* 50(suppl 3):110, 1974.

22. Takaro, T., Hultgren, H.N., Lipton, M.J. et al. The VA cooperative randomized study of surgery for coronary arterial occlusive disease. II. Subgroup with significant left main lesions. *Circulation* 54(suppl 3):107, 1976.

23. Douglas, B.C., Adelman, A.G., Huckell, V.F. et al. Unstable angina: a clinical, angiographic, and surgical profile. *Cardiovasc Med.* 3:167, 1978.

24. Scully, H.E., Gunstensen, J., Williams, W.G. et al. Surgical management of complicated acute coronary insufficiency. *Surgery* 80:437, 1976.

25. Gunstensen, J., Goldman, B.S., Scully, H.E. et al. Evolving indications for preoperative intra-aortic balloon pump assistance. *Am Thorac Surg.* 22:535, 1976.

26. Plotnick, G.D., and Conti, C.R. Unstable angina: angiography, short- and long-term morbidity, mortality, and symptomatic status of medically treated patients. *Am J Med.* 63:870, 1977.

27. Oberman, A., Harrell, R.R., Russell, R.O. et al. Surgical vs. medical treatment in disease of the left main coronary artery. *Lancet* 2:591, 1976.

28. Cohen, L.H., Boyden, C.M., and Collins, J.J. Improved long-term survival after aortocoronary bypass for advanced coronary artery disease. *Am J Surg.* 129:380, 1975.

29. Hurst, J.W., King, S.B., Logue, R.B. et al. Value of coronary bypass surgery. Controversies in Cardiology, Part 1. *Am J Cardiol.* 42:308, 1978.

30. Sheldon, W.C., Rincor, G., Pichard, A.D. et al. Surgical treatment of coronary artery disease: pure graft operations, with a study of 741 patients followed 3–7 years. *Prog Cardiovasc Dis.* 18:237, 1975.

21 Medical and Surgical Therapy of Unstable Angina Pectoris

C. Richard Conti, MD, and
R. Charles Curry, MD

PRELIMINARY RESULTS OF THE NATIONAL HEART, LUNG, AND BLOOD INSTITUTE PROSPECTIVE COOPERATIVE RANDOM TRIAL[1,2]

Before discussing the details of the study, it is important to place the trial in the proper perspective. In 1970, there was overwhelming enthusiasm in this country for emergency myocardial revascularization of patients with the clinical syndrome of unstable angina pectoris.[3] The rationale for emergency surgery was to prevent this group of patients from infarcting jeopardized myocardium and thereby preventing death, at least for a short time. The complication rate was higher in patients with unstable angina pectoris who underwent revascularization than in patients with stable angina who underwent the same operation. The operations were performed at the same institutions by the same surgeons.[4] Little or no data were available in comparable medically treated patients. Thus, the study was designed to try to answer the important question, "What is the best way to manage patients presenting with unstable angina in the early stages of their illness?"[1,2]

301

Participants

The trial began in January 1972 and was supported by the National Heart, Lung, and Blood Institute (NHLBI). Participating centers included Johns Hopkins University, Massachusetts General Hospital, the University of Rochester, the University of Chicago, Duke University, University of Alabama, Stanford University, Cornell University, and the University of Florida. Patient recruitment for the study was stopped in December 1976. The conclusions that will be presented here can be considered preliminary information relating to long-term survival, myocardial infarction rate, and symptomatic status of patients.

Purpose

The purpose of this study was to compare the effectiveness of medical and surgical therapy in the acute management of unstable angina pectoris. The major objective of this study was to obtain the answer to the question, "Is unstable angina best treated by urgent coronary artery surgery or by vigorous medical management?"

The end points of the study were 1) mortality, 2) myocardial infarction, and 3) symptomatic status of the patient.

Patient Population

Clinical selection of patients All patients in the unstable angina study had chest pain that indicated an impending myocardial infarction. As a result, all patients were admitted to the hospital for evaluation and management. We defined unstable angina as follows: 1) angina of recent onset ($\leq$ 4 wk) — either rest angina or angina on minimal effort; or 2) accelerating angina — increased duration, intensity, or frequency of angina or decreased responsiveness to nitrates. Patients who were considered as "medical failures" prior to admission to hospital and patients with recurrent rest angina following a recent myocardial infarction were not included in the trial.

The patients in this study were less than 70 years of age and had a state of health consistent with a further life expectancy of five years. Patients were excluded if a myocardial infarction had occurred less than three months prior to admission. The last episode of chest pain must have occurred less than seven days before admission to the study.

Many of these patients had rest angina that was promptly relieved by the administration of nitroglycerin but frequently would recur after nitroglycerin effects had worn off. In addition to this clinical presentation, all patients demonstrated transient ECG changes associated with pain episodes. These changes included ST-segment elevation or depression, T-wave inversion, or both.

The appearance of new Q waves on the electrocardiogram was grounds for exclusion from the study because of the possibility of an evolving myocardial infarction. During the first 24 hours of hospitalization, three separate enzyme determinations were made. If a rise consistent with myocardial infarction was found, the patients were excluded from the study.

Therefore, this group of patients represented a selected population. All of them were admitted to the hospital or coronary care unit because of a suspected impending infarction; and all survived the first 24 hours without any clinical evidence of myocardial infarction.

Angiographic selection of patients Once the clinical definition of unstable angina pectoris was satisfied, the patient was asked to participate in this study. It was necessary for the patient to consent to coronary angiography within the first 12 to 72 hours as well as coronary artery surgery prior to randomization. Randomization occurred after angiography. To be randomized, patients had to have one or more coronary artery narrowings greater than 70% in the left anterior descending, circumflex, or right coronary artery as well as a left ventricular ejection fraction greater than 30%. Patients were excluded from the random trial if coronary angiography revealed physiologically significant ($\geq 50\%$) left main coronary artery stenosis. These patients were offered surgery. Grounds for exclusion following angiography also included normal or very mild coronary artery disease, distal vessels unsuitable for surgery, or an ejection fraction less than 30%. These patients were treated medically.

Initial Management

During the initial evaluation prior to randomization, all patients (regardless of subsequent randomization) received vigorous medical therapy including one or more of the following: bedrest, sublingual and topical nitroglycerin, long-acting nitrates, propranolol, heparin, and sedation. No patient received intraaortic balloon counterpulsation or intravenous nitroprusside. Following randomization and stabilization with medical or surgical therapy, patients were discharged from the hospital and followed at three-month intervals for the first year and at six-month intervals thereafter.

Results

A total of 288 patients have been randomized, 147 to medical and 141 to surgical therapy. Surgical patients on medical therapy were operated upon usually within eight days after randomization. Long-term medical therapy in the surgical and medical patients was not standardized, but individualized to patient's needs. A large percentage of the patients who did not undergo surgical procedures were continued on propranolol and nitrates. Many of the patients who underwent surgical procedures were not continued on propranolol.

Patients randomized to medicine were similar to those randomized to surgery from the standpoint of clinical presentations, risk factors, ST-segment shifts during pain, previous myocardial infarction, left ventricular end-diastolic pressure, ejection fraction, and left ventricular contraction patterns. Approximately 90% of the patients randomized to either medicine or surgery presented with recurrent rest angina of new onset or progressive from stable angina. Sixty percent of patients had ST-segment depression associated with chest pain, 28% had ST-segment elevation associated with chest pain, and 12% had T-wave changes associated with chest pain episodes.

Analysis of the extent of coronary occlusive disease failed to show any significant difference between the two groups of patients. Twenty-four percent had single-vessel disease, 35% had double-vessel disease, and 41% had triple-vessel disease (≥ 70% narrowing of the coronary artery). The location of physiologically significant coronary occlusive narrowing (> 70% lumen diameter) was analyzed in all three major coronary vessels. There was no significant difference between the medical and surgical patients. The average follow-up of these patients was approximately 30 months as of August 1977.

Incidence of nonfatal myocardial infarction during initial hospitalization and following discharge The myocardial infarction rate during initial hospitalization was 8% in medically treated patients and 17% in those undergoing myocardial revascularization (Table 21-1). When these data are analyzed from the standpoint of one-, two-, and three-vessel disease, the myocardial infarction rate in the medical group compared to the surgical group was equal only in the patients with single-vessel disease.

The incidence of nonfatal myocardial infarction following discharge was approximately equal in both groups of patients (14% medicine and 13% surgery). Patients with double- and triple-vessel disease had a higher infarction rate if they received surgical therapy.

The initial hospital and posthospital myocardial infarction rate in surgically treated patients was not related to completeness of the revascularization procedure. The incompletely revascularized patients had a slightly higher incidence of myocardial infarction, but this was not statistically significant.

The overwhelming majority of myocardial infarctions, early and late, occurred in the area that was perfused by the grafted vessel. Only a few myocardial infarctions occurred in areas perfused by nongrafted vessels.

Mortality during initial hospitalization and following discharge The overall mortality in medically and surgically treated patients was not statistically different during the initial hospitalization phase of management or during an average of 30-month posthospital follow-up period. Early medical mortality was 3% and surgical was 5% (Table 21-2). The later medical mortality was an additional 6% and surgical mortality an additional 5% (Table 21-3). Surgical mortality seemed to be highest in patients with three-vessel disease.

Projected survival curves comparing all patients initially randomized to surgery compared to a similar group who received medical treatment alone revealed no statistical difference. However, as the follow-up period progressed, some medically treated patients were operated on to obtain relief of their symptoms. The actual details of why these patients were

Table 21-1
Myocardial Infarction During Initial Hospitalization*

	No. of Patients	Medical	Surgical
NHLBI[1,2]	288	12/147 (8%)	24/141 (17%)
Pugh et al[5]	27	0/14 (0%)	2/13 (15%)
Selden et al[6]	40	0/19 (0%)	3/21 (14%)
Bertolasi et al[7,8]			
Intermediate	52	2/24 (8%)	4/28 (14%)
Progressive	61	0/27 (0%)	4/34 (12%)
Totals	468	14/231 (6%)	37/237 (16%)

*This and later tables include data from other randomized trials, presented for comparison with the NHCBI data.

Table 21-2
Mortality During Initial Hospitalization

	No. of Patients	Medical	Surgical
NHLBI[1,2]	288	4/147 (3%)	7/141 (5%)
Pugh et al[5]	27	0/14 (0%)	1/13 (8%)
Selden et al[6]	40	0/19 (0%)	1/21 (5%)
Bertolasi et al[7,8]			
Intermediate	52	5/24 (21%)	3/28 (11%)
Progressive	61	1/27 (4%)	3/34 (9%)
Totals	468	10/231 (4%)	15/237 (6%)

Table 21-3
Total Mortality and Myocardial Infarction Rate*

Average Duration of Follow-up	No. of Patients	Death		Myocardial Infarction	
		Medical	*Surgical*	*Medical*	*Surgical*
30 mo (NHLBI)[1,2]	288	13/147 (9%)	14/141 (10%)	32/147 (22%)	43/141 (30%)
18 mo (Pugh et al)[5]	27	1/14 (7%)	1/13 (8%)	1/14 (0%)	3/13 (23%)
4 mo (Selden et al)[6]	40	0/19 (0%)	1/21 (5%)	2/19 (11%)	3/21 (14%)
32 mo (Bertolasi et al)[7,8] Intermediate	52	11/24 (46%)	3/28 (11%)	9/24 (38%)	4/28 (14%)
Progressive	61	2/27 (7%)	3/34 (9%)	2/27 (7%)	4/34 (12%)
Totals	468	24/231 (12%)	22/237 (9%)	45/231 (19%)	57/237 (24%)

*Includes myocardial infarction and deaths during initial hospitalization and following discharge based on original assignment to medical or surgical therapy.

crossed over to surgery are not available at this time, but it is the general impression of the investigators that the major clinical indication for surgery was to relieve angina pectoris. Analysis of a number of vessels involved in these crossover patients reveals that, as the vessel involvement increased from one to three vessels, the percentage crossover increased. For example, 7 of 35 patients with single-vessel disease (20%) crossed over to surgery, whereas 18 of 55 patients with double-vessel disease (33%) crossed over to surgery, and 28 of 57 patients with triple-vessel disease (49%) crossed over to surgery. Thus, a total of 53 of the 147 patients originally randomized to medicine crossed over to surgery (36%).

If the survival curves are replotted comparing randomized medical patients up to the time of crossover against all surgical patients, there is no statistically significant difference. Similarly, if the survival curves of the randomized medical patients who did not cross over to surgery are replotted against all the surgical patients (crossovers included), there is no statistically significant difference in survival. Finally, with the survival curve of patients randomized to surgery, it appears that the crossover patients have a better survival. However, the number in this group is small and does not reach statistical significance. Nevertheless, it seems that the delay in surgery in these patients did not decrease their chance for survival and, in fact, may have increased it slightly.

Mortality and myocardial infarction rate before and after June 1974 Prior to 1974, the early hospital mortality was 3% in medical patients and 6% in surgical patients. After 1974, the medical mortality was 3% and surgical mortality was 4%. There was no significant difference in the early mortality rate of patients with unstable angina regardless of the initial therapy.

The myocardial infarction rate was strikingly different. Before 1974 the myocardial infarction rate for medical therapy was 8% and for surgery 22%. After 1974, the infarction rate for medical patients stayed approximately the same at 9%. For the surgical patients, myocardial infarction rate decreased to 12%.

Effect of complete revascularization on mortality Early and late mortality in patients who were incompletely revascularized was 12% and 9% respectively, compared to 1% and 3% in patients having complete revascularization.

Symptoms Symptomatic status of the patients over the follow-up period was more difficult to analyze than the incidence of myocardial infarction and death. Consequently, an arbitrary comparison was made between the surgical and medical patients who had Class III or IV angina at any follow-up visit over the 30-month period. Thus, an individual patient with severe angina at his six-month follow-up visit, but no angina at his 12-month follow-up visit would be considered a Class III or IV angina.

When results were compared in this fashion, there was a higher incidence of Class III or IV angina in the medical group (45%) compared to the surgically treated patients (15%) (Table 21-4).

Table 21-4
Follow-up of Functional Classes III and IV

Average Duration of Follow-up	Medical (%)	Surgical (%)
30 mo (NHLBI)[1,2]	45	15
18 mo (Pugh et al)[5]	38	0
4 mo (Selden et al)[6]	63	4.7
32 mo (Bertolasi et al)[7,8]		
Intermediate	16.6	3.5
Progressive	18.5	0

During the first year of follow-up, patients randomized to medical therapy had a statistically higher incidence of Class III or IV than did patients randomized to surgery. This was true whether the patients had single-, double-, or triple-vessel disease. During the second year of follow-up, symptoms were greater in the medically treated patients, but the incidence of Class III or IV angina was similar in the medically and surgically treated patients with double- or triple-vessel disease. It is possible that this observation is a result of symptomatic patients crossing from medical to surgery therapy.

Patients who were incompletely revascularized had a higher incidence of Class III or IV angina than those who received complete revascularization. This was true after both the first- and second-year follow-up visit.

COMPARISON OF THE RESULTS OF FOUR RANDOM TRIALS FOR UNSTABLE ANGINA

The NHLBI study is the largest random trial to assess medical and surgical treatment results in patients with unstable angina. There have been three other prospective, randomized studies of treatment for patients with unstable angina. Pugh and colleagues[5] reported results in 27 patients, Selden and colleagues[6] reported results in 40 patients, and Bertolasi and his colleagues[7,8] have studied 113 patients (see Table 21-1). These studies are not entirely similar in the number of patients studied, patient selection criteria, study design, exclusion criteria, or treatment results. A comparison of these four studies partially explains differences in treatment results.

Patient Selection

Selden et al[6] and Pugh et al[5] used a definition of unstable angina similar to that of the NHLBI.[1,2] Bertolasi and his colleagues[7,8] used a different definition. They divided their patients into two subsets: those with intermediate syndrome, and those with progressive angina. Patients with intermediate syndrome are defined based on major and minor criteria. The major criteria are 1) prolonged recurrent rest angina, 2) normal cardiac enzyme level of 50% above basal level, and 3) no heart failure or severe arrhythmias. Minor criteria are 1) poor response to nitrates, 2) transient ECG changes, 3) transient cardiac arrhythmias, and 4) recent onset (less than one month) of angina. Bertolasi's group of patients with progressive angina are similar to the patients with unstable angina who have an accelerated or crescendo pattern of their chest pain syndrome. Some of the patients in the Bertolasi study classified as having an intermediate syndrome would probably have been excluded from the other three studies, as 50% elevation of cardiac enzymes would have been interpreted as evidence for an acute myocardial infarction.

Study Design

The random study designs of Selden and his colleagues and Pugh and colleagues are similar to that of the NHLBI study, ie, all patients were randomized after angiography was performed. In contrast, Bertolasi's patients were randomized into medical and surgical groups prior to angiography.

Exclusion Criteria

Selden's study does not indicate what type of patients were excluded prior to or after randomization. Criteria for exclusion by Pugh and colleagues were similar to those used in the NHLBI study. Bertolasi's paper indicates that patients were excluded because of 1) minimal disease [10], 2) severe angiographic lesions, not otherwise defined [5], 3) refused study [7], and 4) other causes [11]. Bertolasi also notes in his paper that patients with Prinzmetal's angina and recent onset angina were excluded from the trial. Numbers are not given for these latter two groups of patients. It should be noted that in the NHLBI study, approximately 25% of the patients presenting with rest angina had accompanying ST-segment elevation during episodes of chest pain. These patients were not excluded from randomization. The number of patients with ST-segment elevation during unstable angina was not mentioned in the studies by Selden and Pugh. In the NHLBI study, patients were excluded from randomization after angiography, if a physiologically significant left main coronary stenosis was found to be a cause of the patient's chest pain. Patients were also excluded if they had too little disease, too much coronary disease, or severe left ventricular dysfunction. Thus, in comparing the four studies the patient populations were similar, but not exactly the same.

Treatment Results

Treatment results for the four studies are summarized in Tables 21-1 through 21-5. The incidence of nonfatal myocardial infarction during initial hospitalization is summarized in Table 21-1. The overall incidence of myocardial infarction was 6% in the medically treated patients and 16% in the surgically treated patients. All four studies show a higher incidence of acute myocardial infarction following surgery.

A comparison of mortality during initial hospitalization for patients in the four random trials is summarized in Table 21-2. The overall mortality for medically treated patients during the initial hospitalization was 4% and for surgically treated patients 6%. It should be pointed out that Bertolasi's group of medically treated patients with the "intermediate syndrome" had a 21% mortality. This is a mortality rate higher than that found in most modern coronary care units treating patients with documented acute myocardial infarction. Excluding the intermediate group of Bertolasi, all four studies showed no difference in mortality during initial hospitalization regardless of medical or surgical treatment.

Tables 21-3 and 21-4 summarize the total numbers of myocardial infarction and death (including initial hospital mortality and morbidity) in all four random trials. The average follow-up varied (30 months for the NHLBI group, 18 months for Pugh's group, four months for Selden's group, and 32 months for Bertolasi's group). Grouping the data from all four studies, in 468 patients with unstable angina the overall incidence of death appeared to be similar regardless of initial medical or surgical therapy. That is, there were 12% deaths in the medical group and 9% in the surgical group. Similarly, grouping the data from all four studies, the overall incidence of myocardial infarction appeared to be similar regardless of initial medical and surgical therapy — 19% myocardial infarction in the medical group and 24% in the surgical group.

The only discrepancy in the incidence of myocardial infarction and death was in Bertolasi's group with the intermediate syndrome. In an attempt to resolve this discrepancy we reanalyzed our data in the NHLBI study and redefined our patients using Bertolasi's definition of intermediate syndrome. One hundred thirty-one patients were randomized to medicine, and 128 to surgery. There were 11 deaths in both groups of patients (8% mortality for medical therapy and 9% mortality for surgical therapy).

Thus, we were unable to confirm Bertolasi's results suggesting a specific clinical presentation at higher risk compared to other patients with unstable angina.

The symptomatic status of the randomized patients is summarized in Table 21-5. Although the length of follow-up was different in the different groups of patients, all the randomized studies have clearly shown that patients receiving surgical therapy had a lower incidence of functional Class III or IV angina compared to patients on medical therapy.

Table 21-5
Random Trials — Unstable Angina[2,5,6,8]

	Initial Hospitalization		Total*	
	Mortality (%)	Myocardial Infarction (%)	Mortality (%)	Myocardial Infarction (%)
Medical (231)	4	6	12	19
Surgical (237)	6	16	9	24

*Variable follow-up.

ADVANTAGES AND CRITICISMS OF THE NHLBI RANDOM TRIAL

Advantages

Uniformity of definition of the clinical syndrome being evaluated was maintained.

Angiography was performed in all patients to determine surgical suitability *before* randomization.

Transient electrocardiographic changes were required in all patients in order to provide evidence that myocardial ischemia was responsible for the chest pain syndrome. Using this approach, most patients with evolving myocardial infarction are eliminated from randomization by current detection techniques.

Uniformity of data collection   Forms were filled out on each patient.

Statistical considerations   The study design is statistically sound. Therefore, the study eliminates bias in the assignment of patients to treatment groups and assures that medical and surgical treatment groups are identical. In addition, the multicenter trial eliminates regional and local bias, ie, the skill of the medical or surgical team, and provides more patients for the study. In a retrospective or nonrandom study, *all* patients must be included in the study if it is to be meaningful. It is not necessary to study all patients with unstable angina if the patient population is prospectively identified and subsequently randomized.

Ethical consideration   Random trial is ethically sound if the best therapy for the patient is not known at the beginning of the study.

Unique information   A prospective trial provides unique information in medically treated patients. Patients randomized to medicine provide previously unknown data on aggressive modern medical therapy and long-term results in patients who are surgically suitable and comparable to the surgically treated patients.

Criticisms of the Prospective Random Trial

Selected patients   Study does not include all patients with unstable angina pectoris admitted to any one hospital. This criticism is justified only if the results of the random trial are applied to every patient with unstable angina rather than to individual patients with unstable angina who fit the definition for entrance into the study.

Exclusion of patients with left main coronary artery disease   Surgically suitable patients with left main coronary artery disease were excluded from the study, thus eliminating many patients with the clinical syndrome of unstable agina from the random trial. In the experience of most physicians interested in this syndrome, left main coronary artery disease occurs in about 10% of the patients presenting with unstable angina pectoris. Thus, the overwhelming majority of patients with this syndrome are not excluded from the random trial for anatomic reasons.

Improvement of surgical techniques   In any long-term study involving medical and surgical therapy, both medical and surgical therapies generally tend to improve as experience with the therapies increases. Most physicians agree that surgical techniques have improved, and, as a result, surgical mortality and morbidity have decreased. It is also true that medical therapy of unstable angina has improved over the duration of the study. Physicians are now much more aggressive and vigorous in the use of nitrates, propranolol, and other agents when treating patients with unstable angina.

Undetected myocardial infarction   A few patients with evolving myocardial infarction, who are not detected by current standard techniques, may be subjected to surgery and bias the study against surgery (ie, increased mortality and myocardial infarction rate). This is a legitimate criticism. However, any study, random or otherwise, involving acute coronary artery surgery has this problem.

Surgical skill   A final criticism is that the skill and experience of the surgeon or cardiologist may produce different surgical or medical results in the different institutions.

SUMMARY AND CONCLUSION

This study confirms that surgical therapy of patients with unstable angina can be performed with an acceptable mortality and morbidity. Symptomatic improvement in these patients is similar to that observed in patients undergoing revascularization procedures for stable angina.

In contrast to previous reports, however, this study also indicates that intensive medical management of unstable angina results in a better prognosis than previously expected. It is an acceptable alternative to early cardiac surgery since the early mortality and myocardial infarction rate is lower than was once thought. This may be related, in part, to the vigorous use of propranolol and long-acting nitrates, but another factor that may be of equal importance is comparability of the patients. For the first time, long-term follow-up information is available in patients with a similar clinical presentation and a similar degree of anatomic impairment. That is, all patients are surgical candidates. Thus, earlier reports of the results of medical therapy, in which the location, degree, severity, and extent of coronary occlusive disease and the degree of ventricular impairment are not known, may not be relevant. They should not be compared to results of medical therapy in patients with surgically suitable disease.

The early myocardial infarction rate in the surgical patients has decreased, presumably due to better techniques of myocardial protection and more complete revascularization. Long-term medical therapy has been an effective way to control symptoms in many patients, but overall, surgery was better.

Long-term survival seems comparable in both groups of patients. However, the patients crossing over to surgery pose a difficult problem relating to the analysis of survival data. Further follow-up of these patients may clarify this issue.

Patients surviving surgical therapy clearly have fewer symptoms than patients surviving only medical therapy. However, there does not seem to be any evidence to suggest the need for operating on patients on an emergency basis. The early mortality and morbidity in the medically treated patients was quite low. In addition, we were unable to demonstrate that myocardial infarction or death was prevented by surgery. Clinical experience indicates that the majority of the patients with unstable angina, when treated vigorously with pharmacologic agents, have a marked reduction, if not total relief, of their angina syndrome, at least over the short term.

The data suggest that the indication for surgery (relief of symptoms) in patients with unstable angina may be the same as for patients with stable angina. It has not been shown that myocardial infarction or death was prevented by early surgery. Further, the low early mortality and morbidity with medical therapy permits delay of surgery. This may reduce the risk of

314

surgery in patients with persistent, active myocardial ischemia or undetected evolving myocardial infarction.

At the present time, our indications for a myocardial revascularization procedure in patients with unstable angina are as follows: 1) patients with this syndrome who are discovered to have severe anatomic narrowing of the left main coronary artery; 2) patients whose symptoms (pain or life-threatening arrhythmias) are uncontrolled by vigorous medical therapy during the initial hospitalization; 3) patients with multiple-vessel coronary artery disease with persistent chronic angina pectoris despite medical therapy; and 4) patients with surgically suitable coronary artery disease, who are not satisfied with their life-style because of symptoms.

This report contains preliminary data from the NHLBI National Randomized Trial of Unstable Angina. Co-principal investigators and participating institutions are as follows:

Richard Russell, MD, University of Alabama; Michael Wolk, MD, Cornell University; Leon Resnekov, MD, University of Chicago; Robert Rosati, MD, Duke University; Louis Becker, MD, Johns Hopkins University; Adolph Hutter, MD, Massachusetts General Hospital; Theodore Biddle, MD, University of Rochester; John Schroeder, MD, Stanford University; C. Richard Conti, MD, University of Florida; Coordinating Center, Massachusetts General Hospital, Boston, Massachusetts, E.M. Kaplan, MD, J.P. Gilbert, MD, A.M. Hutter, MD, and J.B. Newell, MD; and NHLBI, Bethesda, Maryland: P.L. Frommer, MD, and M.B. Mock, MD.

REFERENCES

1. National Cooperative Study Group. Unstable angina pectoris — National cooperative study to compare medical and surgical therapy. I. Report of protocol and patient population. *Am J Cardiol.* 37:896–902, 1976.

2. National Cooperative Study Group. Unstable angina pectoris — National cooperative study group to compare surgical and medical therapy. II. In-hospital experience and initial follow-up results in patients with one, two, and three vessel disease. *Am J Cardiol.* 42:839–848, 1978.

3. Conti, C.R., Brawley, R.K., Griffith, L.S.C. et al. Unstable angina pectoris: morbidity and mortality in 57 consecutive patients evaluated angiographically. *Am J Cardiol.* 32:745–750, 1973.

4. Gott, V.L. Outlook for patients after coronary artery revascularization. *Am J Cardiol.* 33:431–437, 1974.

5. Pugh, B., Platt, M.R., Mills, L.J. et al. Unstable angina pectoris: a randomized study of patients treated medically and surgically. *Am J Cardiol.* 41:1291–1298, 1978.

6. Selden, R., Neill, W.A., Ritzman, L.W. et al. Medical versus surgical therapy for acute coronary insufficiency: a randomized study. *N Engl J Med.* 293:1329–1333, 1975.

7. Bertolasi, C.A., Tronge, J.E., Carreno, C.A. et al. Unstable angina — prospective and randomized study of its evaluation with and without surgery. *Am J Cardiol.* 33:201–208, 1974.

8. Bertolasi, C.A., Tronge, J.E., Riccitelli, M.A. et al. Natural history of unstable angina with medical or surgical therapy. *Chest* 70:596–605, 1976.

SECTION V

Summation and Conclusions

22 Unstable Angina Pectoris — An Overview

E. Douglas Wigle, MD

Usually, when a symposium and a book result from the consideration of a specific subject in medicine, the book follows a successful symposium. In this treatise on unstable angina pectoris the opposite is true. Drs. Adelman and Goldman planned the book and then, believing they had assembled a highly knowledgeable group of workers in this field, organized a symposium. Fortunately for those attending the symposium, all contributors to this book spoke at the symposium, where the discussion was active and at times provocative, which is quite appropriate for the subject under review.

Drs. Adelman and Goldman have had a long-time interest in the subject of unstable angina pectoris, which led to their planning these proceedings.[1-3] They chose their contributors from Europe and the United States as well as from centers in Canada, where there has been an active interest in this subject.

In this summary and conclusion section, I was originally asked to address myself to the medical management of unstable angina pectoris. I have chosen not do precisely this for two reasons: first, the management of

317

unstable angina pectoris is not solely medical or surgical, but rather a combined approach; second, to discuss management alone would result in my neglecting important aspects of the clinical course, prognosis, pathophysiology, pathology, and other interesting facets of this still evolving syndrome.

DEFINITIONS

For the most part these proceedings concern themselves with four varieties of unstable angina pectoris: recent onset angina pectoris (within one month), crescendo (accelerating) angina pectoris, acute coronary insufficiency, and postmyocardial infarction angina pectoris (within one month). These terms have been repeatedly well-defined in the chapters of this book and will not be repeated here.

Some authors have alluded to variant or Prinzmetal's angina, which is an unstable form of angina pectoris. But the authors have essentially stayed away from this subject as it alone could fill a whole book. Nevertheless, the concept of coronary artery spasm arose principally from studying cases of Prinzmetal's angina; thus it is appropriate to consider it to some extent.

PATHOLOGY

The pathologic studies by Roberts and Virmani (see Chapter 4) and Silver and Butany (see Chapter 5) should provide food for thought for cardiologists and cardiovascular surgeons interested in unstable angina pectoris. It is now clear that the extent of coronary artery disease in stable and unstable angina pectoris is similar. This raises the question as to why patients with similar degrees of coronary artery disease present with different myocardial ischemic pain syndromes. It also leads to consideration of coronary artery spasm (see below). Drs. Silver and Butany report that the myocardial pathology is similar in stable and unstable angina pectoris. Previously, however, Williams et al[4] reported extensive old and recent subendocardial damage in patients who had suffered from recurrent acute coronary insufficiency over longer periods of time, in some cases, years. This fact must be borne in mind when we consider the current evidence for ischemic myocardial damage occurring in patients with unstable angina pectoris. Finally, virtually all participants at the symposium were shocked at Roberts and Virmani's report, which indicated that when the coronary arteries of 22 patients with unstable angina were sectioned into 5-mm segments, 47% of these segments were 76% to 100% narrowed in cross-sectional area. Only 11 of such segments were less than 25% narrowed and none were normal. Roberts and Virmani rightly remind us that a 75%

cross-sectional area reduction is equivalent to a 50% diameter reduction on a coronary angiogram. With statistics such as these cardiologists should be amazed that their surgical colleagues are able to carry out bypass grafts to such diseased arteries. It should be remembered, however, that by the techniques used by Roberts and Virmani, 30% of the length of the coronary arteries from normal controls were narrowed in cross-sectional area by more than 50%. In addition, it is possible that the degree of narrowing might not have appeared so severe if the same patients with unstable angina pectoris had been studied at autopsy, following injection under pressure of their coronary arteries with contrast media. Certainly, coronary arteriograms in patients with unstable angina pectoris do not appear to reflect the degree of coronary artery disease in life that Roberts and Virmani depict in death.

PATHOPHYSIOLOGY

Role of Coronary Artery Spasm in Unstable Angina Pectoris

Maseri et al (see Chapter 6) have cogently summarized their evidence for coronary artery spasm as an important pathophysiologic mechanism in unstable angina pectoris. Dhurandhar et al[1] were among the first to angiographically demonstrate coronary artery spasm in Prinzmetal's angina. Maseri et al have carried out the most extensive and sophisticated studies on the role of coronary artery spasm in variant or Prinzmetal's angina. They are essentially the only investigators to demonstrate spasm in the other forms of unstable angina pectoris. They have also demonstrated spasm at the onset of an acute myocardial infarction.[5] In Prinzmetal's angina, an attack of pain associated with coronary artery spasm (spontaneous or induced by ergonovine) is associated with a transmural thallium perfusion defect. In acute coronary insufficiency, spontaneous or induced spasm is associated with a more diffuse subendocardial perfusion defect. Maseri et al have rightly drawn attention, however, to the fact that in a single patient with unstable angina pectoris, attacks of myocardial ischemic pain may be associated with ST-segment elevation or depression on the ECG. In this symposium they also showed that normalization of a previously inverted T wave or peaking of a normal T wave may be the ECG reflection of spasm.

Of great clinical importance is the demonstration by Maseri et al that myocardial ischemic pain is a late event in an episode of unstable angina pectoris. Thus, evidence of left ventricular dysfunction (decrease in negative and positive left ventricular dp/dt, elevation of left ventricular end-diastolic pressure) and ECG evidence of ischemia precede the ischemic pain and in many instances occur in its absence. Accompanying these changes is a decrease in oxygen saturation of the coronary veins draining the areas of myocardial ischemia. All of the above characteristics of myocardial ischemia in unstable angina pectoris occur prior to any increase in heart rate or blood pressure, ie, in the absence of any increase in oxygen demand.

These studies, combined with the angiographic demonstration of spontaneous or induced coronary artery spasm, have tremendously increased our knowledge and understanding of the pathophysiology of unstable angina. This is beginning to profoundly affect therapy. Based on these observations Maseri et al now divide angina pectoris into primary and secondary types. Secondary angina results from an increase in myocardial oxygen demand as a stable and predictable effort-induced angina. Primary angina pectoris occurs in the absence of an increase in oxygen demand as in many cases of unstable angina pectoris. It also occurs in Prinzmetal's angina, where a decrease in oxygen supply due to diminished coronary blood flow occurs as the result of coronary artery spasm or other factors, such as platelet aggregates. Maseri et al note coronary artery spasm in a high proportion of their cases of unstable angina pectoris (80% to 90%). Others, such as Mizgala (see Chapter 9), believe that spasm is responsible for only a small proportion (3% to 5%) of cases of unstable angina. Thus the incidence of spasm as a cause of unstable angina must be resolved, as must the basic mechanisms responsible for spasm. The possible role of prostaglandins, prostacyclins, and/or platelets, and possibly other factors, requires clarification.

Evidence of Ischemic Myocardial Damage in Unstable Angina Pectoris

It now seems clear that myocardial damage does indeed occur in a significant percentage of patients with unstable angina pectoris. This was certainly evident in earlier pathologic studies of patients who had unstable angina over prolonged periods of time.[4] In this symposium, McLaughlin and Morch (see Chapter 7) reviewed the evidence from myocardial imaging studies that indicate that myocardial damage does occur in unstable angina. In this respect the positive technetium pyrophosphate studies are particularly convincing. Parker and Leach (see Chapter 3) refer to the recently reported studies of colleague Dr. Paul Armstrong. Armstrong[6] studied 199 patients with unstable angina pectoris, none of whom had evidence of infarction by conventional clinical, ECG, or daily CPK enzyme criteria. When frequent (4/hr), CPK analyses were carried out in these same patients, 19% had significant rises signifying myocardial damage that was undetected by the conventional studies. Furthermore, those patients demonstrating CPK elevations by frequent sampling had a poorer prognosis at one year than those who did not.[6] Baigrie (see Chapter 8) and Weisel et al (see Chapter 18) have detected a rise in CK-MB isoenzyme in some of their patients with unstable angina pectoris. They found that the risk of surgery is higher in patients with preoperative myocardial damage. The evidence seems clear, therefore, that a certain percentage of patients with unstable angina pectoris do in fact have myocardial damage during their myocardial ischemic pain episodes. The above studies should provide a stimulus for further research to identify the most sensitive techniques for recognizing subclinical myocardial damage. Further research could also define the characteristics of episodes of pain that may likely result in a type of myocardial damage that is not detected by current techniques.

Clinical Course

Feinstein[7] recently pointed out that "what used to be called the natural history of a disease can now seldom be observed because of frequent interventions by various forms of treatment. Consequently, the phrase 'clinical course' has become better than 'natural history' as a descriptive label for the sequence of events that occurs in a diseased host both before and after therapy." This is perhaps particularly true in unstable angina pectoris.

The contributions of Cairns (see Chapter 1), Parker and Leach (see Chapter 3), Mizgala (see Chapter 9), Baigrie (see Chapter 8), and Conti and Curry (see Chapter 21), as well as others in this symposium have outlined various studies of the clinical course of patients with unstable angina pectoris. The studies in the 1960s indicating myocardial infarction rates of 22% to 80% and death rates of 16% to 60% within three months of onset of unstable angina were truly alarming (see Chapters 1 and 9). Although later studies in the 1960s and early 1970s revealed an improved clinical course, there continued to be great concern about the results of medical therapy. This led to the belief that surgery was required on an urgent or emergency basis in a great number of these cases in the mid-1970s. Fortunately, controlled trials[8-10] (Conti and Curry, Chapter 21) have now indicated that in the majority of cases, aggressive medical therapy is at least the equal of surgical intervention in the acute phase of unstable angina. Out of these various studies have come a number of prognostic indicators in patients with unstable angina pectoris. Some factors pointing to a poor prognosis are: left main coronary artery stenosis, extent of coronary artery disease, poor ventricular function, previous stable angina pectoris or myocardial infarction, acute coronary insufficiency (particularly with pain unresponsive to medical therapy), myocardial damage by frequent enzyme sampling, and certain electrocardiographic patterns.

Treatment

Following this symposium and the controlled clinical trials that have been carried out it seems clear that intensive medical therapy is the initial treatment of choice in unstable angina pectoris. Patients with new onset angina and crescendo angina should be admitted to the hospital, preferably with ECG monitoring available. Not many of them appear to require the facilities of a coronary care unit, although if such is available, so much the better. Patients with acute coronary insufficiency, postmyocardial infarction unstable angina, and Prinzmetal's angina should definitely be admitted to a coronary care unit. All patients with unstable angina should have daily ECGs for at least three days, an ECG during and after any pain episode, continuous ECG monitoring for two to three days, and cardiac enzymes determined more than once a day in an attempt to detect evidence of myocardial necrosis. Technetium pyrophosphate scanning is valuable for the same reasons and correlative studies are required to determine whether frequent enzyme sampling techniques or technetium scanning is more sensitive in detecting evidence of necrosis in this population of patients. Patients should be in a quiet, relaxed situation with oxygen therapy and sedation where appropriate. Therapy with β-adrenergic blocking agents and oral vasodilators should be administered soon after hospital admission. Some participants in this symposium give the former intravenously, some orally, but in either case the dose is sufficient to reduce the resting heart rate to 60 beats/min or less. Isosorbide dinitrate should be given in maximum tolerable doses and its vasodilator effect may be augmented by nitroglycerin paste applied to the skin. With evidence of heart failure, digitalis glycosides and diuretics should be given. In these circumstances they can lessen myocardial oxygen consumption and hence the ischemic pain. Maseri et al (see Chapter 6), and Michels et al (see Chapter 10) have been impressed with the use of the calcium-blocking agents in unstable angina pectoris for relief of ischemic pain due to coronary spasm. Maseri et al have mainly used verapamil with significant success but this drug should not be given with a β-blocking agent for fear of inducing heart failure. Nifedipine, however, apparently can be given as a calcium-blocking agent in the presence of propranolol without inducing heart failure. When patients so treated break through with further ischemic chest pain, Michels et al and Mizgala have been very impressed with the use of continuous intravenous nitroglycerin infusions and/or nifedipine infusions to further stabilize the patient in a pain-free state. The use of these latter interventions has markedly reduced the need for the intraaortic balloon pump in these situations, although its use is still required for stabilization of some patients with unstable angina.

Patients who break through the initial therapy sometimes require intravenous infusions of nitroglycerin and/or nifedipine or the intraaortic balloon pump to stabilize their clinical state. These patients should undergo coronary arteriography and bypass surgery, if they are operable, during the same hospital admission. The coronary arteriography should be carried out continuing whatever intervention has stabilized the patient. Even under these circumstances the surgery rarely has to be done as an emergency but can usually be scheduled on an urgent or semiurgent basis. The realization that coronary bypass surgery is rarely an emergency today and the knowledge that intravenous nitroglycerin, nifedipine, or the intraaortic balloon pump can usually stabilize patients with unstable angina pectoris has been a great relief to cardiac surgeons.

Bardet and Bourdarias (see Chapter 19) have stressed the early use of the intraaortic balloon pump and urgent surgery in the management of postmyocardial infarction unstable angina pectoris and their results support their enthusiasm. It is possible that some of these patients could initially be managed with intravenous nitroglycerin and/or nifedipine infusions without having to resort to the balloon pump during subsequent invasive investigations and ultimate surgery, where possible.

There is general agreement that patients with unstable angina pectoris who have recurrent pain on full medical therapy should be assessed for bypass surgery during the same hospitalization. How to manage the patients who become pain-free on medical therapy becomes somewhat of a problem in terms of future management. One of the biggest questions to be answered is "Should all of these patients undergo coronary arteriography and, if so, when in the course of their management?" Michels et al and Mizgala discharge these patients on full medical therapy and readmit them to the hospital about three months later for a complete work-up including coronary arteriography. One reason for doing this is to identify the 10% of these patients who will have left main coronary artery stenosis and the further 10% of these patients who will have normal coronary arteries. Controlled trials have demonstrated that survival in significant left main coronary artery disease is improved by surgery.[11] Baigrie, on the other hand, only carries out coronary arteriography in unstable angina pectoris that has initially responded to medical therapy, when there is pain breakthrough on follow-up. Thus not all patients are investigated, as 30% to 40% (or more) will become asymptomatic on continued medical therapy according to Mizgala and Michels et al. Still other centers carry out coronary arteriography on all patients with unstable angina pectoris during the initial hospital admission. Obviously, choosing which course to follow depends on whether or not bypass surgery is expected to prolong life and reduce infarction rate. It also depends on the results of surgery in the particular center.

The controlled trials of medical vs surgical therapy in the initial phases of unstable angina pectoris indicate that there is no difference in the early (one month) or late (30 months) mortality rate between the two modes of therapy; nor is there any difference in the late myocardial infarction rate.[8-10] (See also, Conti and Curry, Chapter 21.) Early myocardial infarction, however, is more common in the surgical group, but this difference is lessening with time. Conti and Curry's report indicates that 45% of the medically treated patients have Grade III or IV angina on follow-up whereas only 15% of the surgical group have such incapacitating symptoms. Thirty-six percent of patients initially randomized to medical therapy have crossed over to surgical therapy because of the incapacitating angina during the 30-month follow-up period. Patients initially treated medically who subsequently cross over to surgery have a survival rate no worse than, and possibly better than, those initially randomized to surgery.

SUMMARY

The "intermediate" myocardial ischemic pain syndromes of coronary artery disease, now known as unstable angina pectoris, have undergone intensive study in the last decade. The result is evolution of a much clearer picture of pathology, pathophysiology, prognosis, clinical course, and modes of therapy. With the recent evidence that spasm is an important pathophysiologic mechanism and that myocardial necrosis does in fact occur in some 20% or more of these patients, new therapeutic challenges confront us.

It is clear that aggressive medical therapy is the initial treatment of choice. Subsequent surgical therapy is timed for relief of myocardial ischemic pain refractory to medical therapy or for coronary anatomic situations for whch surgery offers an improved prognosis.

REFERENCES

1. Dhurandhar, R.W., Watt, D.L., Silver, M.D. et al. Prinzmetal's variant form of angina with arteriographic evidence of coronary arterial spasm. *Am J Cardiol.* 30:902–905, 1972.

2. Scully, H.E., Gunstensen, J., Williams, W.G. et al. Surgical management of complicated acute coronary insufficiency. *Surgery* 80:437, 1976.

3. Chesnie, B.M., Adelman, A.G., Douglas, B.C. et al. Results of aorto-coronary bypass surgery in patients with unstable angina. *Can J Surg.* 22:127–140, 1979.

4. Williams, W.G., Aldridge, H.E., Silver, M.D. et al. Preinfarction angina—what is it? Edited by J.C. Norman. In *Coronary Artery Medicine and Surgery: Concepts and Controversies.* New York: Appleton-Century-Crofts, 1975, pp 344–348.

5.. Maseri, A., L'Abbate, A., Baroldi, G. et al. Coronary vasospasm as a possible cause of myocardial infarction: a conclusion derived from the study of "preinfarction" angina. *N Engl J Med.* 299:1271–1277, 1978.

6. Armstrong, P.W., Chiong, M.A., and Parker, J.O. The spectrum of unstable angina. *Circulation* 60(suppl II):II-248, 1979.

7. Feinstein, A.R. Clinical epidemiology. III. The clinical design of statistics in therapy. *Ann Intern Med.* 69:1287-1312, 1968.

8. Pugh, B., Platt, M.R., Mills, L.J. et al. Unstable angina pectoris: a randomized study of patients treated medically and surgically. *Am J Cardiol.* 41:1291-1298, 1978.

9. Selden, R., Neill, W.A., Ritzman, L.W. et al. Medical versus surgical therapy for acute coronary insufficiency: a randomized study. *N Engl J Med.* 293:1329-1333, 1975.

10. Bertolasi, C.A., Tronge, J.E., Carreno, C.A. et al. Unstable angina — prospective and randomized study of its evaluation with and without surgery. *Am J Cardiol.* 33:201-208, 1974.

11. Hultgren, H.N., Pfeifer, J.F., Angell, W.W. et al. Unstable angina: comparison of medical and surgical management. *Am J Cardiol.* 39:734-740, 1977.

23 A Surgeon's View of the Symposium

Ronald J. Baird, MD

It is impossible to have a meaningful scholarly discussion unless we can define our terms. The problems arising from the lack of a precise and generally accepted definition of unstable angina were evident throughout this symposium. In general, the term was used to describe patients in five clinical situations:

1. Patients with recent onset of angina. (This includes a multitude of patients.)
2. Patients whose effort-induced angina is increasing in frequency or severity. (This is a loosely defined group open to the bias of patient and physician.)
3. Patients who have begun to suffer from angina at rest. (The duration of the anginal episode was variously defined as from over ten minutes to over one-half hour.)
4. The onset of any form of angina within one month of proved myocardial infarction.
5. The various forms of variant angina. (Coronary artery spasm may be separate or may apply in any of the above groups.)

In accepting this broad range of syndromes, each author could generally apply them to his own study; but there was no way to compare effects of therapy in the various reports meaningfully, mathematically, or scientifically with each other. The fact that they were talking about very different patient populations was evident in the clinical reviews of Drs. Parker, Mizgala, Hugenholtz, Weisel, Keon, Cohn, Bardet, and Conti. Precise classification into various subgroups (based on clinical, electrocardiographic, and biochemical data) as presented by Weisel et al and Parker and Leach is the route that must be taken before deciding on the optimum therapy for any patient.

The contributions by Roberts and Virmani, and Silver and Butany, on the pathology of the coronary arteries and the ischemic myocardium were illuminating and humbling to the clinician. There was no specific coronary or myocardial pathology that distinguished the stable from the unstable patient. Also, the clinician almost invariably underestimated the extent and severity of the reduction in cross-sectional area of the involved arteries. A significant obstruction was variously defined in the clinical papers as a 50% to 80% reduction in angiographic diameter. Once again, it was impossible to compare patient populations when definition of the subject was so imprecise. There was general agreement with Conti and Curry that clinicians must begin to define the coronary pathology precisely in terms of cross-sectional area and the length of the stenotic lesion.

The contribution of Maseri, L'Abbate, and Chierchia was the most exciting presentation and was highly relevant to our future understanding of the pathophysiology of myocardial ischemia. We knew that ischemic episodes could be painless, detected only by the cardiogram. We have now been shown that coronary sinus sampling can detect ischemic episodes that may not be reflected in the cardiogram. Whether this is related to spasm of certain major coronary arteries, as they believe, or to transmural and regional shifts in myocardial supply and demand, is conjectural. However, it seems likely that coronary sinus monitoring will become an important part of evaluation of anginal instability.

We were also excited by the rapid and promising advances in knowledge available from myocardial imaging as presented by McLaughlin and Morch and in the therapeutic effectiveness of the new calcium antagonists as presented by Mizgala.

The contribution by Teasdale was both appropriate and pertinent. In this era of effective myocardial protection, with electromechanical arrest and myocardial temperatures consistently under 20°C, the incidence of perioperative myocardial infarction is closely related to the overall effectiveness of the anesthesiologist and her team. Tachycardia and systolic hypertension before, during, and after induction must be avoided.

What about surgeons and their spectrum of competence and experience? The striving for excellence through careful analysis and frequent reporting of results is praiseworthy. It has been an essential element in the rapid advance of cardiac surgery to its present level of safety. In precisely described congenital or valvular cardiac abnormalities, improved results from a technical or procedural n,cdification in one center have been followed by rapid assimilation and emulation in others.

The obstructive coronary artery lesions and their myocardial sequelae have been less clearly defined. The cardiac surgical community has suffered from the "albatross" of the Veterans Administration Multicenter Trial of surgery for stable angina and the subsequent vigorous criticism of its results. When speaking on the basis of different patient populations and evolved technology in the late seventies, it was unseemly that clinicians should have been so critical of the results achieved by their colleagues in an earlier period. The argument that "my surgeons are better than your surgeons" is not constructive, nor is it conducive to better results.

From 1977 to 1980, over 3000 patients received coronary artery operations in three of the University of Toronto hospitals. About 1000 procedures were for unstable angina. I have been aware of minor criticism directed at each institution at various times over this period. Some aspects criticized were patency, morbidity, mortality, and participation of residents in the operative procedure. This line of criticism was also heard in the symposium where some discussants stressed the need for "surgical groups which would deliver a 1% mortality rate for patients with unstable angina." No one has asked the same for the coronary care unit. I believe it is appropriate to remind our colleagues that cardiac surgeons are very aware of the technical and procedural controversies that are still unsettled in the field of coronary artery repair. Current discrepancies in results relate far more to different patient populations and categories of disease than to supposed variations in regional or individual surgical competence.

With the recent improvements in intraoperative lighting, magnification, suture materials, and care of both the ischemic heart and the harvested venous conduit, the possibilities of surgical misadventure are minimal. With the techniques of the proximal and distal vascular anastomoses now relatively standardized, surgical errors mainly relate to misjudging the correct length of the conduit or to being too vigorous in complete revascularization. Error also results from attempting to attach a bypass to an artery that is too small or too diseased. Such misadventure is now infrequent.

The rapid recent advance in our knowledge of the pathophysiology and therapy of coronary obstructive processes and myocardial ischemic syndromes will surely continue. That which is murky, ill-defined, and controversial today will be less so in the future. I congratulate Drs. Adelman and Goldman on their success in drawing together our current knowledge and in pointing the way for future advances in our understanding and management of unstable angina.

INDEX